Clinical Management of Scars

Clinical Management of Scars

Editor: Asher Hill

MURPHY & MOORE
www.murphy-moorepublishing.com

www.murphy-moorepublishing.com

MURPHY & MOORE

Cataloging-in-Publication Data

Clinical management of scars / edited by Asher Hill.
p. cm.
Includes bibliographical references and index.
ISBN 978-1-63987-114-8
1. Scars. 2. Scars--Treatment. 3. Skin--Diseases. 4. Dermatology. I. Hill, Asher.
RL110 .C55 2021
616.5--dc23

Murphy & Moore Publishing,
1 Rockefeller Plaza,
New York City, NY 10020, USA

ISBN 978-1-63987-114-8 (Hardback)

Contents

Preface IX

Chapter 1 **Scar Resurfacing** 1
Fiona M. Wood

Chapter 2 **Invasive Techniques in Scar Management: Skin Substitutes** 7
F. W. Timmermans and E. Middelkoop

Chapter 3 **Facial Scars Reconstruction** 14
Luc Téot

Chapter 4 **Invasive Techniques in Scar Management: Fat Injections** 21
F. Bassetto, C. Scarpa and V. Vindigni

Chapter 5 **Usefulness of Local Flaps for Scar Contracture Release** 31
Rei Ogawa

Chapter 6 **Specific Attention Areas in Scar Management: Management of Atrophic Scars** 39
Matteo Tretti Clementoni and Ernest Azzopardi

Chapter 7 **Emerging Technologies in Scar Management: The Role of Allogeneic Cells** 49
Clarisse Ganier and Sonia Gaucher

Chapter 8 **Specific Attention Areas in Scar Management: Specific Scar Management Depending on Anatomical Features (Face, Hair, Breast, Hand, Joints, Foot)** 54
Julian Poetschke and Gerd G. Gauglitz

Chapter 9 **Management of Scars in Skin of Color** 62
Huidi Tchero

Chapter 10 **Additional Invasive Techniques in Scar Management** 69
E. de Bakker, M. C. E. van Leeuwen, O. W. M. Meijer and F. B. Niessen

Chapter 11 **Scar and Scarring in the Elderly** 76
Hester Colboc and Sylvie Meaume

Chapter 12 **Scars After Breast Reconstruction** 82
Wouter B. van der Sluis

Chapter 13 **Atrophic Scars: Reinforcing the Flap Mattress Using Adipocyte Transfer in Paraplegic Patients at Risk of Pressure Ulcer Recurrence** 86
Luc Téot

Chapter 14 **Hyperpigmented Scar** 89
Julian Poetschke and Gerd G. Gauglitz

Chapter 15 **Secondary Lip Correction in a Cleft Lip Patient** 92
Wouter B. van der Sluis and Johan P. W. Don Griot

Chapter 16 **Vacuum Massage in the Treatment of Scars** 95
Peter Moortgat, Jill Meirte, Ulrike Van Daele, Mieke Anthonissen, Tine Vanhullebusch and Koen Maertens

Chapter 17 **Management of Scarring Following Aesthetic Surgery** 103
Alexandra Chambers

Chapter 18 **Clinical Case: Earlobe Keloid** 113
Luc Téot

Chapter 19 **Scars in Pediatric Patients** 117
Anne Le Touze

Chapter 20 **Clinical Case Reports: Scar Prevention by Laser Treatment in Mastopexy with Implant** 125
Vincent Hunsinger, Martin Lhuaire, Ibrahim Dagher and Laurent Lantieri

Chapter 21 **Genital Scars** 132
Ursula Mirastschijski

Chapter 22 **Psychological Impact of Living with Scars Following Burn Injury** 153
Nancy E. E. Van Loey

Chapter 23 **Makeup Therapy for Scars** 159
Joëlle Nonni

Chapter 24 **Effectiveness of Corticosteroid Tapes and Plasters for Keloids and Hypertrophic Scars** 165
Rei Ogawa

Chapter 25 **Burn Hypertrophic Scar in Pediatric Patients: Clinical Case** 171
Roohi Vinaik, Joel Fish and Marc G. Jeschke

Chapter 26 **Emerging Technologies in Scar Management: Laser-Assisted Delivery of Therapeutic Agents** 176
Juhee Lee and Jihee Kim

Chapter 27 **Minimally Invasive Technologies for Treatment of HTS and Keloids: Fractional Laser** 183
M. Tretti Clementoni and E. Azzopardi

Chapter 28 **New Drugs for Scar Treatment** 190
Sun Hyung Kwon, Jagannath Padmanabhan, Dominic Henn, Kellen Chen and Geoffrey C. Gurtner

Chapter 29 **Emerging Technologies in Scar Management: Remodeling of Post-surgical Linear Scar Using Microplasma Radiofrequency** 197
Wei Liu

Chapter 30 **Minimal Invasive Technologies for Treatment of HTS and Keloids: Medical Needling** 205
Antigona Aliu and Matthias Aust

Chapter 31 **Shock Wave Therapy for Wound Healing and Scar Treatment** 216
Peter Moortgat, Mieke Anthonissen, Ulrike Van Daele, Jill Meirte, Tine Vanhullebusch and Koen Maertens

Chapter 32 **Suture Edge Tension Control Technologies for Scar Improvement** 222
Luc Téot, Sergiu Fluieraru and Christian Herlin

Permissions

List of Contributors

Index

Preface

It is often said that books are a boon to mankind. They document every progress and pass on the knowledge from one generation to the other. They play a crucial role in our lives. Thus I was both excited and nervous while editing this book. I was pleased by the thought of being able to make a mark but I was also nervous to do it right because the future of students depends upon it. Hence, I took a few months to research further into the discipline, revise my knowledge and also explore some more aspects. Post this process, I begun with the editing of this book.

The fibrous tissue which replaces the normal skin following an injury is termed as a scar. It is an integral part of the wound repair process. Scar tissue and the normal tissue are made up of the same protein, but the fiber composition differs. Generally, the functional quality of scar tissue is inferior to the original tissue. However, in cases such as bones, there is no functional or structural deterioration after healing. There are various types of scar tissue, namely, hypertrophic, atrophic, keloid and stretch marks. Hypertrophic scars are raised above the surrounding skin due to the overproduction of the collagen by the body. Keloid scars are able to grow indefinitely into large neoplasms. The objective of this book is to give a general view of scars and their clinical management. It is a compilation of chapters that discuss the most vital concepts and emerging trends in this field. Those in search of information to further their knowledge will be greatly assisted by this book.

I thank my publisher with all my heart for considering me worthy of this unparalleled opportunity and for showing unwavering faith in my skills. I would also like to thank the editorial team who worked closely with me at every step and contributed immensely towards the successful completion of this book. Last but not the least, I wish to thank my friends and colleagues for their support.

Editor

1

Scar Resurfacing

Fiona M. Wood

Contents

Overview

The Mechanism of the Initial Skin Injury and Clinical Pathway of Healing

The Timing of the Intervention

The Techniques for Preparing the Scar Wound Bed for Resurfacing

The Techniques of Wound Repair for Resurfacing

Post-Intervention Scar Management

Conclusion

References

Overview

Established scarring can have an impact on the function and aesthetics of the skin related to the volume of the fibrous tissue, the vascularity of the area, the colour mismatch with the adjacent normal skin and disruption of the skin adnexal structures. Resurfacing is a technique which involves the disruption of the epidermal surface of a scarred area with removal of a varying volume of the underlying scarred dermal element, followed by a controlled repair of the surface.

The aim of resurfacing is to improve the character of the scarred area with a resulting scar more closely matching the surrounding uninjured skin. This can be focused on improving the texture of the surface, the pigment match or reduction of the volume of scar. Resurfacing will not address scar contracture or the absence of skin adnexal structures, with the exception of full-thickness excision and reconstruction with full-thickness skin graft or flap repair. The character of the skin varies across body sites such that the specialist nature of the skin site must be considered when planning any intervention. A complex scar reconstruction may be undertaken as a combined procedure with strategies designed to address the range of issues including resurfacing.

The timing and technique of the procedure are guided by the preceding clinical situation and specifically by the understanding of the conditions at the time of wound healing and subsequent scar development [1]. It is essential to understand that the opportunity to improve the scar depends upon the opportunity to better control the wound healing at the time of the resurfacing intervention.

There are a number of considerations to be taken into account when planning the interventions to improve the scar quality by control of the secondary wound healing:

- The mechanism of the initial skin injury and clinical pathway of healing, with specific reference to the initial techniques of wound repair, the time to healing and the presence of infection and other comorbidities influencing wound healing
- The time from the initial insult, considering if the scar is fully mature or there are symptoms of the scar, or epithelial stability compromise, such that early intervention is being driven in an immature active scar
- The techniques available for the intervention in terms of the scar intervention and subsequent wound repair and post-intervention scar management
- Counselling that it is possible to improve the scar but not to eradicate the scar with the current stage of knowledge of wound healing

For the scar resurfacing intervention to translate into an improved scar outcome, it is important to understand the clinical opportunities which offer an improvement on the initial treatments which have resulted in the unacceptable scar. For example, if the plan is to repeat the same procedure, such as a surgical shave and split-thickness skin graft, then there has to be a significant difference in the clinical situation to advise that such a strategy offers the opportunity of scar reduction. This may be appropriate as in a mature scar there is control over the timing of the intervention such that it is not associated with the inflammation of the acute episode. Alternatively, there may be the use of a new method of scar reduction such as laser or a method to reduce the time to healing such as a cell-based therapies.

The chapter aims to outline strategies for scar improvement by disruption of the scar surface and control of the secondary healing process. In the context of this discussion, it is essential to articulate clearly the potential gains on a risk matrix that is realistic for the patient. The more severe a scar is, the greater the potential for improvement, as compared to a good-quality scar when the risk of worsening the scar may sensibly limit the interventions.

The Mechanism of the Initial Skin Injury and Clinical Pathway of Healing

It is well known that scar outcome is related to the mechanism of injury such that burn injury is frequently associated with an aggressive scar outcome. The surface area of the body involved in the injury is also a driver of the outcome with the challenges in healing large surface areas in a timely fashion. Further, the body site of the injury is also influential with areas such as the presternal and deltoid regions and areas of skin tension being associated with poor scar outcome.

The time to healing is a key element in the scarring process and can be affected by local and [1] systemic factors, infection, necrotic tissue, haematoma and comorbidities such as diabetes, nutritional deficiency, drugs such as steroids and retinoid in acne treatment. The clinical history is key in understanding what can be optimised to improve the quality of healing and what factors may have been influential in the scar quality. Resurfacing is an elective procedure, and therefore, the preoperative optimisation of the patient's condition is possible and needs attention. The history of infection is of importance in ensuring the intervention is covered by the appropriate antibiotics or the risk of triggering secondary problems such as herpes is considered with the appropriate prophylaxis.

The knowledge of the initial intervention will also assist in the understanding of how resurfacing can be used in the post-acute phase to rehabilitate the scarred area [2]. Sharp dissection and haemostasis followed by careful approximation of the opposing surfaces with a suture designed to minimise inflammation are setting up the healing for the best outcome possible. In a wound such as a burn requiring cover of surface area, matching the repair to the defect in depth and body site with a focus on time to healing will again set up the best possible outcome. The concept of scar minimisation by meticulous attention to detail at the time of the initial intervention is covered in detail in ► Chap. 23.

Despite the best efforts, the post-intervention period has influence on the outcome with infection control and techniques of wound support and post-healing scar management having an ongoing role.

The knowledge of the clinical pathway, both initially and the proposed interventions, is essential when considering the following question:

- Is it possible to re-wound the scar and control the healing in such a way as to significantly reduce the risk of scar recurrence?

The Timing of the Intervention

The natural history of scarring is such that in the majority of cases, the scar severity will plateau between 6 and 12 weeks with subsequent remodelling leading to a mature scar construct by 52 weeks. However, the scar will continue to improve over the subsequent years. In order to have control over the extent of scar re-excision, it may be prudent to wait until the scar is mature prior to intervention. The scar may well improve over time to the point that it is acceptable. The progress towards maturation can be influenced by a range of non-invasive strategies highlighted in the chapters in section VIII. When considering resurfacing interventions, it is important to consider what aspects of the scar are of concern and how this could be influenced by time and conservative strategies.

However, there may be indications such as unstable epithelial surface, unsightly mismatched skin surfaces, or symptoms related to the scar such as itching which drives the decision for earlier intervention.

On the other hand, concern that a scar may be too old to consider treatment is unfounded, with improvement in the quality being achieved after many years.

Timing is an element in the risk matrix that needs to be considered in the context of the patient's symptoms and concerns. Early intervention may be explored related to specific techniques such as the re-suture a scar mismatch in height or laser to reduce pruritus, whereas in a florid vascular scar, more aggressive early intervention may add to the overall scarring pruritus, whereas in a florid vascular scar, more aggressive early intervention may add to the overall scarring [3]. The discussion with the patient needs to include the options such as time with the risks and benefits. It is useful to have a scar assessment tool which assists in understanding the character of a scar and facilitates the discussion and clinical decision-making.

The assessment of the scar can be done in a number of ways, e.g. surface scanning focusing on specific aspects such as stiffness or colour [4], subjective standard assessment systems, validated questions [5] and clinical photography. When embarking on scar revision, the documentation of the scars is essential in tracking progress over time; the options are explored in detail in section VII.

The Techniques for Preparing the Scar Wound Bed for Resurfacing

The prerequisite to prepare the scar for resurfacing is the removal or disruption of the epithelial layer by techniques including chemical, laser, dermabrasion and sharp dissection [6].

Chemical peels have been widely used aiming to remove the surface epithelium to a limited depth such that rapid healing by secondary intention is achieved with limited improved scar outcome.

There has been an expansion of the laser techniques used to remove or to disrupt the epithelial surface as explored in the chapters in section IX. Again, laser in isolation can be used with surface damage limited to a superficial level such that the healing by secondary intention is rapidly achieved. The use of fractional laser with discrete microthermal zones has been shown to initiate scar remodelling within the dermis. Further, the ablative lasers can be a tool used to prepare the wound bed for secondary interventions as described below.

Dermabrasion can be achieved with manually using abrasive sand papers, or mechanically with rotating brush or burr. The depth of tissue removal can be controlled, and the contour can be guided using adjuncts such as injection or surface coating with agents such as methylene blue. Surface irrigation is necessary to mitigate against heat damage and to remove the debris from the surface.

The sharp dissection tools range from freehand scalpels to mechanised guarded blades allowing serial shaving of the scar surface. Again, the depth of the tissue excision is dictated by the strategy of consequent wound healing [7]. In situations of superficial shave, the aim may be controlled healing by secondary intention. However, the use of sharp dissection lends itself to debulking of the scar volume such that the wound bed does not retain the capacity to heal within a timeframe that would limit the secondary scar risk [8].

The extent of the excision of the fibrotic dermal layer can range from total scar excision to minimal removal of the tissue. With the retention of the scarred bed, the overall scar result relies on the remodelling, driven by the interaction of the cells of the new epidermal layer and those in the retained scar construct.

The Techniques of Wound Repair for Resurfacing

In the situation of total scar excision, a full-thickness skin replacement is the ideal reconstruction and is considered in ▶ Chap. 37, using flap repair, and ▶ Chap. 39 exploring the use of skin substitutes.

In some instances, an appropriate donor site for a full-thickness skin graft may allow full-thickness reconstruction, or the use of tissue expansion can facilitate local flap repair with the most similar skin characteristics. In complex scar reconstruction, the functional restriction may require the introduction of tissue from a remote uninjured body site using local or free tissue transfer explored in ▶ Chaps. 37 and 40.

In a scar which has been prepared using limited removal of the epidermal surface, healing by secondary intention may be appropriate. In these cases, specific attention to detail is required to protect the healing wound surface [9]. The key to limiting the risk of worsening the scar is the time to healing. There are many strategies employed to facilitate healing with advanced technology dressing systems, both synthetic and biologically based.

When the scar has been de-bulked, then secondary repair of the surface should be considered as prolonged healing by secondary intention will be associated with an increased scar risk. The use of thin split-thickness skin graft can result in an improvement of the scar in terms of contour and colour. However, this can be unpredictable with some split-thickness skin grafts associated with abnormal pigmentation. There is also the drawback of the donor site availability in terms of area and site specificity.

Matching the donor and recipient site is a key element in improving the potential outcome from scar resurfacing. For example, the use of full-thickness skin grafts to release scar contractures of the palm of the hand will frequently afford an excellent functional release but is associated with significant mismatch in terms of the skin characteristics. The ability to match donor site is most frequently limited by the surface area required. The donor site itself can be resurfaced such that a thick split-thickness or full-thickness harvested area is secondarily covered by a thin split-thickness skin graft aiming to reduce the overall donor site morbidity.

The use of tissue expansion techniques may also be used to address the donor site limitation. The concept of tissue expansion can be extended beyond the full-thickness skin construct, to the cells essential for re-epithelisation. The development of the processes of cultured epithelial autograft was specifically to address the need of large surface area skin cover in major burn injuries. The techniques of laboratory-based tissue expansion can provide epithelial cells as sheets or suspension from a limited donor site which will retain the epithelial characteristics of the donor site. The drawback of such cell-based therapies is the reliance on the laboratory environment and the time taken to achieve the expansion via the tissue culture process.

The first steps of the cell-based expansion process have been incorporated into a medical device as a lab in a box, ReCell™. The technique of harvesting at the point of care of the cells of the dermal-epidermal junction, for delivery as a cellular suspension, provides a method with an expansion ratio of up to 1–80. The technique uses the wound bed as the tissue culture environment with the cellular suspension adhering to the prepared wound surface and the cells migrating and differentiating into an intact epithelium. The use of the cell suspension from the dermal-epidermal junction allows the transfer of keratinocytes, melanocytes and papillary dermal fibroblasts in their normal ratio [10]. The use of such a cellular suspension in resurfacing is particularly useful in treating hypopigmentation. The melanocytes within the suspension will re-establish in the prepared wound, and re-pigmentation is seen over the subsequent 6–12 weeks. The introduction of the cell suspension facilitates the epithelial repair reducing the time to healing and therefore the risk of secondary scarring.

There is also interesting basic science evidence that the interaction between the keratinocytes and fibroblasts has influence on the phenotype of the fibroblasts impacting on collagen deposition [11].

The use of cell-based therapies is an opportunity to expand the surface area of wound cover possible for a given donor site with the appropriate cell phenotype. The seeding of the cells onto a de-bulked scarred wound bed reduces the time to achieve an intact epithelial surface with the potential to introduce melanocyte and keratinocyte characteristics to match the area. The introduction of an uninjured cell phenotype has a theoretical impact on the scar remodelling as the scar matures.

Whatever method of scar resurfacing is used, the objective remains constant, to improve the area of scar such that the scar blends better into the surrounding skin.

Post-Intervention Scar Management

The wound healing is only the first phase in the process of scar remodelling post resurfacing, and attention to detail at all stages is essential. The post-intervention dressing systems may involve a range of products focused on providing an environment of healing with infection control and protection of the fragile wound surface.

Further, the protection of the healed epithelial surface and control of the environment are important as the dressings are removed and the surface exposed. At this stage, it may be prudent to consider the non-invasive conservative strategies for scar minimisation such as silicones and massage as explored in the chapters of section VIII. At all stages, hygiene is an essential element to prevent secondary infection and breakdown whilst the cell surface is fragile and immature.

For decades, pressure garments have been used in the attempt to control scar progression particularly post burn injury. The mechanism of action is debated, but it remains a widespread practise. The fabrics used vary in terms of the pressure delivery and the moisture wicking characteristics. A light pressure fabric can be used to protect the area in the early stages post healing if well designed to avoid trauma and sheering.

Sun protection is also important not only to prevent sunburn of course but also to avoid the overstimulation of the melanocytes with the risk of hyperpigmentation in the resurfaced area. Simple advice such as wearing a hat and topical sunblock needs to be considered as part of the post-intervention information given to the patient. The advice will need to be tailored to the patient in relation to their environment.

Conclusion

The clinical decision to undertake a scar resurfacing procedure needs to bring together the needs of the patient and the characteristics and history of the scar, along with the tool box of potential interventions (◘ Table 36.1).

The choice of the specific resurfacing technique will then consider the triangle of care to specifically address the patient's needs in the context of the clinician's knowledge and experience along with the technology environment available (◘ Fig. 36.1). The diagnosis of the scar with the inclusion of an assessment tool will give clarity to the clinical discussion with the focus on the aspects of the scar causing the concern.

Understanding the natural history of the scarring process will help in giving advice to the patient, explaining the opportunities of conservative therapies and time to improve the scar. Then, choosing the technique that will give most benefit for least risk is the key to safely improving the scar. There are many ways of resurfacing, but understanding the need for bulk reduction, repigmentation or stabilising the epithelium of the scar will drive the clinical decision.

In the clinical counselling, being realistic that the scar may be reduced and blended to the surrounding skin rather than eradicated facilitates decision-making for the patient.

◘ Table 36.1 Understanding the clinical details of the scar and the impact of the symptoms on the patient to drive the most appropriate clinical intervention for the individual

a

Scar Assessment to guide intervention

Clinical history	**Scar symptoms**
• Mechanism of original scar process	• Itching
• Timeframe of scar development	• Pain
• Time to healing	• Stiffness
• Technique used to achieve healing	• Dryness
• Presence of infection	• Epithelial instability
• Systemic health and nutrition	• Thickness
	• Vascularity
	• Colour

b

Scar Resurfacing

Techniques to prepare the scar for resurfacing	**Techniques to control secondary wound healing**
• Sharp dissection	• Cell based therapies
• Dermabrasion	• Advanced dressing systems
• Laser techniques	• Infection control
• Chemical preparation	• Systemic optimisation

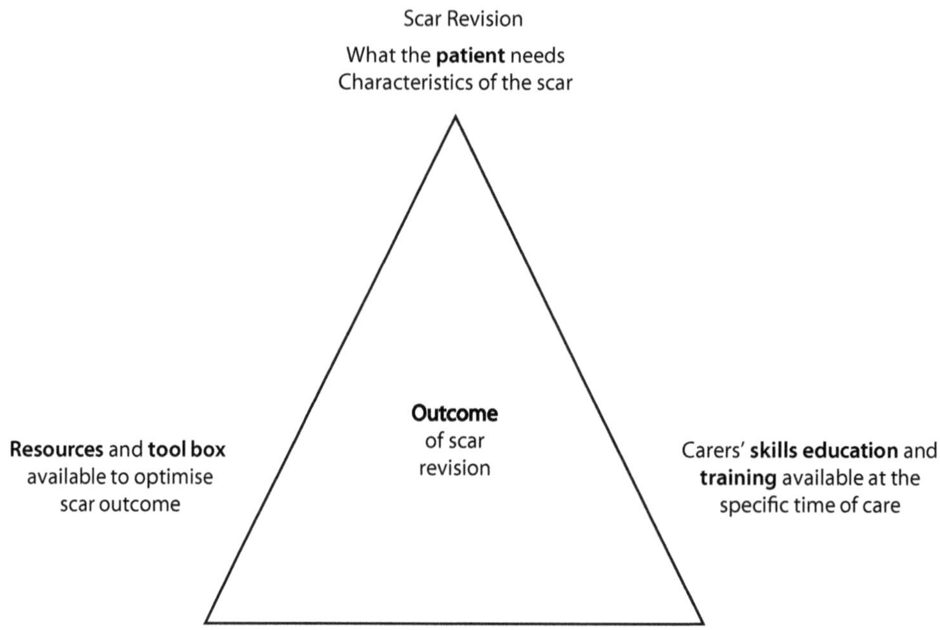

Fig. The triangle of care bringing together essential considerations for clinical decision making

Take-Home Messages

- Clinical history of the patient and the scar is pivotal in the decision-making process.
- Scar assessment is key in tracking the impact of the scar intervention over time.
- Be clear on what elements of the scar need to be treated.
- Focus the intervention on the outcome required.
- The time to healing is a key element driving scar outcome.
- Meticulous attention to detail needs to be continued to the time of scar maturity.
- Education of the patient along the clinical journey is essential for a successful outcome.

References

1. Finlay V, Burrows S, Burmaz M, Yawary H, Lee J, Edgar D, Wood F. Increased burn healing time is associated with higher Vancouver Scar Scale score. Scars Burns Heal. 2017;3:2059513117696324.
2. Hess C. Checklist for factors affecting wound healing. Adv Skin Wound Care. 2011;24(4):192.
3. Akaishi S, Ogawa R, Hyakusoku H. Keloid and hypertrophic scar: neurogenic inflammation hypotheses. Med Hypotheses. 2008;71(1):32–8.
4. Gankande TU, Duke JM, Danielsen PL, HM DJ, Wood FM, Wallace HJ. Reliability of scar assessments performed with an integrated skin testing device – the DermaLab Combo®. Burns. 2014;40(8):1521–9.
5. Simons M, Price N, Kimble R, Tyack Z. Patient experiences of burn scars in adults and children and development of a health-related quality of life conceptual model: a qualitative study. Burns. 2016;42(3):620–32.
6. Pugliese E, Coentro JQ, Raghunath M, Zeugolis DI. Wound healing and scar wars. Adv Drug Deliv Rev. 2018;129:1–3.
7. Onur Erol O, Atabay K. The treatment of burn scar hypopigmentation and surface irregularity by dermabrasion and thin skin grafting. Plast Reconstr Surg. 1990;85(5):754–8.
8. Bradley DT, Park SS. Scar revision via resurfacing. Facial Plast Surg. 2001;17(04):253–62.
9. Tarijian A, Goldberg D. Fractional ablative laser skin resurfacing: a review. J Cosmet Laser Ther. 2011;13(6):262–4.
10. Wood FM, Giles N, Stevenson A, Rea S, Fear M. Characterisation of the cell suspension harvested from the dermal epidermal junction using a ReCell ® kit. Burns. 2011;38(1):44–51.
11. Ghaffari A, Kilani RT, Ghahary A. Keratinocyte-conditioned media regulate collagen expression in dermal fibroblasts. J Investig Dermatol. 2009;129(2):340–7.

2

Invasive Techniques in Scar Management: Skin Substitutes

F. W. Timmermans and E. Middelkoop

Contents

Background

Permanent Wound Coverage
Epidermal Cells/Cultured Epidermal Autografts CEA
Dermal Substitutes
Cellular Dermal Substitutes

Full-Skin Substitutes

Subcutaneous Fat

Regulatory/Safety Issues

Conclusion

References

Background

Modern wound care demands a high focus on quality of healing. Skin substitutes can play an important role in achieving the best possible outcome for each patient. Although skin substitutes were primarily developed for use in acute wound care, they have since then started to play an important role in secondary scar revision surgery. Initially, epidermal cell cultures were developed with a focus on efficient wound closure of large wound surfaces. Long-term results, however, indicated that several structures that played a role in stabilizing the connection between epidermis and dermis did not fully regenerate [1]. Thus the role and importance of the dermal component of skin regeneration became more apparent. This eventually led to the development of dermal substitutes. Various biomaterials were tested for their capacity to stimulate dermal regeneration, with various degrees of success. Synthetic as well as biological materials were extensively tested. Where synthetic materials demonstrated to actively stimulate wound healing in chronic circumstances such as diabetic wounds, biological biomaterials proved to be more beneficial for treating acute wounds. These biological materials were mainly composed of purified extracellular skin matrix components such as collagen, elastin, and/or proteoglycans. Long-term clinical results of several of these materials have since then become available. Further development of the field resulted in the addition of cells to these synthetic and biomaterial constructs. Various cell sources were investigated, with specific attention to different sources of stem cells, as well as allogeneic versus autologous cell sources [2–4]. Alongside the clinical studies, outcome analysis on different skin and scar parameters was further developed. This provided insight into the different skin characteristics that were influenced by the use of skin substitutes. Besides acute wound treatment, scar treatment using fat-derived mesenchymal stem cells is also subject of further research. Initial studies have demonstrated beneficial effects on scar maturation after lipofilling. This technique aims at regeneration of the subcutaneous fat layer underneath the dermal layer of the skin. Nowadays, all these developments allow us to use these different biomaterials as acellular dermal substitutes in state-of-the-art reconstructive surgery and acute wound treatment. New advancements are found in the development of full skin constructs, using autologous epidermal as well as dermal cell sources. At present, autologous (i.e., from the patient) cells are still the mainstay in the successful use of cellular substitutes. This is an advantage in terms of the absence of potential immunological reactions, but at the same time, the long culture times needed to prepare these constructs are definitely a disadvantage of using cellular substitutes in the acute trauma setting. Furthermore, the long-term regenerative capacity of these cellular skin constructs still remains to be fully established.

Permanent Wound Coverage

Wound closure normally proceeds by migrating epidermal cells from both wound edges and skin appendages such as sebaceous glands and hair follicles. As wounds grow deeper and larger, the skin loses its ability to provide enough epidermal cells to close the wounds in a reasonable time frame. This time frame of healing is considered to be adequate if the wound is closed within 3–4 weeks. Prolonged exposure to pathogens and fluid loss represent immediate dangers in delayed healing and might potentially lead to bacterial contamination, sepsis, and death in the worst cases. Biological processes such as wound contraction are initiated that aimed at speeding up wound closure. This is paradoxically an undesired action in terms of the final quality of the wound-healing process. Therefore, most large and deep wounds require surgical assistance to promote timely wound healing and adequate wound closure. The main purpose of surgery is to bring a new source of viable epidermal cells to the wound in order to speed up the wound closure. Skin grafts are the most well-known and most used methods for epidermal transfer and permanent wound coverage.

Epidermal Cells/Cultured Epidermal Autografts CEA

The keratinocytes in the epidermal layer of the skin form the first barrier of the skin. A standard technique for closure of large wounds is transplantation of skin using a split-thickness skin graft (STSG). The protective properties of the epidermal layer are best conserved in the form of split-thickness skin grafts, which usually comprise the whole of the epidermis and a very thin layer of dermis (approximately 0.1–0.2 mm). Coverage of larger wound areas is possible using meshed STSGs, where expansion rates up to 1:6 are possible (◘ Fig. 37.1). However, scar formation in the mesh interstices is apparent, and therefore larger expansions with fewer donor sites were needed. This pushed Rheinwald and Green, as early as 1975, into being the first to show that keratinocytes could be extracted, in vitro cultured into sheets, and that they were suitable for grafting [5]. This can easily be considered the first step in the tissue engineering of the skin. The usage of cultured cells marked a leap forward in the treatment

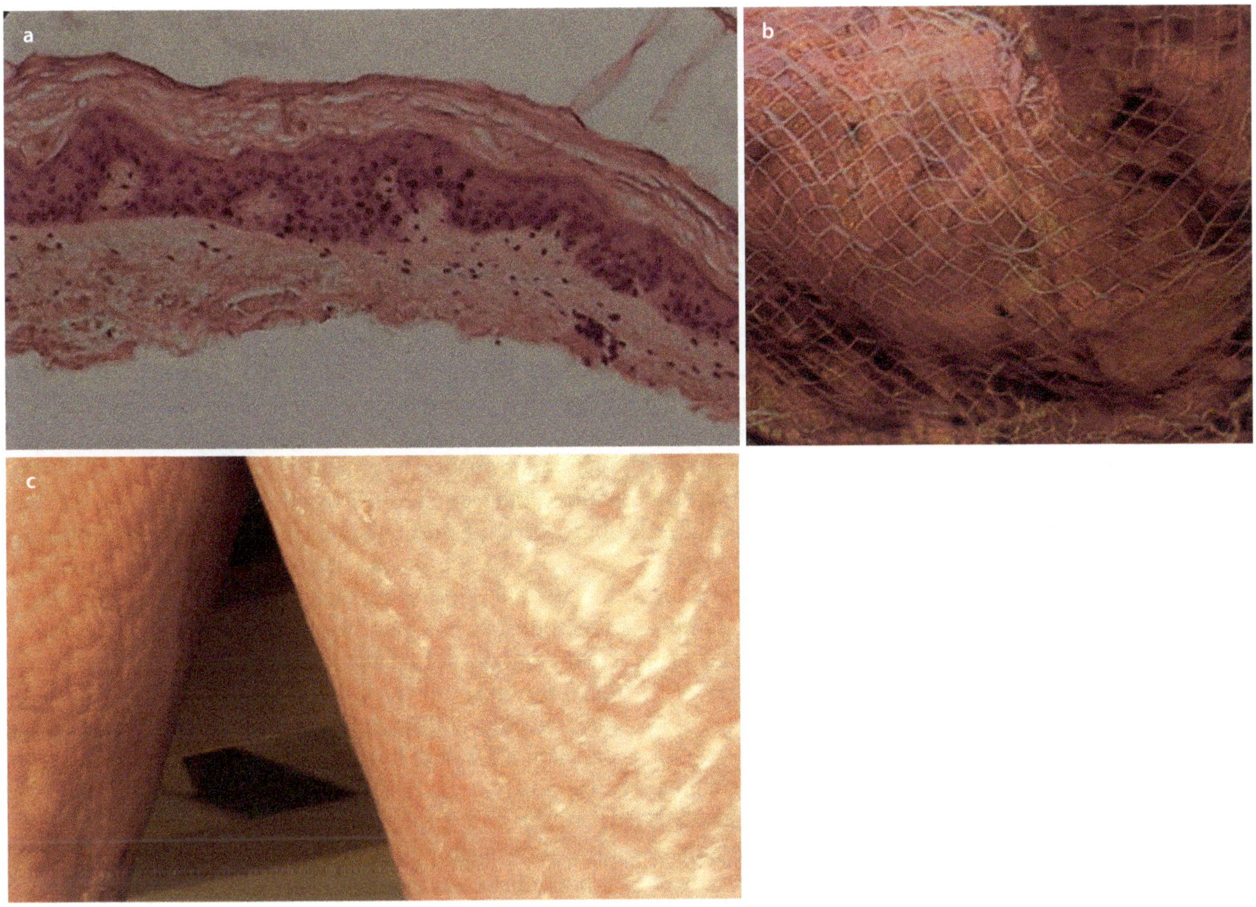

Fig. a Microscopic image of hematoxylin eosin staining of human split skin. Note that only a very thin layer of dermis is present. b Split-skin mesh graft with wide expansion to cover larger wound area. c Typical scar pattern showing mesh pattern of the graft in the scar

of burn patients as larger areas of wounds could be covered with very small donor sites of healthy skin.

The development of cell culture techniques opened up the possibility to maintain viable cells outside of the human body. Initially, cultured keratinocyte layers (cultured epithelial autografts or CEA) opened opportunities to cover large parts of the body without the necessity for substantial donor sites. This greatly improved the survival chances of severely burned patients. However, early studies of CEAs on wound beds showed insufficient regeneration of dermal–epidermal junctions between the epidermis and the underlying tissue, which even after many years resulted in a vulnerable and weak skin barrier [1]. Thus, it was discovered that substitution of dermal tissue is also of great importance in creating and maintaining a well-functioning new skin. These insights sparked the development of more complex skin substitutes.

Although CEAs have been used for over 40 years now, they did not provide the definitive solution for the treatment of large wounds. Specific downsides such as variable graft-take rates, high manufacturing costs, production and transportation logistics, insufficient dermal–epidermal junction regeneration, and often having to compete with readily available split-skin grafts have limited most of the further development of CEAs [6].

A more recent development in the application of epidermal cells is in the form of in situ cell therapy, called the ReCell® system (Avita Medical, Cambridge, UK). With only a small donor site of split skin (approximately 1 cm^2), this device allows the isolation of a single-cell suspension that can be sprayed on a wound bed. The cell suspension consists of approximately 65% keratinocytes, 30% fibroblasts, and 3–5% melanocytes. This system avoids the time-consuming and costly cell culture step. The cells in the cell suspension can adhere to the wound bed and promote tissue regeneration by both cell proliferation and growth factor stimulation. This technique is sometimes used in combination with expanded meshed autografts to accelerate wound healing. The combination of these two treatment options has shown to improve cosmetic outcomes of scars and pigment abnormalities. In situ cell therapy can also be used as a means to promote repigmentation of depigmented skin in patients with vitiligo and congenital melanocytic naevi [7]. Whether these effects are due to actual cell survival and proliferation or to growth factor and cytokine secretion is presently still unclear.

Dermal Substitutes

Skin substitutes aiming at dermal regeneration are dermal constructs designed to either temporarily or permanently replace dermal defects. In all cases, the aim of skin substitutes is to provide protection against microorganisms, reduce pain, promote wound healing, and assist in recreating the barrier function of the skin [8]. This method has become increasingly important for the treatment of burns, open wounds, chronic wounds, and deep tissue donor sites, as it has been shown to improve and accelerate skin regeneration, reduce scar contracture, and minimize donor site morbidity. All these different treatment indications resulted in the development of a wide range of skin substitutes with different characteristics such as mono- or bilayered compositions, temporary or permanent fixture, and cellular or acellular skin substitutes.

Tissues

A biological approach used in the design of permanent skin substitutes was to start with real human tissue. One of the early developed acellular allogeneic skin substitutes is Alloderm®. Alloderm® is harvested from cadaver donors as skin grafts, which are then washed with hypertonic saline to remove cell remnants. After removal of the epithelial layer, the remaining dermal layer is treated to inactivate viruses and then freeze-dried to be used on demand. This provides a nonantigenic dermal scaffold with basement membrane proteins, which are known to promote wound healing and angiogenesis. After rehydration of the Alloderm®, coverage with an ultrathin split skin would suffice as a full coverage treatment option. Recently, Alloderm® has seen a rise in its use for breast reconstructive surgery, whereas the use of Alloderm® on wounds and burns remains limited. Glyaderm® is a similar product based on allogeneic dermis preserved in glycerol instead of freeze-drying. Initial studies on burn patients have been performed with favorable results [9].

Dermal Scaffolds

Some of the most well-known and most used dermal scaffolds are Integra® and Matriderm®. Although both materials consist of bovine collagen combined with extracellular matrix components, their mode of application is generally different. Integra® was the first dermal substitute of its kind in the early 1980s and was created with the apparent goal of minimizing fluid loss and bacterial contamination and promoting cell migration into the wound bed. It does so through its two-layered composition and its two-stage procedure. The deeper layer of Integra® is made out of a combination of bovine collagen and glycosaminoglycan chondroitin-6-sulfate, whereas the top is made with a 0.2-mm-thick polysiloxamine polymer membrane with vapor-transmitting characteristics similar to normal epithelium. This membrane is intended to be placed on the full-thickness wound, and the outer silicone membrane will function as a temporary epidermal replacement and will need to be replaced by a split-skin graft after 2–3 weeks of sufficient ingrowth of vasculature into the deeper dermal scaffold. Due to the combination with a silicone layer as temporary epidermal coverage, Integra® can immediately function as a barrier to limit fluid loss and protect from microbial contamination of the wound, while providing the required extracellular scaffolding for cell ingrowth and proliferation of fibroblasts and endothelial cells. In the second stage, after vascular ingrowth, the silicone layer is replaced by a thin split-skin graft. This product has gained widespread use in the clinical treatment of deep partial-thickness and full-thickness burn wounds, full-thickness skin defects of other etiologies, chronic wounds, and soft tissue defects. The results of Integra® within burn care have been generally favorable and have shown improved quality of healing. However, the staged procedure leaves the wound open for a prolonged period of time and thus bears a risk of submembranous bacterial infections resulting in loss of the biomaterial. Other similar bilayered substitutes are Renoskin®, Pelnac™, and Hyalomatrix® [10].

Matriderm® is usually applied in a one-step procedure as this dermal scaffold allows immediate coverage with a thin split-skin graft. It consists of an extracellular matrix scaffold made out of purified, freeze-dried bovine collagen mixed with 3% elastin hydrolysate. An autologous split-skin graft can be applied directly onto the Matriderm®. Clinical research showed a somewhat slower take of the graft, which reflects the interpositioning of the unvascularized scaffold between the wound bed and the split-skin graft. Nevertheless, the outcome in terms of scar quality was shown to be superior over split-skin graft treatment even after a 12-year follow-up [11].

Both Matriderm® and Integra® have been used for acute and reconstructive purposes and as a means to improve scar quality. These dermal scaffolds initially lack cellular compounds and do require the body to incorporate the exogenous matrix into the wound environment through cell migration and remodeling, which is mediated by macrophages and fibroblasts. Fibroblasts, similar to keratinocytes, also secrete various cytokines and growth factors. But besides promoting cell proliferation, inducing angiogenesis, and modulating the inflammatory process, they also produce a new extracellular matrix, which helps to reconstruct the three-dimensional dermal structure of the skin. Other one-layered scaffolds are Novomaix® (freeze-dried collagen with elastin fibers) and Permacol® (a porcine collagen matrix which is now primarily used in hernia and abdominal wall surgery) [10].

Cellular Dermal Substitutes

Cellular dermal and composite skin substitutes are the most recent products of skin substitute research. Dermal skin substitutes are primarily created to guide dermal regeneration and are used in combination with autologous split-skin transplants. This treatment is aimed at providing an underlying layer of dermal tissue where normally fibrotic scar tissue would be formed. One of the disadvantages of an acellular dermal scaffold is the relatively slow ingrowth of blood vessels and other cells into the scaffold, which can hamper the take and even minimize the survival of the covering split-skin autograft. The general understanding is that the inclusion of dermal cells in the scaffolds improves these outcomes and at the same time promotes the wound-healing process. DenovoDerm™, Hyalograft 3D®, Dermagraft®, and TransCyte® are a few of these known cellular dermal skin substitutes. The first two are, respectively, made of autologous fibroblast seeded in bovine collagen and hyaluronic acid scaffolds, and the latter two are respectively made of allogeneic fibroblasts seeded in a polyglactin and nylon scaffold. Other experimental studies have looked into using adipose-derived regenerative cells in combination with Integra®, and some attempts have been made to create skin substitutes with nanotechnology. However, the effectiveness and safety of these methods still need to be demonstrated outside of the experimental stages of development.

Most of the cellular dermal substitutes are produced using living neonatal fibroblasts. Examples include TransCyte® and Dermagraft®. TransCyte is produced by culturing neonatal fibroblasts on a nylon mesh, where the cells deposit collagen, other matrix proteins, and growth factors. After freezing, the cells are no longer alive, but the matrix proteins and growth factors remain and can actively promote healing, e.g., for deep partial thickness acute wounds. Dermagraft®, however, is composed of living allogeneic neonatal fibroblasts cultured on a polyglactin scaffold. The neonatal cells provide the extracellular matrix compounds and growth factors needed for efficient tissue regeneration. The allogeneic compounds in the skin substitute will subsequently stimulate granulation tissue formation that enables secondary closure or eventual coverage with a split-skin graft. Compared to the autologous counterparts, allogenic skin substitutes have thus far predominantly been successfully used for the treatment of chronic diabetic ulcers.

Full-Skin Substitutes

Several research groups have developed full biological skin substitutes comprising of both dermis and epidermis, while containing either allogeneic or autologous fibroblasts and keratinocytes. Apligraf® was the first of this kind to become commercially available. Apligraf® consists of cultured allogenic human foreskin-derived neonatal fibroblasts in a bovine type I collagen matrix over which allogenic human foreskin-derived neonatal epidermal keratinocytes are then cultured and allowed to stratify. The allogeneic character of this skin substitute ultimately results in the rejection of the keratinocytes, which eventually requires an autologous split-skin coverage for definite would closure. Therefore, Apligraf® is less suitable for large acute wounds but has found its main use in the treatment of chronic wounds. Orcel® is a similar product with a similar composition. The allogenic cells are considered to survive up to 2–3 weeks in the wound bed, and the overall effectiveness of these composite skin substitutes is thought to be based on the excretion of a mix of growth factors and cytokines.

Some novel autologous composite skin substitutes are DenovoSkin™ and Permaderm®. Both of these composite skin substitutes are made with a bovine collagen scaffold. Another described full-skin substitute is the TissueTech Autograft System™, which is essentially the combination of a dermal skin substitute (Hyalograft 3D®) with a CEA (Laserskin®). A major advantage of autologous composite skin substitutes is its one-stage character. Except for the initial skin biopsy from which the autologous cells are harvested and cultured, no secondary procedures such as split-skin transplantations are required. Most of these are newly developed skin constructs, which are still undergoing trials, and none are commercially available at present. Besides regulatory obstacles (see below), other downsides to the further development of autologous composite skin substitutes are the high production costs, long preparation time, and the necessity for a well-organized production-to-clinic transfer. Nevertheless, these are important developments, since in the end, these advancements may lead to clinically applicable regenerative full-skin substitutes, comprising of not only dermal and epidermal structures but also vasculature, skin appendages, and even nerves.

Subcutaneous Fat

In recent years, there has been an apparent shift from merely thinking about reconstructing the dermis and epidermis, to the inclusion of the subcutis. It has become more clear that the subcutaneous fat layer plays an essential role in the gliding and mobile functions of the skin. This characteristic is especially important in anatomical locations where the skin is relatively thin, such as the back of the hand or the tibia. Scars in these areas can easily fuse to underlying tendons or bones if subcutaneous fat is missing. Recent studies have noted beneficial effects on scar quality of lipo-injection with the patient's own fat, harvested by liposuction. Lipofilling of these scars showed an increase of elastic fibers at the dermopapillary layer, which could account for the improvement of scar quality [4, 12–14]. The sustainability of a mere single treatment of autologous fat grafting in mature adherent scars showed to promote a lasting improvement in scar elasticity and tactile pliability [15]. Although there is not enough solid clinical evidence yet, the data gathered so far indicate that fat grafting could become a new treatment modality in improving scar quality and outcome after burns. Further research should aim at elucidating the best indications, timing, and techniques as well as frequencies of application.

Regulatory/Safety Issues

Further development of cell therapy and tissue engineering for better clinical outcomes with regard to wound healing and the reduction of scar formation is a common recommendation in studies on the use and development of skin substitutes. However, new regulations have become effective during the last decade, which designate cell-based therapy as advanced therapy medicinal products (ATMPs). Practically, this means that cell-based therapies in Europe are under direct assessment of the European Medicines Agency (EMA, a monitoring institute of the European Union), which is dedicated to the scientific evaluation and supervision of market access of medicinal products. In the USA, the Food and Drug Administration (FDA) is the relevant authority, where the Office of Cellular, Tissue, and Gene Therapies (OCTGT) exerts the tasks to evaluate and supervise market access of ATMP products.

The European Regulation (EC) No. 1394/2007 provides the overall framework on production and use of ATMPs within the European Union. According to this regulation, an ATMP is a "medicine for human use that is based on genes, cells or tissue engineering." When elaborating on the definition of tissue-engineered products, such products may contain or consist of engineered cells or tissues, with the purpose to regenerate, repair, or replace a human tissue, and it may contain viable or nonviable cells or tissues of human or animal origin. This means that most of the skin substitutes with living cells (both autologous and allogeneic), adipose tissue, and matrices containing human and/or xenogeneic material fall under the regulatory issues associated with this regulation. Scaffolds made of isolated and/or purified animal or human-derived proteins, however, are classified as medical devices. One of the main features of these regulations is that the production of ATMPs for human use must take place under *Good Manufacturing Practice* (GMP) conditions. This is translated into high standards of production facilities, which is only possible in a select few centers and represent a considerable administrative burden for importing and exporting ATMPs across international borders. These strict regulatory and production requirements imply intensive collaboration between centers for the further development of ATMP' and for successful commercial exploitation of these novel treatment options.

Conclusion

Acellular skin substitutes have gained a solid position in the treatment options for acute and chronic wounds as well as scar revisions, with improved outcomes in skin quality over standard split-skin graft treatment. Autologous cellular skin substitutes still hold a promise for the future. Tissue repair and regeneration through the use of autologous cells promote superior healing over the known methods. There are still some drawbacks in the production and application of tissue-engineered skin constructs, but further research, automated production process, and harmonizing our treatment practices will bring us closer toward a scarless future.

Take Home Messages

- Acellular dermal substitutes have proven their efficacy in reaching better scar quality compared to split-skin grafting for acute and reconstructive treatment.
- Acellular dermal substitutes can be used in a one-step procedure, providing immediate wound coverage, or two-step approach, which allows prevascularization of the dermal component prior to epithelial grafting.
- Epidermal cell sprays can be used to treat pigment disorders in scars and/or to increase epithelialization rate during acute wound healing
- Fat grafting is used successfully on adherent scars as autologous fat injection to improve scar elasticity and regenerate a gliding layer underneath a scar.
- Cellular dermal and full-skin substitutes are in clinical trials for treatment of acute and reconstructive wounds.

References

1. Desai MH, et al. Lack of long-term durability of cultured keratinocyte burn-wound coverage: a case report. J Burn Care Rehabil. 1991;12:540–5.
2. Boyce ST, Lalley AL. Tissue engineering of skin and regenerative medicine for wound care. Burns Trauma. 2018;6:4. https://doi.org/10.1186/s41038-017-0103-y.
3. Akershoek JJ, et al. Cell therapy for full-thickness wounds: are fetal dermal cells a potential source? Cell Tissue Res. 2016;364:83–94. https://doi.org/10.1007/s00441-015-2293-6.
4. Leonardi D, et al. Mesenchymal stem cells combined with an artificial dermal substitute improve repair in full-thickness skin wounds. Burns. 2012;38:1143–50. https://doi.org/10.1016/j.burns.2012.07.028.
5. Rheinwald JG, Green H. Serial cultivation of strains of human epidermal keratinocytes: the formation of keratinizing colonies from single cells. Cell. 1975;6:331–43.
6. Brockmann I, et al. Skin-derived stem cells for wound treatment using cultured epidermal autografts: clinical applications and challenges. Stem Cells Int. 2018;2018:4623615. https://doi.org/10.1155/2018/4623615.
7. Lommerts JE, et al. Autologous cell suspension grafting in segmental vitiligo and piebaldism: a randomized controlled trial comparing full surface and fractional CO2 laser recipient-site preparations. Br J Dermatol. 2017;177:1293–8. https://doi.org/10.1111/bjd.15569.
8. van der Veen VC, van der Wal MB, van Leeuwen MC, Ulrich MM, Middelkoop E. Biological background of dermal substitutes. Burns. 2010;36:305–21. https://doi.org/10.1016/j.burns.2009.07.012.
9. Pirayesh A, Hoeksema H, Richters C, Verbelen J, Monstrey S. Glyaderm((R)) dermal substitute: clinical application and long-term results in 55 patients. Burns. 2015;41:132–44. https://doi.org/10.1016/j.burns.2014.05.013.
10. van Zuijlen P, et al. Tissue engineering in burn scar reconstruction. Burns Trauma. 2015;3:18. https://doi.org/10.1186/s41038-015-0017-5.
11. Bloemen MC, van Leeuwen MC, van Vucht NE, van Zuijlen PP, Middelkoop E. Dermal substitution in acute burns and reconstructive surgery: a 12-year follow-up. Plast Reconstr Surg. 2010;125:1450–9. https://doi.org/10.1097/PRS.0b013e3181d62b08.
12. Byrne M, O'Donnell M, Fitzgerald L, Shelley OP. Early experience with fat grafting as an adjunct for secondary burn reconstruction in the hand: technique, hand function assessment and aesthetic outcomes. Burns. 2016;42:356–65. https://doi.org/10.1016/j.burns.2015.06.017.
13. Pallua N, Baroncini A, Alharbi Z, Stromps JP. Improvement of facial scar appearance and microcirculation by autologous lipofilling. J Plast Reconstr Aesthet Surg. 2014;67:1033–7. https://doi.org/10.1016/j.bjps.2014.04.030.
14. Bruno A, et al. Burn scar lipofilling: immunohistochemical and clinical outcomes. J Craniofac Surg. 2013;24:1806–14. https://doi.org/10.1097/SCS.0b013e3182a148b9.
15. Jaspers MEH, Brouwer KM, van Trier AJM, Middelkoop E, van Zuijlen PPM. Sustainable effectiveness of single-treatment autologous fat grafting in adherent scars. Wound Repair Regen. 2017;25:316–9. https://doi.org/10.1111/wrr.12521.

3

Facial Scars Reconstruction

Luc Téot

Contents

Objectives of the Chapter

Techniques

Critical Analysis of the Literature

References

Objectives of the Chapter

The objective of the chapter is to present the different reconstruction techniques, distinctly describing the ones recruiting autologous skin and subcutaneous tissues, transferred from surrounding color-matching donor site areas as well as techniques suitable for a complete face transplantation from a living human donor, with this homologous transfer being realized using microsurgical revascularization.

The aim is to minimize as far as possible the consequences of facial scars, which induce a loss of the dynamic aspect of the face and loss of the specific mimics of each human character to express different emotions. Consequences of the different surgical strategies are described, including local, regional, and systemic potential complications.

Techniques

1. Skin Resurfacing

   Used in postburns scars involving retractions and loss of skin capacity, the resurfacing using dermal substitute and partial thickness skin grafts is the easiest technique to perform. Excision of the scars is done via a long meticulous surgical debridement, preventing to severe venous and arterial pedicles, resecting the hard thick scar tissue, which may be strongly adherent to the muscular and aponeurotic structures of the face around the orifices, mouth, nose, and ears. The neck is extensively freed from retracting scars, allowing a restauration of the movements up and down and laterally on each side. Covering using dermal substitute has become more and more popular in burns surgery since the initial works on Integra [1].

2. Pedicled-Expanded Deltopectoral Flaps

   Among the commonly used donor sites, the deltopectoral site was conceived as one of the most suitable donor tissues for the reconstruction in the face and neck for its adjacent site and match in color and texture [2]. This technique uses an island flap, which is prepared and expanded to the size of the surface to be covered over the face and the distance of the flap pedicle to the distal end of the flap. This is a two-staged procedure. The size and projection of the silicone expander should precisely be determined before the first surgical step. Thanks to a limited incision outside the future face flap which will be drawn over the dorsal skin, a large expander will be inserted in a cavity created subcutaneously between the subcutaneous fat and the underlying muscle aponeurosis. The expander is chosen based on its capacity of inducing a predetermined skin projection, surface of the projected area, and length and width. The expander is connected via a silicone tubing to a valve which is also inserted under the skin at a limited distance from the expander edges. After a period of 2 weeks, the expander filling will start, and the amount of liquid determined on the rate of filling and the needed projection to obtain the desired skin expansion. Usually the skin expander is overexpanded to 1.5 of its volume, in order to obtain an even skin expansion. Possible complications may include extravasation of the expander (in case of rigid silicone angle), a too rapid expansion inducing a local devascularization and stretch marks, the long distance from the back to the face and the postop edema sometimes causing flap tip necrosis

   But a good skin compliance, normal contours, and emotional expression are usually noted after the reconstruction.

3. Prefabrication

   In 2000, the main author proposed the neofabrication of a cervico-deltopectoral flap used as an island flap after skin perfusion boosting. This technique, called prefabrication, was developed on the principle that when a vascular carrier (a fascia including an artery and a vein) is inserted between the expanded skin and the silicone balloon, the expanded skin territory can be extended and its neovascularization amplified. The technique was published in 2000 in *The Lancet*, opening the way to the creation of flaps larger than the normal anatomy allows it [3].

   Technically, the radial forearm facial flap (20 cm × 6 cm) is harvested with the radial artery and the vein, which are microsurgically branched on the facial vessels artery and vein using a limited incision. The fascia is inserted subcutaneously over the clavicular bone anteriorly, the trapeze muscles posteriorly, and the deltoid muscle laterally. A transfixient suture is needed at the distal end of the fascia in order to prevent any gliding possibility.

   Depending on the surface to cover, the amount of expansion and size and capacity of the expander may vary. When the complete face should be covered, a 2-liter skin expander will be inserted between the vascularized fascia and the underlying structures. The valve and tubing are positioned posteriorly on the back.

   A progressive filling of the skin expander is realized twice a week, with a regimen allowing to get the surface of the face (25 cm × 30 cm) on the shoulder after 3–4 months. An arteriogram is realized before the second stage in order to confirm the viability of the fascia and its capacity to revascularize the extra skin obtained thanks to the skin expansion. This arteriogram shows all the new arterial ramifications emerging from the radial transplanted artery, a sign which was interpreted by the radiologists as a certi-

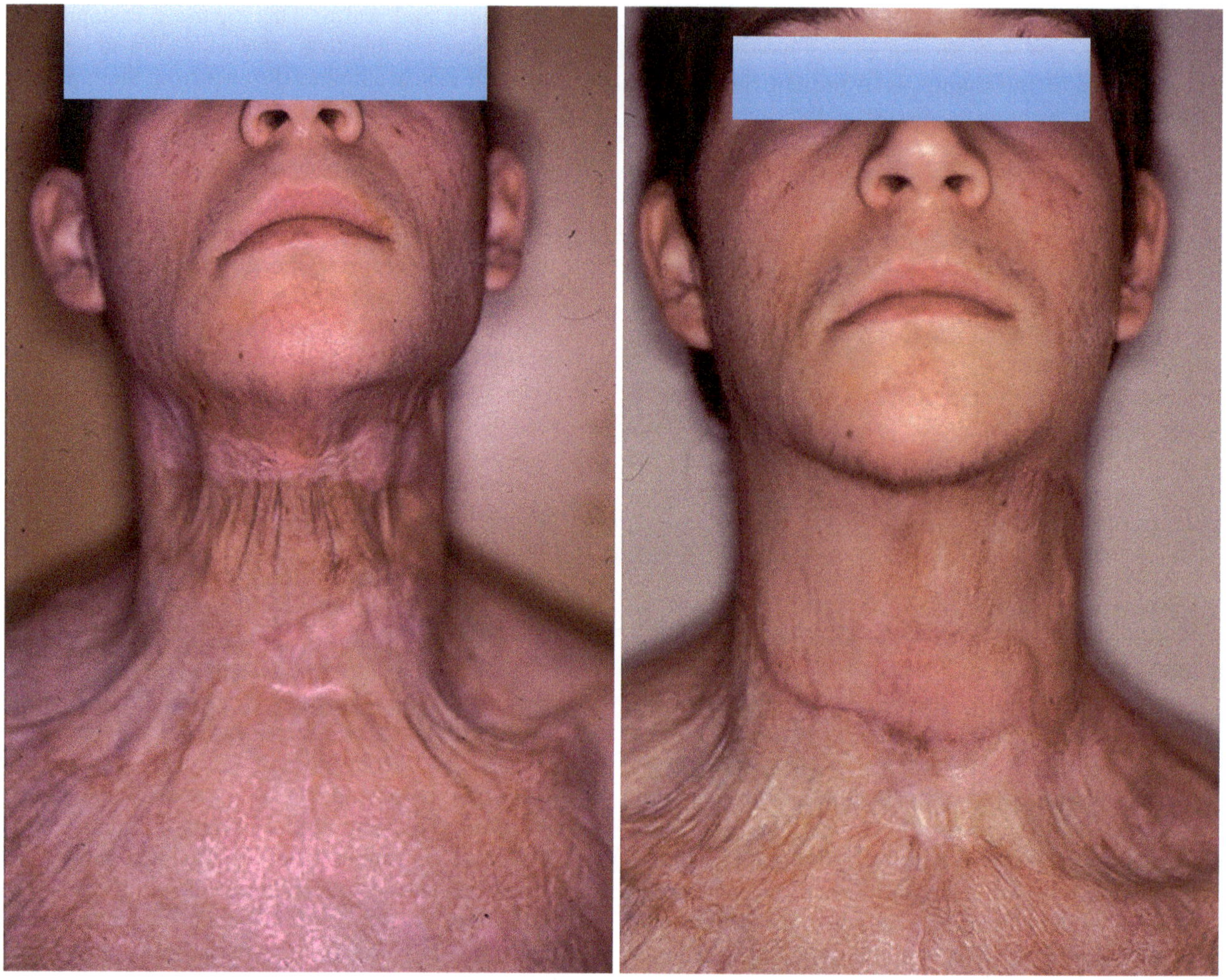

■ **Fig.** Before and after prefabricated flap on the neck of a young male presenting a contractile postburn scar

tude that the fascial vessels were inducing the new flap vascularization.

During the second step, a flap large enough to cover the entire face (if needed) is designed over the expanded skin. The dissection starts from lateral to medial over the shoulder, with a particular attention not to harm the vascular pedicle. Once the flap is harvested and the flap pedicled on the arteriovenous pedicle, all facial scars are removed deep to the fascia, in order to get a maximum surface covered by the new flap. Orifices (mouth, eyes, nostrils) are opened in front of the anatomical corresponding zones.

Long-term results are good, with the transplanted skin depth remaining adapted to the volume of the face, thanks to the precompression realized during the skin expansion (■ Figs. 38.1, 38.2, 38.3, 38.4, 38.5, 38.6, and 38.7).

This technique allows to get a precompressed large piece of skin, well vascularized and conformable. The whole face can be covered with a large viable piece of skin. There is no need for complementary drugs.

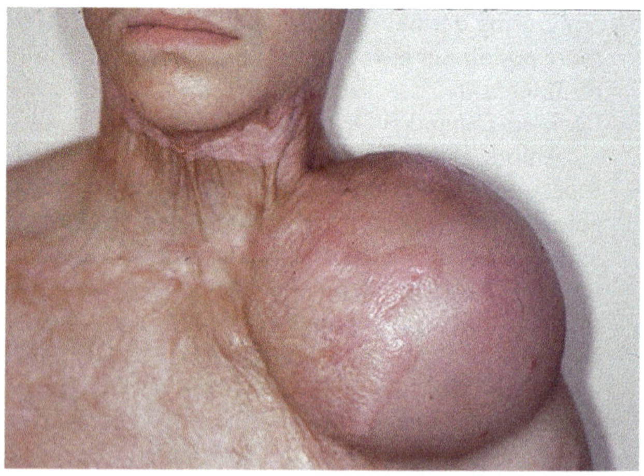

■ **Fig.** Aspect of the expanded skin flap before the second procedure

4. Superthin Flaps

   The "superthin flap" concept was introduced by Ogawa et al. in 1994 [4], based on the subdermal vascular network (SVN).

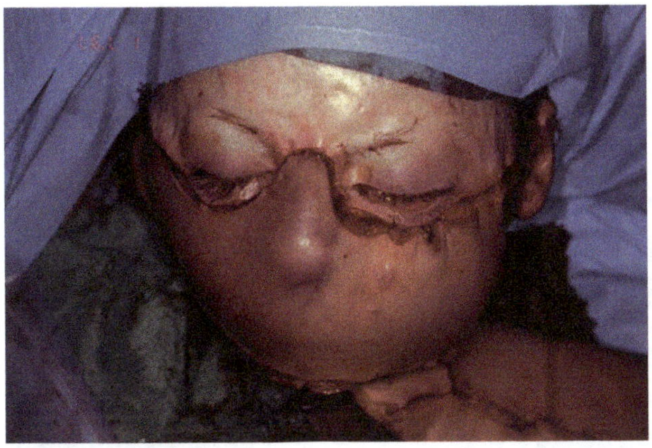

Fig. During the second procedure, the orifices (mouth, nose,) must be reopened adequately

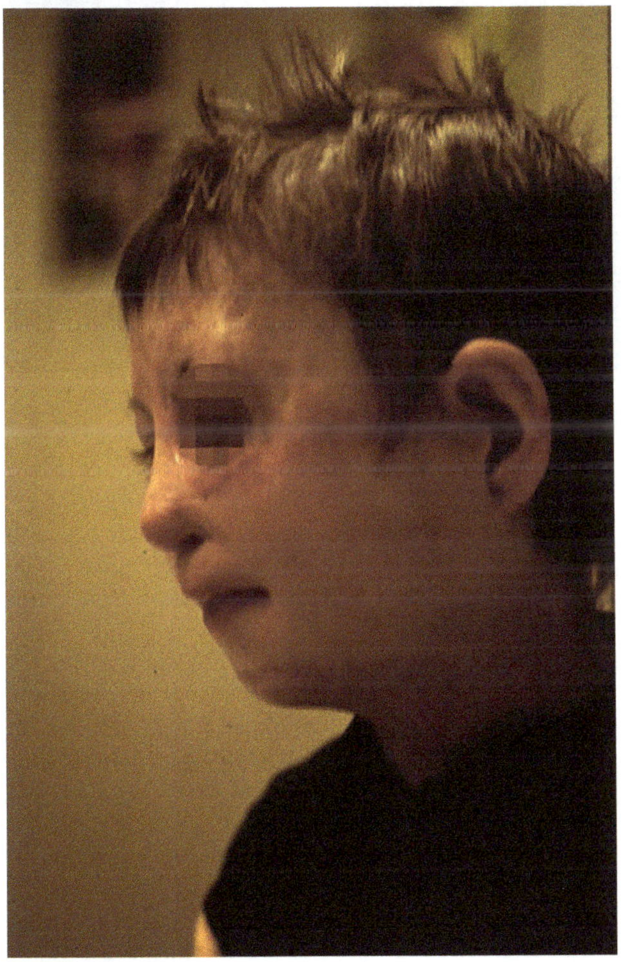

Fig. One year postoperative aspect

Superthin flaps were used in different clinical situations. Twenty-one expanded flaps were used to reconstruct 21 face or neck scar cases in 9 males and 12 females. In the first operation, an expander was inserted on the fascia of the pectoralis major muscle, and then about 1000 cc of saline was injected during a 2-month period. In the second operation, the flap was thinned primarily and applied to the recipient site. Three weeks after the second operation, the pedicle of the flap was cut down and sutured.

In 2007, the authors reported an expanded "superthin flap" for reconstruction of the face and neck for the first time in a patient.

In their series the authors reported different flap sizes, ranging from 4 cm × 14 cm to 10 cm × 22 cm. Expanded volume ranged from 800 cc to 1200 cc. All flaps survived completely, and scar tissues were replaced with normal skin. Flaps did not shrink after the operations, and contractures did not recur. The main advantages of the expanded flaps are the potential to create large thin flaps with a texture and color matching with the recipient area. The donor site can be closed primarily; and microsurgery is not required. However, the disadvantage of the method is the requirement for two or three operations.

The advantages and limits of the techniques are using skin expansion with or without microsurgery. This technique may be considered safe in terms of skin manipulations, the obtained tissue being conformable enough to redrape the whole face without lymphatic accumulation. Edema can be maintained at a low level, especially when using complementary compressive techniques comparable to the ones used in postburn-grafted faces. However, the second stage (flap positioning) after skin expansion is crucial in order to prevent distal regions of the flap to be partially devascularized and become distally necrosed, a complication issuing to a potential tissue loss. The transferred tissues are coming from areas where the dermal component is thicker than desired for facial tissues like the eyebrows or lips, but the global aspect of the transplanted face is compatible with a normal life, thanks to a daily adapted makeup and some retouching on the eyebrows and the lips. The skin has been submitted during skin expansion to a pressure which limits the depth and gives a thin texture. However, in most of the cases, complementary surgical retouches will be needed for refining the red lips, nasal skin depth and nostrils, columella, and eyebrows, reshaped using liposuction, fat transfer, and mucosal surgery

5. Facial Allotransplantations

Historical Aspects

The Pioneers

The first clinical case was realized in November 27, 2005, in Amiens (France); the patient presented a disfiguration after a severe dog bite. She was submitted to the world's first partial face transplant This disruptive approach established loss of quality of

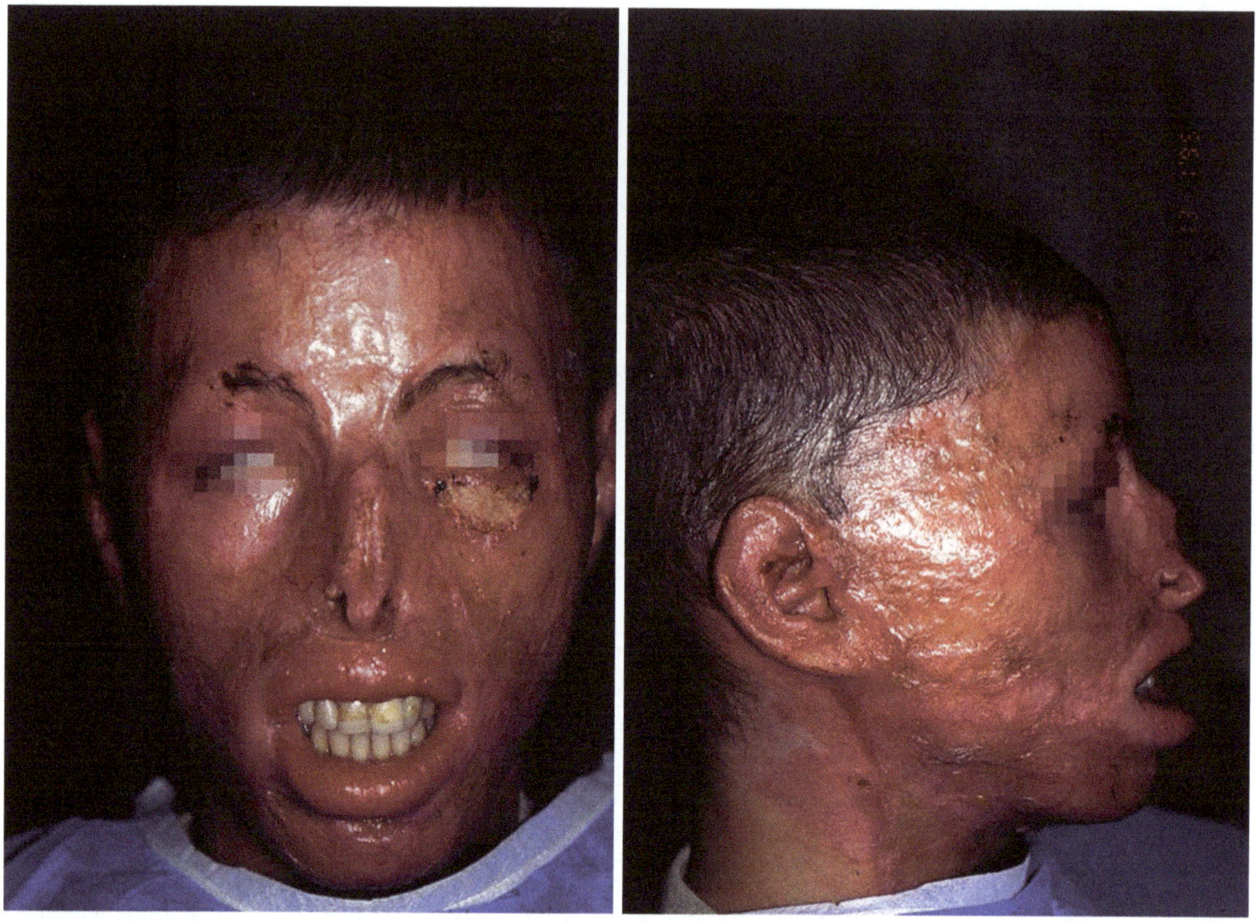

Fig. Preoperative aspect face and profile female 28 years old

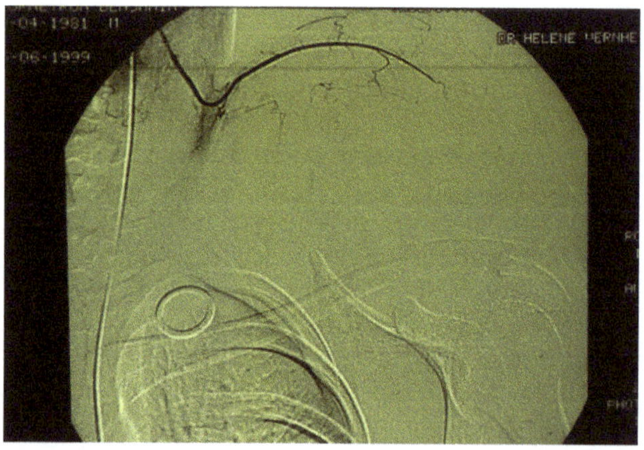

Fig. Arteriogram before the second procedure. Note the good vascularization of the pedicle and the branches covering the freshly expanded skin area

life and social exclusion due to scarring as a medical consideration comparable to a life-threatening situation, as it imposed an immunosuppression for life.

In 2015, 12 partial and 5 full facial transplants were recorded in the literature. Procedures included partial and near-total facial myocutaneous flaps and complex osteomyocutaneous grafts [5]. Fifteen patients received fully vascularized grafts, and 2 patients died of transplant-related and infectious complications

Facial transplantation was proposed to restore quality of life and enable social reintegration. Results publishing the first facial transplants created some polemics all over the world. The main discussions were concerning the long-term aesthetic and functional outcomes where more precisely defined outcomes are expected. In addition, significant technical, medical, and ethical issues remain to be solved, such as the secondary late failure and need for a second transplantation, recently reported by two authors [6, 7].

In 2018, Ozkan et al. [8] presented their long-term experiences with a series of five face-transplanted patients in terms of surgical aspects and postoperative outcomes. Possible salvage strategies in case of difficulties were also described. Five patients, four receiving full-face transplantation and one undergoing partial transplantation were included. The

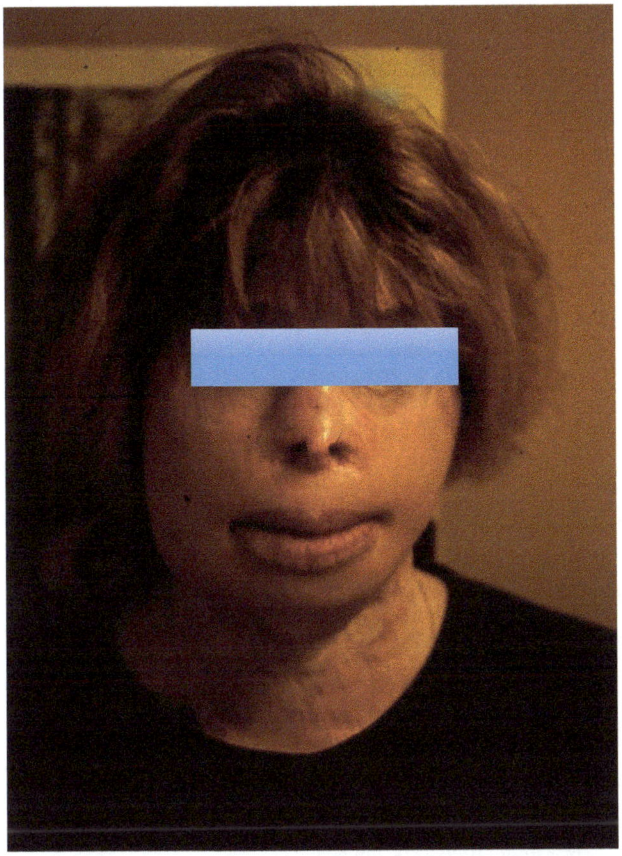

Fig. Four years postoperative, the quality of life has strongly improved. This young woman married, had a child, and returned to work

patients were aged between 19 and 54 years. Two had extensive burn scars to the face, and three had suffered gunshot injuries. The posttransplant induction immunosuppressive regimen included ATG plus tacrolimus, mycophenolate mofetil, and prednisone.

Patient files included their etiologies, preoperative preparations, surgical techniques, immunosuppressive regimen, postoperative courses, revisional surgeries, together with challenges including acute rejection episodes, and immunosuppressive drug complications.

No re-surgery due to vascular compromise was required in any case. One of the five patients was eventually lost due to complicated infectious and metabolic events 11 months posttransplantation. The other four patients were still alive, with a mean follow-up time of 53 months, and had satisfactory functional transplants and cosmetic appearance.

Potential complications may be linked to compliance and psychological maturity of the patients, the risk of opportunistic infections, and malignancies.

These situations need be resolved for it to be accepted as a safe procedure.

Advantages and Limits of the Homologous Transplantation

After more than 50 transplants, the concept of "face transplantation" has emerged even if several considerations should be mentioned: the immunological science used for these transplantations is derived from the ones used in organ transplantation, and the antirejection regimen should be adapted to the rejection levels of the transferred tissues, their rejection capacities depending on their structure and vascularization (skin, muscle, aponeurosis), etc. The number of cases already realized all over the world is limited, and each case has his/her own multifactorial problems, linked to their own medical history, the preoperative difficulties during transplantation, the rate of opportunistic infections, and the compliance of the patient [9].

The ethical discussions ended with a mandatory preliminary authorization for transplantation in most of the countries where they were realized. This frame has limited the number of cases but opened a disruption in the "no-harm" principle, due to the risk of potential complications induced by immunosuppression in a non-vital medical situation. However, the intense need for more social inclusion of these abandoned patients has transformed the conservative approaches into more progressive possibilities.

Critical Analysis of the Literature

The scarce literature concerning large face reconstruction is the reflection of the limited number of patients presenting a scar incompatible with a minimal social life or the difficulty to find surgical teams able to sustain a complex program including microsurgery, multiple actors, and adapted rehabilitation and care. The choice between the two strategies may be led by other considerations, like the ethical problem of submitting the patient to immunosuppression for the rest of his/her life. Several authors have considered this as a progress opening the way to a large diffusion; others have simply refused to consider that facial tissues would be compared to any organ transplant performed on a daily basis all over the world like the kidney, pancreas, lung, or heart.

In conclusion, extensive facial scars remain a difficult challenge for reconstruction. Even in highly sophisticated teams, the capacity of a homologous facial transplantation needs to be prepared. The technique demands a permanent immunosuppression, and even if the ethical problem was more or less solved, the opportunistic infections remain a risk, and the long-term consequences are unknown in terms of life-threatening issues. The techniques imposing a long-term preparation like skin expansion plus or minus microsurgical revascularization are more usual. The specificity of the transferred tissues is less fine than with a complete homologous transfer and will need complementary techniques (fatty tissue removal or fat injections, makeup, etc.). A more EBM-based approach is needed to compare the results and mainly quality of life after allotransplantation versus auto transfers.

Take Home Message

Face disfiguration represent difficult cases where the technical capacities of restoring a normal face using long and complex surgical techniques have to be weighed to the motivation and understanding of the patient. Psychological testing should be realized before proposing surgery, in order to prevent disillusions and bad feelings afterward and to drive the patient toward the right choice to do. All potential complications have to be explained, as well as the length and risks of each procedure, keeping in mind that some strategies will need several procedures and that the final result will only be visible a long time after the last procedure.

References

1. Nuri T, Ueda K, Fujimori Y. Ten-year follow-up after treating extended burn scar contracture with an autologous cultured dermal substitute. Plast Reconstr Surg Glob Open. 2018;6(6):e1782. https://doi.org/10.1097/GOX.0000000000001782.
2. Ma X, Li Y, Li W, Liu C, Liu H, Xue P, Cui J. Reconstruction of facial-cervical scars with pedicled expanded deltopectoral flap. J Craniofac Surg. 2017;28(6):1554–8. https://doi.org/10.1097/SCS.0000000000003901.
3. Teot L, Cherenfant E, Otman S, Giovannini UM. Prefabricated vascularised supraclavicular flaps for face resurfacing after post-burns scarring. Lancet. 2000;355(9216):1695–6.
4. Gao JH, Ogawa R, Hyakusoku H, Lu F, Hu ZQ, Jiang P, Yang L, Feng C. Reconstruction of the face and neck scar contractures using staged transfer of expanded "Super-thin flaps". Burns. 2007;33(6):760–3.
5. Garrett GL, Beegun I, D'souza A. Facial transplantation: historical developments and future directions. J Laryngol Otol. 2015;129(3):206–11. https://doi.org/10.1017/S0022215114003478.
6. Morelon E, Petruzzo P, Kanitakis J, Dakpé S, Thaunat O, Dubois V, Choukroun G, Testelin S, Dubernard JM, Badet L, Devauchelle B. Face transplantation: partial graft loss of the first case 10 years later. Am J Transplant. 2017;17(7):1935–40. https://doi.org/10.1111/ajt.14218.
7. Lantieri L: report of a facial transplantation failure and need for second procedure. Dublin 2018, Make Better Summit.
8. Özkan Ö, Özkan Ö, Ubur M, Hadimioğlu N, Cengiz M, Afşar İ. Face allotransplantation for various types of facial disfigurements: a series of five cases. Microsurgery. 2018;38(8):834–43. https://doi.org/10.1002/micr.30272.
9. Giatsidis G, Sinha I, Pomahac B. Reflections on a decade of face transplantation. Ann Surg. 2017;265(4):841–6. https://doi.org/10.1097/SLA.0000000000001760.

4

Invasive Techniques in Scar Management: Fat Injections

F. Bassetto, C. Scarpa, and V. Vindigni

Contents

Adipose-Derived Stem Cells: Their Biological Properties

The Guidelines

The Procedure

The Free Fat Grafting and Scars

The Skin Texture, Thickness, and Pliability
The Fibrosis
The Volume and Contour
Pain: The Analgesic Effect
The Possible Applications

The Ancillary Procedures to Increase the Overall Survival of Adipose Cells

The Plasma-Rich Platelet
The External Volume Expansion
The Future

Something to Discuss: The Oncological Point of View

Conclusion

References

Background

Since the end of the nineteenth century, fat grafting has become one of the most promising treatments for aesthetic and reconstructive purposes. Its very first application dates back to 1889 when Van der Mullen used fat grafting to treat a diaphragmatic hernia; some years later, in 1893, Neuber A. treated posttraumatic depressed facial scars with a small-dimension autologous fat graft taken from the forearm. Neuber, indeed, noticed that the application of small pearls of fat, compared with the bigger ones, could bring to better aesthetic results. Later, in 1910, Lexer reported the application of the autologous fat grafting for facial rejuvenation; in fact, he uses the fat as a filler for periorbital and facial wrinkles. During his experience, Lexer noted that, in order to obtain a good aesthetic results, the fat should not be damaged during the taking procedure.

In the same period, authors reported their experience with the engraftment of fat tissue, and in 1911 Brunning noticed that fat graft could be reabsorbed.

From 1912 to the Second World War, many studies have reported on the application of lipofilling for "aesthetic purpose" as treatment of the scars; but in the meantime, researchers such as Wasserman in 1926, and later Neuhof, Shapiro, and others, demonstrated that the fat grafting was a "living tissue" in which there were present preadipocytes which could later become mature adipocytes. They also noted that even if there were a degenerative process for the first months after the implantation, later there was the presence of a regenerative process with a full transformation of the preadipocytes in mature adipocytes after 5 months.

But it has been only during the end of the twentieth century that the real features and potentiality of the autologous fat graft started to become clear. In fact, it was only during that period that researchers started to demonstrate the presence of stem cells, the adipose-derived stem cells, which could survive after the transplantation and regenerate the adipose tissue. Nowadays, it is a common opinion that there are three zones that arrange the autologous fat grafting: (1) the outer one called "surviving zone," (2) the intermediate one called the "regenerating zone," and(3) the inner one called the "necrotic zone."

As the name suggests, the intermediate zone or regenerating zone can replace the dead adipocytes in necrotic/center area; this process is allowed by the presence of the so-called stromal vascular fraction (SVF). The SVF indeed consists in a multiple cellular lineage composed by fibroblasts, pericytes, endothelial cells, and mesenchymal stem cells which composed the "adipose-derived stem cells" (ADSCs) and which can promote wound healing stimulating the reepithelization and neo-angiogenesis.

But how can ADSCs do this?

Adipose-Derived Stem Cells: Their Biological Properties

Obtained by a lipo-aspiration procedure, ADSCs can be found in large quantities, representing a fraction of 1/500–1/1500 cells for a total of 5000 per cell each gram of fatty tissue taken, with stem potential 500 times higher than the medullary equivalent.

The adipose-derived stem cells have both a regenerative and a volumetric effect due to multiple mechanisms:

1. They produce a sort of filler effect because of the direct differentiation of the preadipocytes to mature adipocytes. This differentiation is promoted by an auto-paracrine stimulation too.
2. They have an antioxidant effect and protect against damage due to ischemia reperfusion, reactive oxygen species (ROS), and hypoxia.
3. They induce angiogenesis promoting the perfusion of the treated area, supporting existing vascular structures, and having a paracrine promotion of angiogenesis.
4. They modulate inflammation suppressing the T- and B-cell proliferation via NFkB-mediated mechanism; they also produce IL6 and IL8. These cytokines can recruit monocytes and macrophages in the site of injury because of their chemoattractive role.
5. They modulate the granulation tissue and other processes as fibrosis and/or reepithelization. In fact, they upregulate type I procollagen a1mRna, and they stimulate the migration of keratinocytes and fibroblasts.
6. They secrete lymphangiogenic factors.
7. They recruit systemic endogenous stem cells via a home chemokine gradient to the area of injury.

The Guidelines

As every procedure, the free fat grafting also has to follow some guidelines. From 2007 to 2014, the US Food and Drug Administration and the American Society of Plastic Surgeons (ASPS) and American Society for Aesthetic Plastic Surgery (ASAPS) proposed many guidelines [1, 2], but it has been only in 2016 that there have been clear guidelines. In fact, FDA defined the adipose tissue as a "structural tissue" because it is a "connective tissue that stores energy in the form of lipids, insulates the body, and provides cushioning and support for subcutaneous tissues and internal organs"; but this definition restricted its use. Nowadays, the guidelines can be summarized as follows:

1. *The graft should be taken and used in the same patient at the same session. Delayed grafting is not allowed.*
2. *The graft should be minimally manipulated.* Based on the definition given by FDA, the minimal manipulation is "a process that doesn't alter the original features of the tissue, which maintains its utilities." *The graft shouldn't be sizing*. Even if centrifugation is consid-

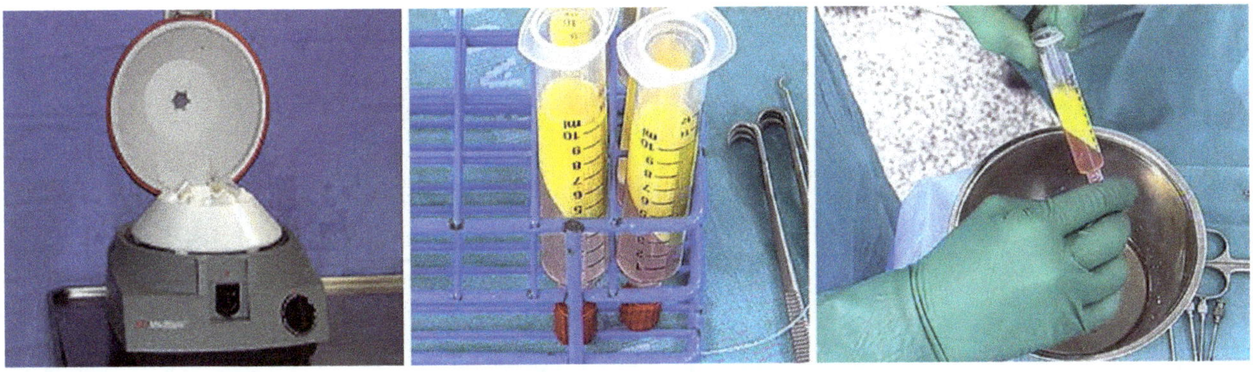

Fig. 39.1 Centrifugation

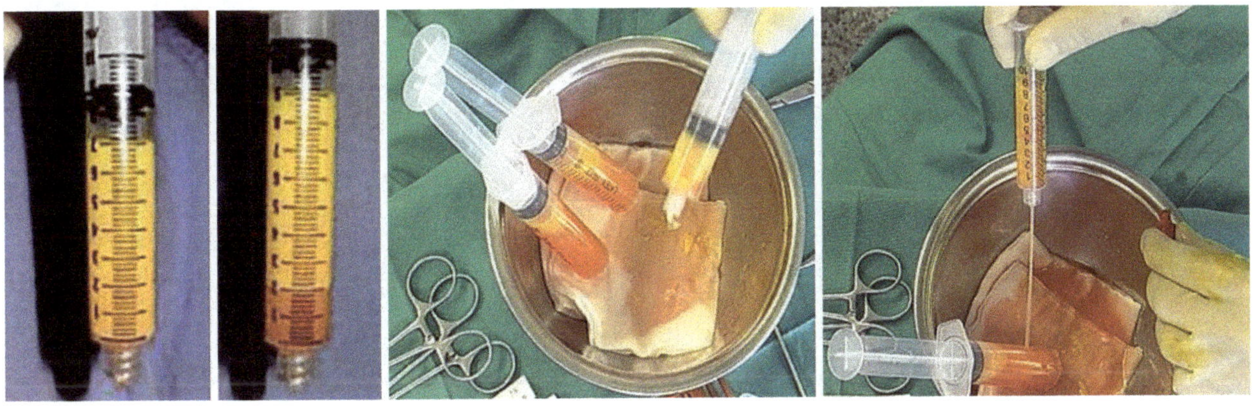

Fig. Decantation

ered a sizing procedure, nowadays the immediate centrifugation at low speed (3000 rpm for 3–5 minutes) is allowed, but decantation and mechanical purification are preferable, because they don't alter any features of the tissue (Figs. 39.1 and 39.2).

3. *The manufacturing of the graft may not involve combination with another article, except for water, crystalloids, or a sterilizing, preserving, or storage agent. Enzymatic process is not allowed. Separation and reinjection of the stromal vascular fraction are not allowed.* Till some years ago, enzymes were permitted to be used as collagenase in order to "upgrade" an adipose stem cell (ASC)-poor fat. In fact, the collagenase could disrupt the link between the ASC permitting to add some freshly isolated stromal vascular fraction in order to obtain a so-called ASC-enriched fat. Nowadays, this enzymatic process is considered manipulation, so it cannot be allowed. Also, today it is possible to prepare the adipose tissue with a tumescent solution, and the lipoaspirate obtained can be added with sterile saline without altering the tissue. This process guarantees the keeping of the original features of the tissue, but it doesn't help us in increasing the engraftment of the free fat graft; so, as we will see later, we can use some ancillary procedures to increase the survival of the fat grafting, as plasma-rich platelet.
4. *The graft has to be harvested with sterile technique; the contact with air has to be minimal.* In order to perform this process, a so-called closed system has to be used that is featured by a sterile disposable canister for collecting, separating, concentrating, and transferring the fat graft (Fig. 39.3).
5. *The graft has to be taken with small cannulas (3–4 mm) and injected with 2–2.5 mm cannulas in a retrograde way (retrograde fat distribution).* Actually this is not a new guideline; indeed it was there already in 1893 when Neuber A. treated scars noticing that small-dimension fat graft could be more effective than bigger one (Fig. 39.4).

The Procedure

Set up by Coleman in 1925, in order to improve overall adipose cell survival, the procedure is featured by a tumescent technique lipo-aspiration with cannulas or micro cannulas from regions as, for example, the abdomen, medial thighs, hips, and trochanteric region. The fat taken can be centrifuged for 3000 rpm for 3–5 minutes or decanted in order to separate the oily part, which can be calcified if injected, from the seric part and the "real" fat. After being separated, the adipose tissues are injected, with small cannulas, in other regions as, for example, the face. The lipofilling

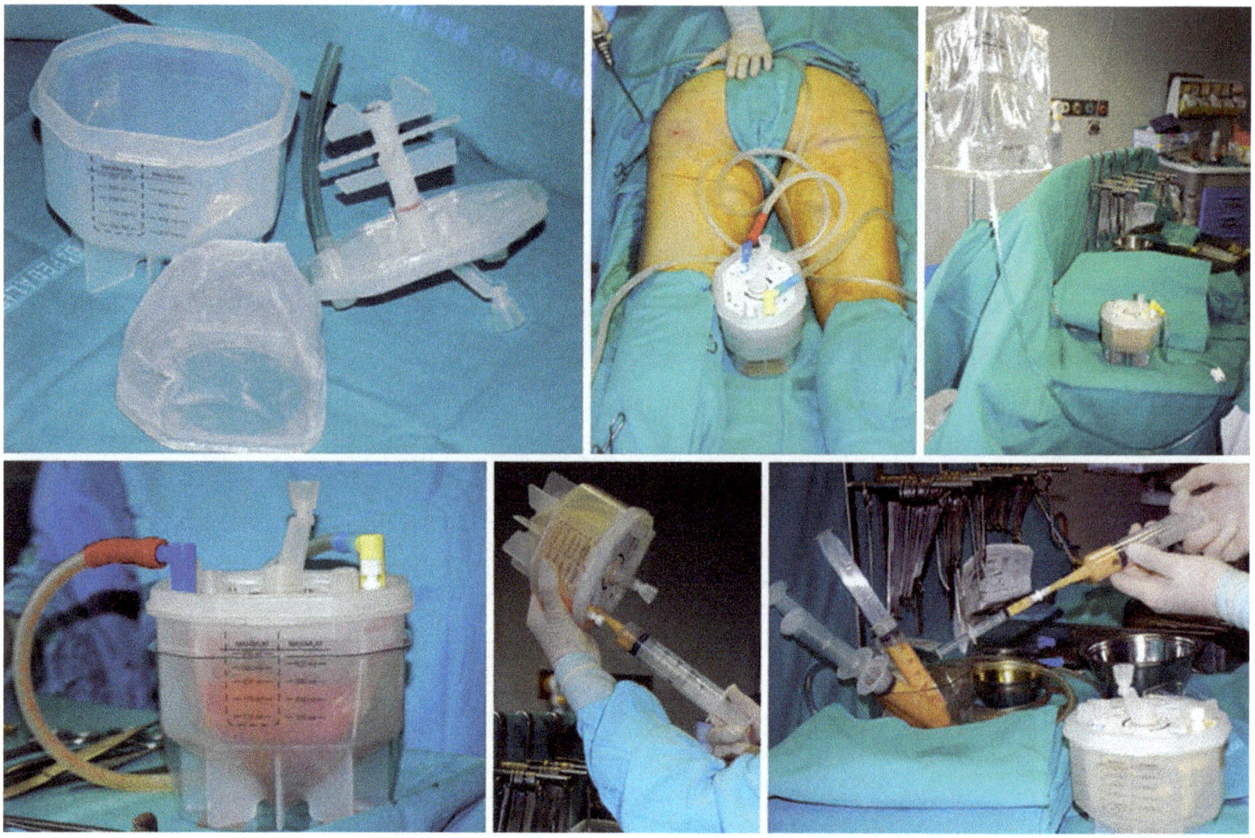

Fig. Closed system

Fig. The cannulas

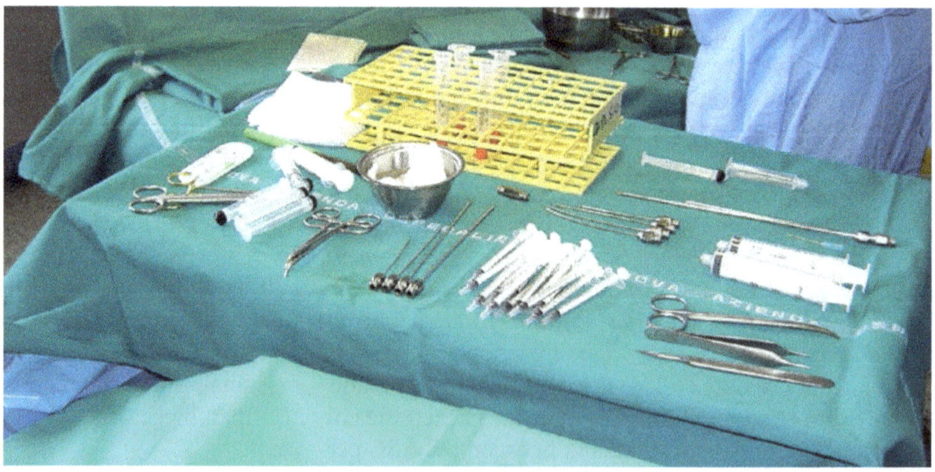

procedure can be executed under general or locoregional anesthesia; it depends on the volume of adipose tissue that we have to take and on the area that has to be injected. The procedure is not free of peri- and postoperative complications such as infection, hematoma, or calcifications.

It also has to be also considered that the free fat grafting can be physiologically reabsorbed. Unfortunately, the engraftment percentage is a subjective parameter, and it varies from 10% to 70% and in some comes till a total reabsorption. This feature can be brought to multiple sessions in order to obtain the correct volume.

The Free Fat Grafting and Scars

Considering its biological properties, we can propose the free fat grafting both to stimulate wound healing and to treat or prevent scarring, because it can act and improve more than one feature of a scar:

1. *The skin texture, thickness, and pliability*
2. *The volume and contour*
3. *The fibrosis*
4. *The pain*

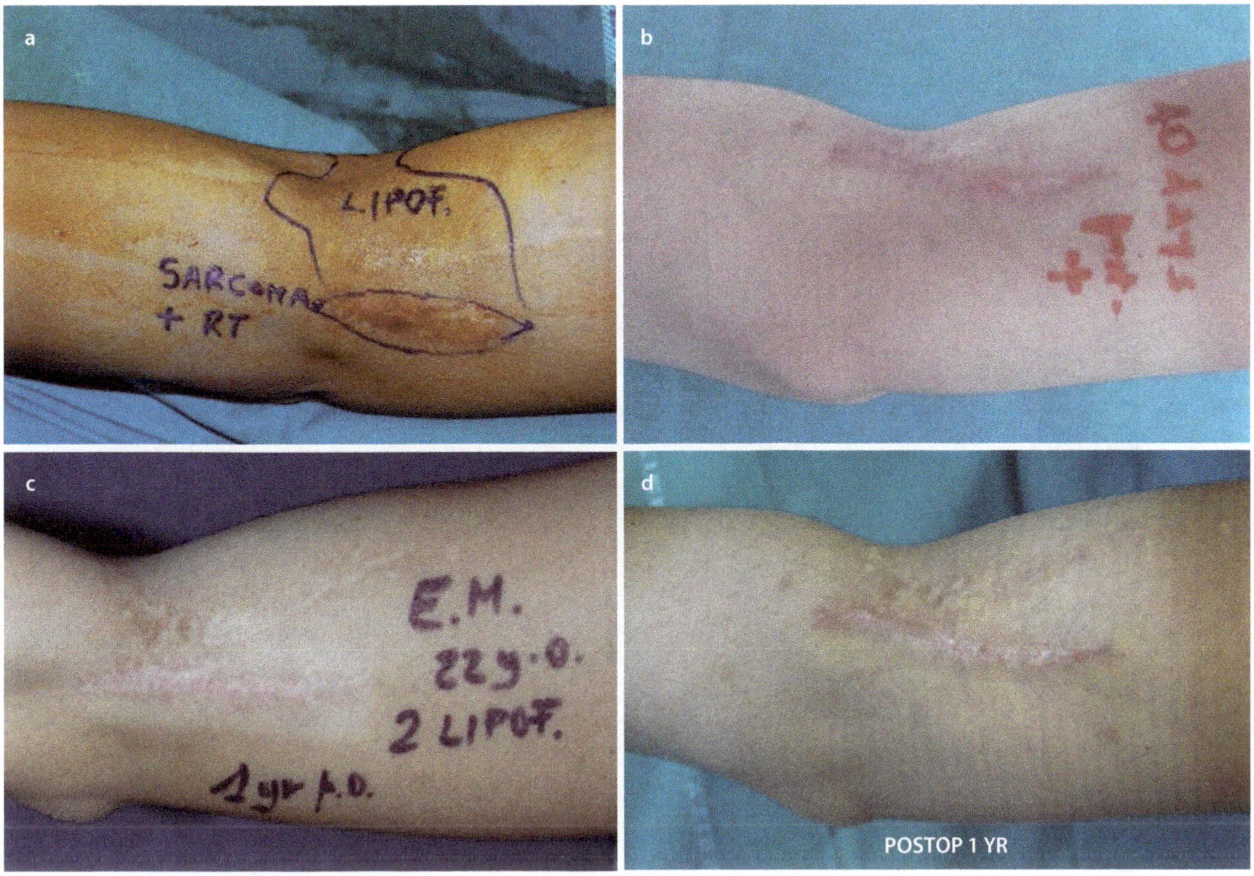

Fig. Skin texture and color: **a** Pre-lipofilling after radiotherapy for sarcoma; **b** 40 days postop; **c** preop second lipofilling; **d** post-second lipofilling at 1 year

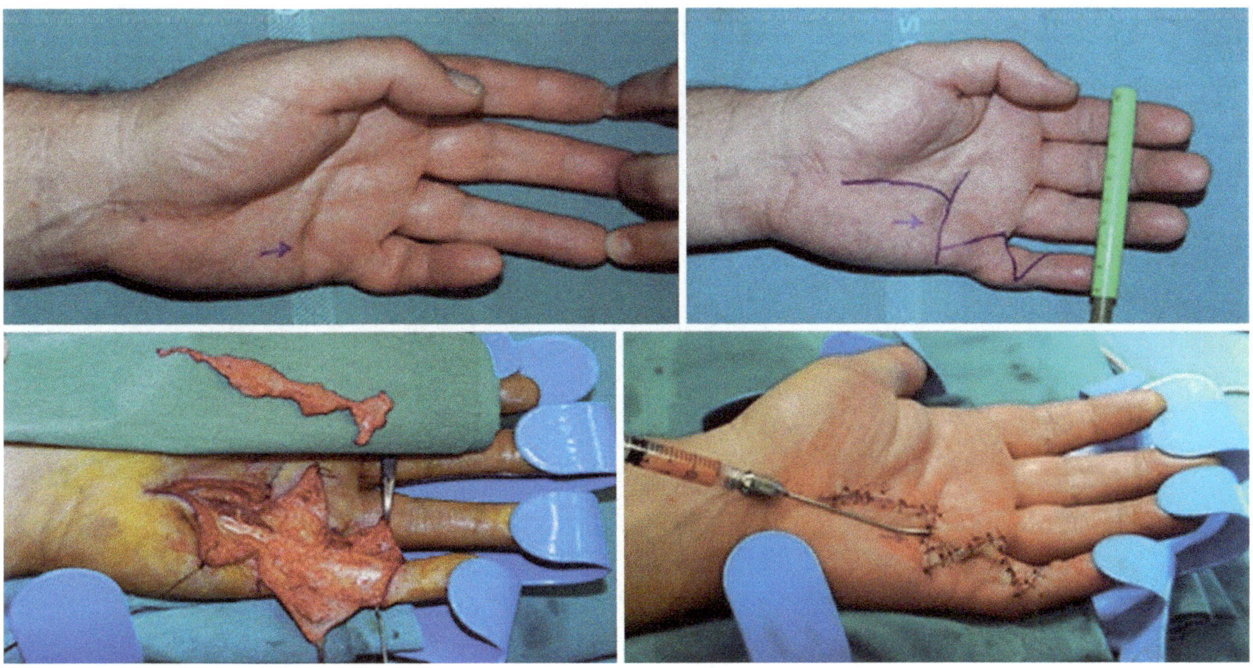

Fig. Fibrosis control in Dupuytren's disease

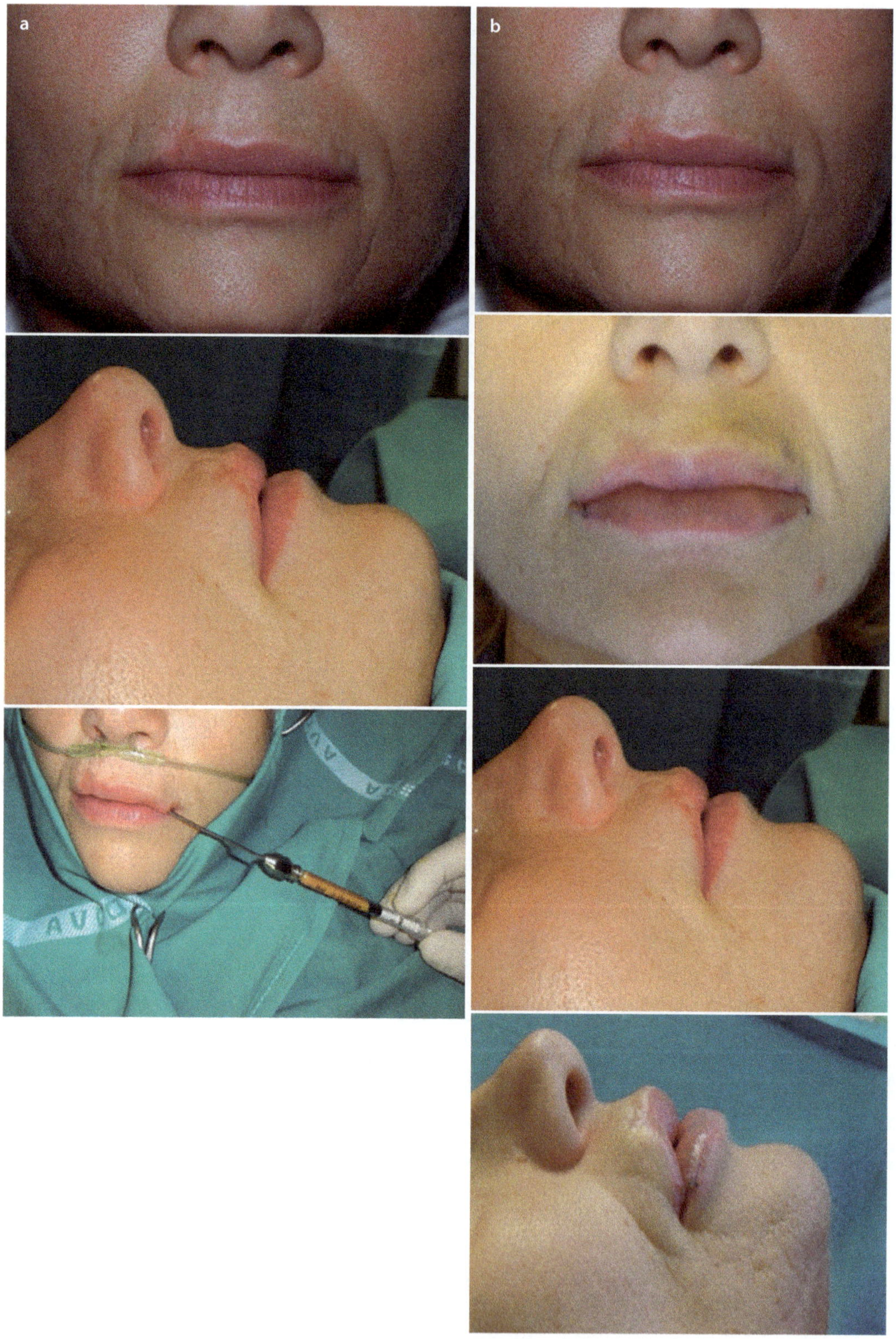

Fig. a Volume and contour: dog bite scar; pre-lipofilling; interoperative. b Volume and contour: postoperative results

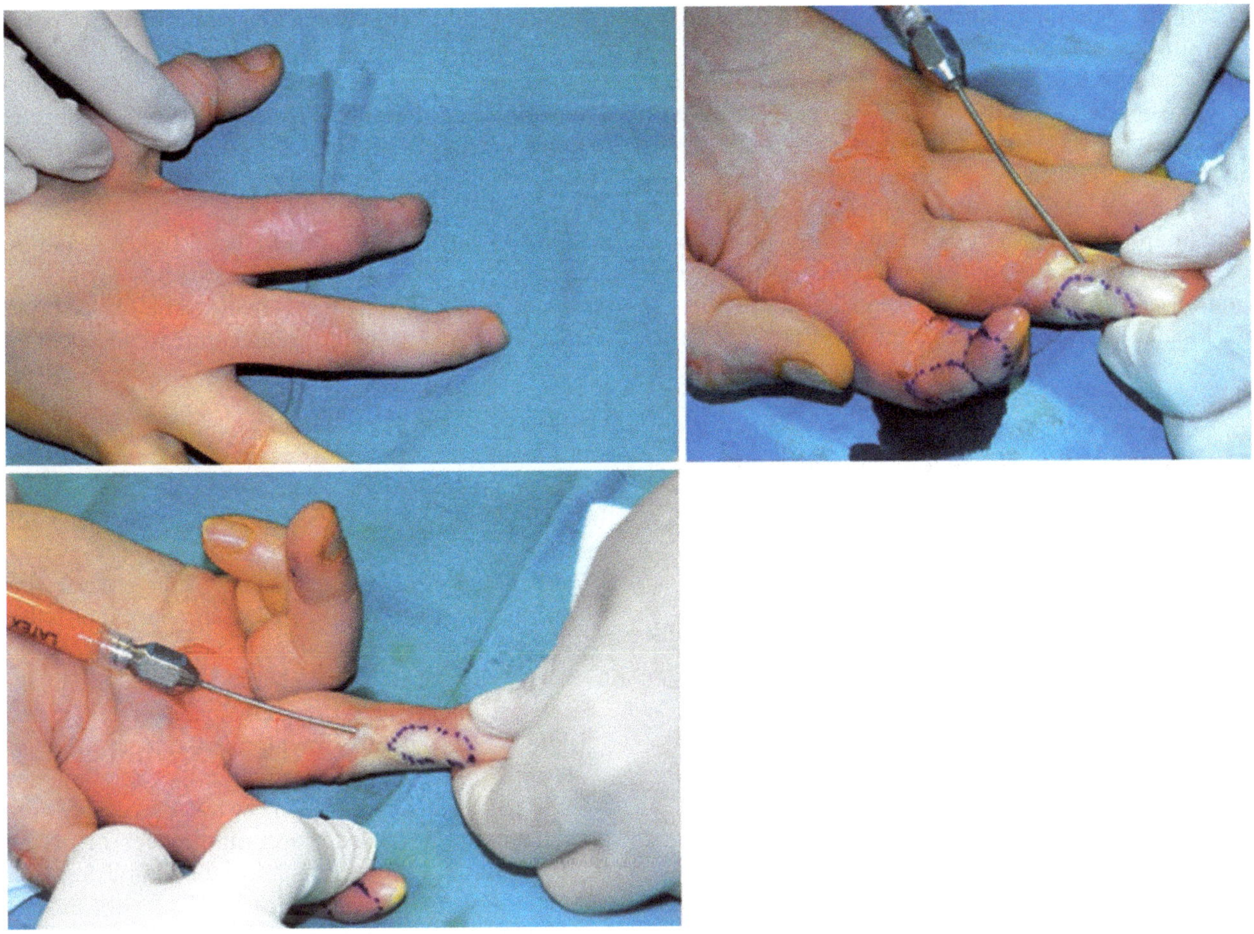

Fig. Pain and nerve release: posttraumatic nerve entrapment

The Skin Texture, Thickness, and Pliability

As demonstrated in 2009 by Mojallal et al. in an experimental mouse model, the transplantation of human adipose tissue to nude mice brought to an improving in the thickness of dermis. These results were obtained, thanks to a stimulated neosynthesis of type I collagen fibers, with a consequent composition of a denser extracellular dermal matrix. This skin feature improved its texture, thickness, and pliability.

Some years later, in 2013, Klinger M. et al. performed a study on humans, and they noted that the areas treated with free fat grafting assumed features that were similar to normal skin in terms of elasticity and softness. In order to demonstrate these features, they also used a durometer evaluation that demonstrated a significant reduction of skin hardness.

But why do ADSCs behave this way? As we said earlier, ADSCs can modulate and reduce inflammation; studies demonstrated that there is also an improvement in melanin secretion. These last utilities can also modify the skin color, thereby reducing the erythema and improving normal color of the skin.

The Fibrosis

Related to skin thickness, fibrosis can be due to diseases as, for example, connective tissue diseases or Dupuytren's disease or treatment such as radiotherapy. We used lipofilling in the treatment of a specific connective tissue disease called scleroderma or systemic sclerosis. This systemic connective tissue disease is featured by a progressive skin fibrosis especially on the face and in particular in the perioral region which brings to the so-called microstomia. The patients affected (usually female) report a bad lips sensation and progressive mouth dryness, difficulty in speaking, oral hygiene, and feeding. In our experience, the application of fat grafting in perioral region has improved the symptoms reducing skin stiffness and improving opening the mouth.

Regarding the use of lipofilling in Dupuytren's disease, this pathology is due to a fibrotic degeneration of the longitudinal fibers of palmar aponeurosis, with the consequent involvement of subcutaneous septa, the loss of subcutaneous fat, and the adherence of dermis to palmar aponeurosis. In this case the autologous adipose tissue is used as adjuvant therapy to prevent the formation of new fibrotic tissue (◘ Fig. 39.7).

Finally, regarding radiotherapy, the fibrosis is a sort of adverse event that rises years after the end of radiotherapy treatment and that it is due to the presence of an important post irradiated fibro-necrotic tissue featured by local dystrophic fat lobules, smaller but thicker vessels, and a perivascular fibrosis. In this case the fat grafting reduces the necrotic areas and improves neoangiogenesis with a consequent increasing in skin quality. It is supposed that these results are due to the intrinsic ability of the ADSCs to secrete growth factors, as angiogenic ones, as we said earlier.

The Volume and Contour

As we said earlier, the free fat grafting has a trophic/volumetric effect. As Mojallal noticed the autologous free fat grafting has to be considered as a *dynamic filler*. In fact, the "fat filler" doesn't have only an immediate effect of restoring volume, but it has the ability to produce adipogenesis with the consequent transformation of the preadipocytes in mature adipocytes. This can bring to an increased volume of the soft adipose tissue. The plasticity that features the adipose tissue makes it a good filler to restore the contour too, not only in posttraumatic scars but also in postoperative deformities and/or congenital malformation or adult progressive and self-limited deformation as, for example, in Parry-Romberg syndrome (the adult hemifacial atrophy).

Pain: The Analgesic Effect

According to Coleman who demonstrated the positive effect of free tissue transfer on neuralgias, Riyat et al. published in 2017 a review in which they noticed as the lipofilling had an analgesic effect, demonstrated with tests as, for example, POSAS or McGill Pain Questionnaire, on 966 patients. This effect seems to be due to multiple aspects: first of all, there is a mechanical release. To perform the injection, we have to insert the cannula under the scar in the space of the dermo-hypodermal junction, and then we proceed to distribute the fat in a retrograde way to reproduce a sort of a weblike matrix. This procedure can mechanically release fibrotic adherence and nerve entrapment, but most of all, the presence of the adipose stem cells can stimulate the nerve repair mediated by the brain-derived neurotrophic factor (BDNF), an adipose-derived neurotrophin which is fundamental in nerve growth and repair. But this is not the only mechanism to improve analgesic effect: as we said earlier, fat tissues are featured by an anti-inflammatory effect which is mediated both by the TGFβ production that can modulate and suppress T-cell function and by the production of IL 10 a cytokine which is abundantly produced by ADSCs and is known to inhibit Cd4 and CD8 lymphocytes reducing the inflammation response.

The Possible Applications

Based on the aforementioned effects, we can propose the free fat grafting for the treatment and prevention of multiple kinds of scars such as the following:

1. The treatment of atrophic and/or depressed scar, for example, in case of acne or previous removal of bulky neoformations. In case of atrophic and/or depressed scar, the free fat grating can be used both for a volumetric effect, indeed it fills the empty spaces, and for regenerative effect, indeed it can improve the skin texture.
2. The treatment of retracting scars which can limit not only the aesthetic point of view but also many functions as the flexor extension of the neck or of the elbow. In this case we can associate fat grafting with surgery as z-/w-plasty or flaps.
3. Unstable posttraumatic scars in order to obtain both scar stabilization and to improve wound healing.
4. Fibrotic diseases such as Dupuytren's disease and connective tissue diseases such as scleroderma, as we said previously.
5. Fibrotic irradiated tissue.
6. Fibrotic response to foreign bodies named periprosthetic fibrotic and, often, contracted capsule: this response can be described as a pathological and excessive deposition of collagen fibers around a mammary implant, in this case, the lipofilling.
7. Postsurgical deformities.
8. Nerve release in case of neuromas or posttraumatic pain.

The Ancillary Procedures to Increase the Overall Survival of Adipose Cells

The Plasma-Rich Platelet [10]

Known as PRP, it is a product obtainable by a blood draw of at least 20 cc. It is featured by a high concentration of platelet >300–350 × 10^3 platelets/μL, (three to five times than normal) and the production of growth factors, including *PDGF*, *TGF β*, *VEGF*, *IGF-1*, *FGF*, and *EGF*, released by the α granules of the activated platelets. These factors promote tissue repair, modulate inflammatory processes and neoangiogenesis, and ultimately regulate homeostasis of tissue and regenerative process. The PRP is easily obtainable without morbidity for the patient, and it can be associated to free fat grafting during the same session, in order to increase the percentage of engraftment and to improve the overall adipose cell survival.

The External Volume Expansion [11]

In order to improve on-site adipogenesis and overall adipose cell survival, a new technique called external volume expansion (EVE) is being used in these years. This procedure is based on tissue expansion combined with the mechanobiology principles which explain how mechanical forces, such as the ones produced by the application of the negative pressure therapy, can be transduced in the cells in order to stimulate processes as cellular shaping, proliferation, and differentiation. In fact, studies demonstrated that the EVE application can increase cell proliferation, deep dermis capillary density, and adipogenesis due to the edema and inflammation response which are proadipogenic factors.

The Future

Recently the fat graft has been proposed for the treatment of keloids or hypertrophic scars. Keloid is a fibroproliferative disorder which is known as pathological scar, and it is featured by an excessive production and deposition of extracellular dermal matrix due to prolonged inflammatory and proliferative phases of wound healing. Nowadays, there is not a gold standard treatment for pathological scars; it is actually based both on prevention with compressive garments or silicone gel or sheets both on topical injection of keloid with anti-inflammatory drugs as corticosteroids. Based on the anti-inflammatory properties of the free fat grafting and on its ability to stimulate neoangiogenesis and a better skin quality, it has been proposed to use it in the treatment of hypertrophic/keloid scars, for example, in postburn patient. Even if the first impressions are absolutely positive, unfortunately, as Lee G et al. noted in 2017, there is a lack of high-level literature about this field, so further studies are required.

Something to Discuss: The Oncological Point of View

Even if the adipose tissue transfer has multiple benefit effects, recently it has been supposed that the pluripotent adipose-derived stem cells and the neoangiogenesis stimulated by growth factors can bring to the onset of a new neoplasia or a recurrence if the free fat graft is injected in a recipient site which is recently affected by a cancer, especially in a breast that has undergone a nipple-sparing mastectomy or a partial mastectomy (quadrantectomy). Many studies have been performed in order to demonstrate the safety of the fat grafting in such patients, but nowadays, even if a correlation between lipofilling and neoplasm or its recurrence has not been demonstrated, it is preferable to propose the free fat transfer after 2 years free of disease.

Conclusion

In light of our experience, the free fat grafting is considered an effective and promising treatment for scars. The biological properties of ADSCs combined with an easy and quick procedure, a low morbidity for the patients, and a high compliance make lipofilling an ideal treatment to propose. Unfortunately, the treatment has some limitations. First of all it cannot be proposed to a very slim patients; in fact we need fatty areas to obtain ADSCs; secondly, as we said earlier, the percentage of reabsorption of fat grafting subjectively varies from 10% to 70% till the complete reabsorption in extreme cases. This negative feature can result in multiple treatment sessions in order to obtain the right volume, but unfortunately it is not possible to set the number of sessions required since the beginning.

Fortunately, new studies and new research on cell therapy help us to avoid or reduce this problem, as we saw that the use of the external negative pressure therapy and/or the combination of free fat grafting with the plasma-rich platelet can improve the fat engraftment and the overall adipose cell survival with consequent better morpho-functional results.

Take Home Messages

- The fat grafting contains stem cells called adipose-derived stem cells.
- The adipose-derived stem cells are pluripotent cells.
- The fat grafting is an easy procedure with low morbidity rate.
- The fat injection has both a volumetric and a regenerative effect.
- The fat injection stimulates neo-adipogenesis and neoangiogenesis, and it modulates inflammation and fibrosis.
- The fat grafting can be reabsorbed.
- We can use external volume expansion and/or the combination with plasma-rich platelet to improve engraftment and overall adipose cell survival.

References

1. US Department of Health and Human Services. Tissue guidances: human cells, tissues, and cellular and tissue-based products (hct/ps) from adipose tissue: regulatory considerations; draft guidance. www.fda.gov/BiologicsBloodVaccines/GuidanceComplianceRegulatoryInformation/Guidances/Tissue/ucm427795.htm. Accessed 8 June 2015.
2. American Society of Plastic Surgeons and the Plastic Surgery Foundation. Docket #FDA-2014-D-1856 (HCT/Ps). www.plasticsurgery.org/Documents/Legislation-Advocacy/Regulatory/asps-response-hctp-draft-guidance.pdf. Accessed 7 July 2015.
3. Bassetto F, et al. Adipose-derived stem cells to modulate scar tissue: from biological basis to clinical application. In: Shiffman MA, Di Giuseppe A, editors. Stem cells in aesthetic procedures. art, science and clinical techniques. Berlin: Springer; 2014.
4. Bassetto F, et al. Fat grafting in the treatment of skin fibrosis and scars. J Wound Technol. 2014;24:17–19.
5. Mojallal A, et al. Improvement of skin quality after fat grafting: clinical and observation and an animal study. Plast Reconstr Surg. 2009;124:765.
6. Lee G, et al. Autologous fat grafting in keloids and hypertrophic scars: a review. Scars Burn Heal. 2017;3:2059513117700157.
7. Riyat H, et al. Autologous fat grafting for scars, healing and pain: a review. Scars Burn Heal. 2017;3:2059513117728200.
8. Bassetto F, et al. Fat grafting in wound healing and scar control. J Wound Technol. 2016;31:54–55.
9. Klinger M, et al. Autologous fat graft in scar treatment. J Craniofac Surg. 2013;24:1610Y1615.
10. Osaid H Alser, Ioannis Goutos (2018). The evidence behind the use of platelet-rich plasma (PRP) in scar management: a literature review. Scars, Burns & Healing 4:205951311880877.
11. Lujan Hernandez J, et al. Induction of adipogenesis by external volume expansion. Plast Reconstr Surg. 2016;137(1):122–31.

5

Usefulness of Local Flaps for Scar Contracture Release

Rei Ogawa

Contents

Background

Selection of Local Flaps

Transposition Flaps

The Square Flap Method

Propeller Flaps

Conclusion

References

Background

Local flaps are useful for reconstructing scar contractures on mobile areas such as the joints, the neck, the axilla, the digital web, and the mouth commissure. They are superior to skin grafts because the latter can contract, thereby leading to secondary contractures. Moreover, the color and texture match of local flaps is better than that of grafted skin. Consequently, local flaps generally provide superior aesthetic outcomes. Thus, if there is healthy skin adjacent to the scar contracture, local flaps should be the first choice. Based on the type of movement needed to place the flap, local flaps can be classified as advancement flaps, rotation flaps, and transposition flaps. A more recent advance is to design these flaps as perforator flaps. The inclusion of perforators in the flap provides great freedom in terms of flap shape and the movement and rotation arc of the flap: the propeller flap method is a particularly good example of such flaps. Moreover, flap combinations such as the bilobed flap and the square flap method can expand the possibilities offered by local flaps.

Selection of Local Flaps

Several approaches that elongate the scar and thereby release linear contractures have been reported. Z-plasty is one of the best-known options when it comes to releasing linear contractures [1]. The theoretical final scar length for the 60° angle z-plasty is approximately 1.73 times the original length of the scar. W-plasty also allows contracture release to some degree due to its so-called accordion effect: this reflects the fact that zigzag-shaped scars elongate in an accordion-like fashion over time [2]. However, these methods are mainly used for "linear" contractures. If the scar is wide, the scar cannot be removed and then sutured primarily. In this case, the scar should be divided by a local flap to obtain contracture release.

In terms of local flap selection, it is necessary to choose between a skin-pedicled flap and an island flap. We showed recently [3] that 6 months after surgery, skin-pedicled flaps associate with greater scar extension rates than island flaps (◘ Fig. 35.1). Notably, skin-pedicled and island flaps, respectively, extended the scar by 1.53- and 1.28-fold 6 months after surgery. Thus, local flaps, especially skin-pedicled flaps, elongate the scar as effectively as z-plasty. It should be noted that if the scar is large, it is effective only by dividing the scar with the local flap. However, the flap size can be slightly smaller than the deformity size (although how much smaller depends somewhat on how extensible the flap type is): it is not necessary that the flap is as big as the open wound after scar division or scar removal.

In the case of the local flap design, it can be affected not only by the ease of the technique but also by the geometry of the scar and open wound tissues. Thus, selecting between the skin-pedicled flap and the island flap should be performed on a case-by-case basis. However, the greater extensibility of the skin-pedicled flap means that it should be the primary choice in the

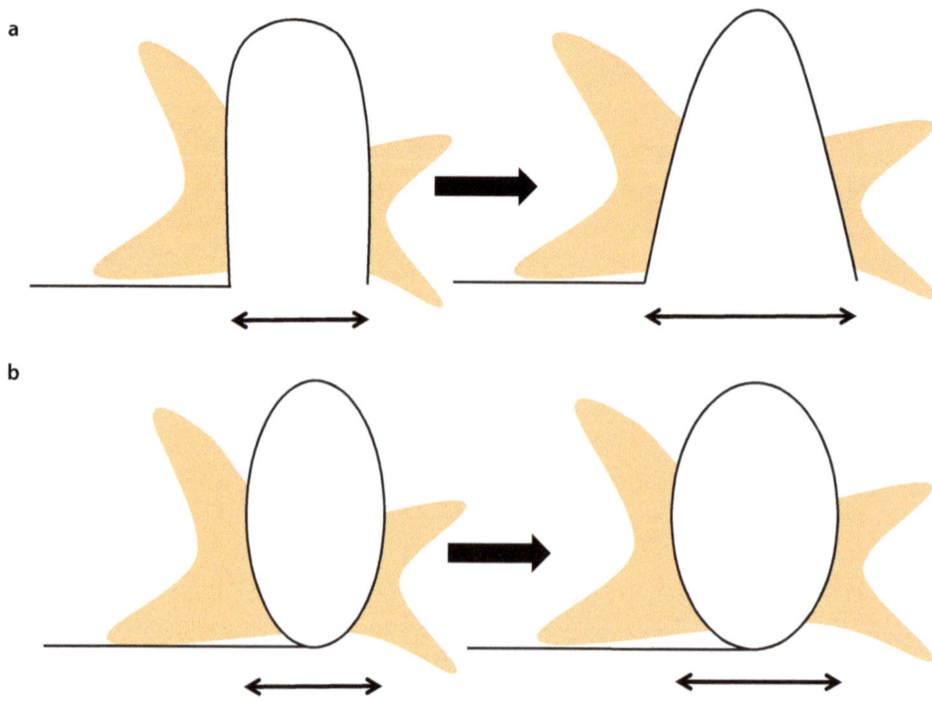

◘ **Fig.** Comparison of skin-pedicled and island flaps in terms of extensibility. **a** Skin-pedicled flap. **b** Island flap. Skin-pedicled flaps have a greater extension rate than island flaps because they include healthy skin, which can expand after surgery. By contrast, the inelastic scar tissue all around the island flap limits its extensibility

case of scar contracture release [3]. This greater extensibility is probably because the entire perimeter of the island flap is surrounded by new scar, whereas the skin-pedicled flap maintains a connection with normal skin. Since normal skin is highly elastic (much more elastic than scar tissue), it may promote the elongation and enlargement of the skin-pedicled flap. Moreover, at a theoretical level, the circular shape of the island flap also limits its extensibility. However, it should be noted that island flaps have technical advantages over skin-pedicled flaps: they are relatively simple to transfer to the recipient site, and they can employ the remaining healthy skin around the scars without any waste.

Transposition Flaps

The transposition flap is one of the classical and most representative of the local flaps. Its contracture-releasing effect is very high because the flap has a skin pedicle. The healthy skin of the flap expands over time after surgery; as a result, the rectangular shape of the flap becomes triangular (◘ Figs. 35.2, 35.3, 35.4, and 35.5). This effect reflects the release of tension via the skin pedicle.

If the flap has to be large, perforators can be attached, and a supercharged transposition flap can be designed [4]. The perforator is then anastomosed to the recipient site. This perforator-supercharged transposition flap is

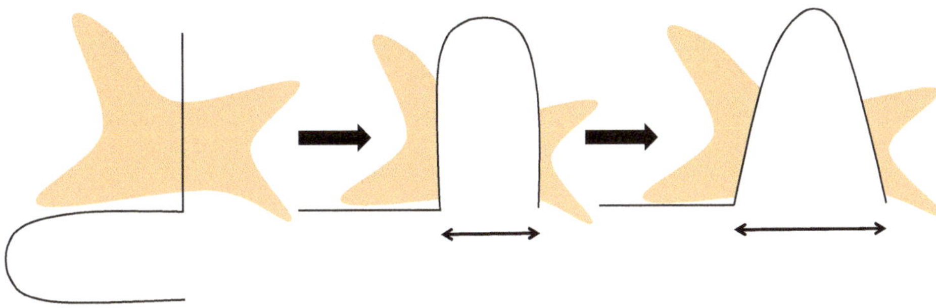

◘ **Fig.** Transposition flap. Transposition flaps should be designed parallel to the contracture line. After surgery, the skin pedicle can expand over time

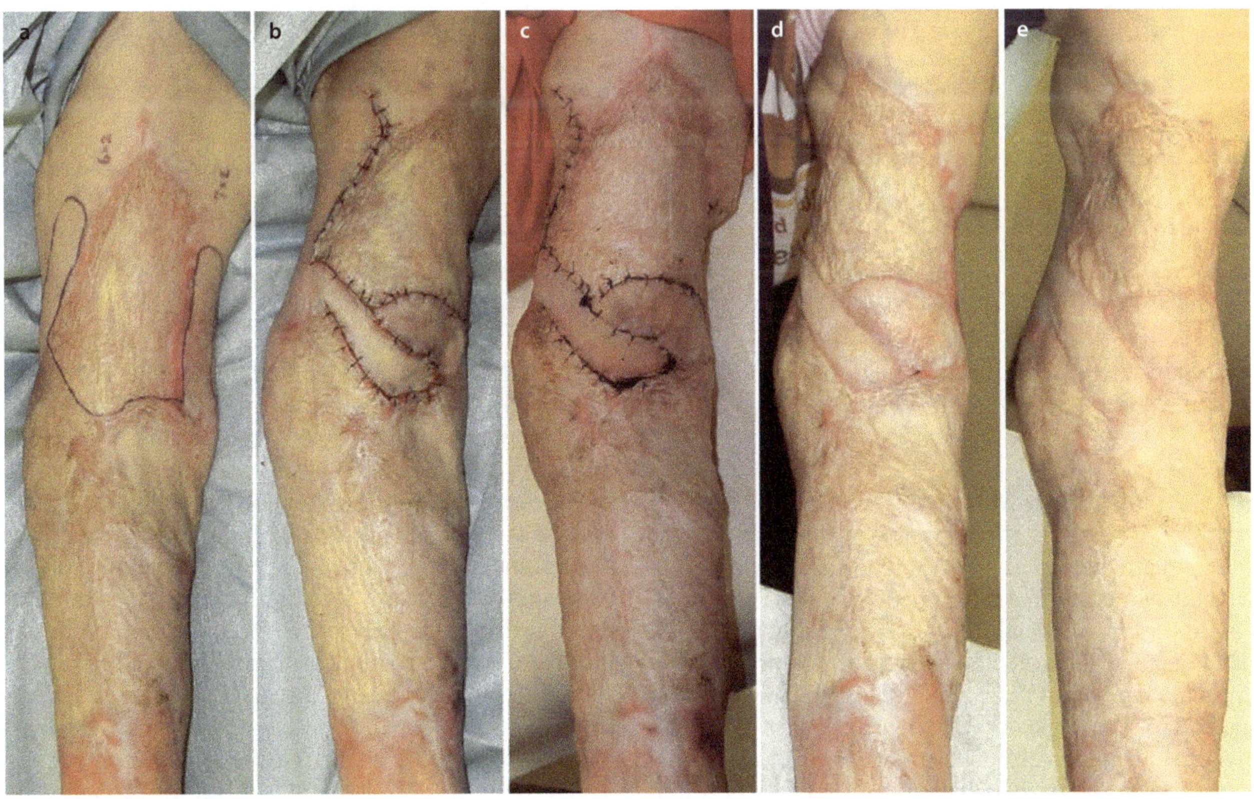

◘ **Fig.** Reconstruction of a scar contracture on the cubital fossa. **a** Preoperative view. **b** View immediately after the operation. **c** Two weeks after the operation. **d** Two months after the operation. **e** Ten months after the operation. Bilateral transposition flaps were harvested. No flap ischemia was observed. The contracture was released by about 10 cm

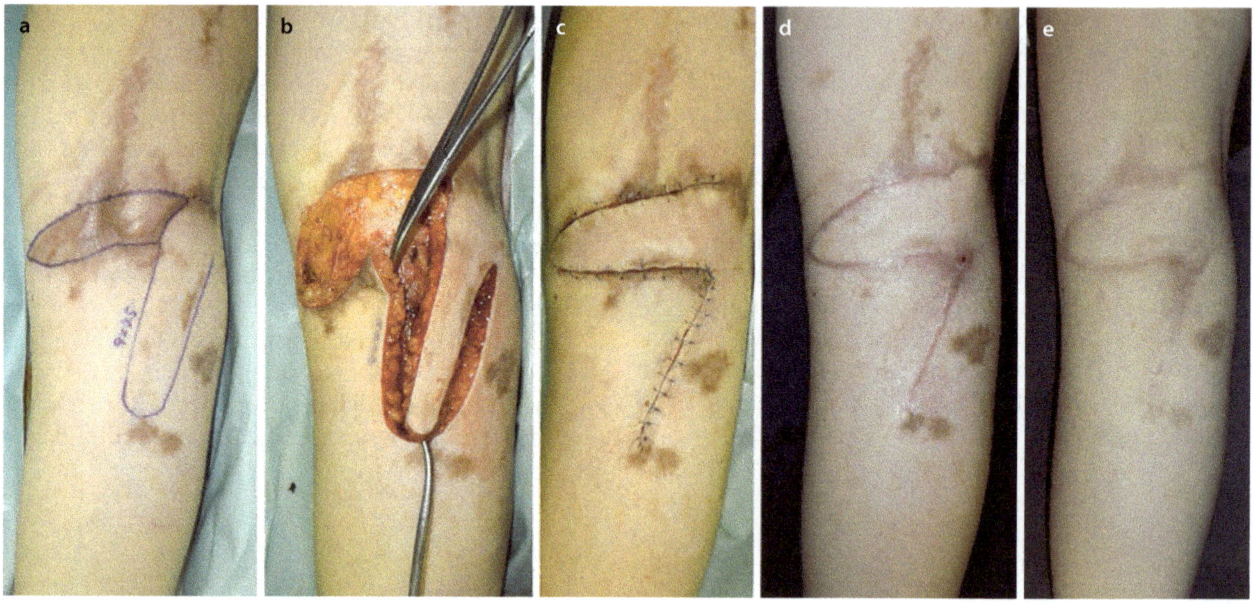

■ **Fig.** Reconstruction of a scar contracture behind the knee. **a** Preoperative view. **b** Intraoperative view. **c** View immediately after the operation. **d** One year after the operation. **e** Two years after the operation. A transposition flap was designed next to the scar contracture behind the knee. The contracture was released completely

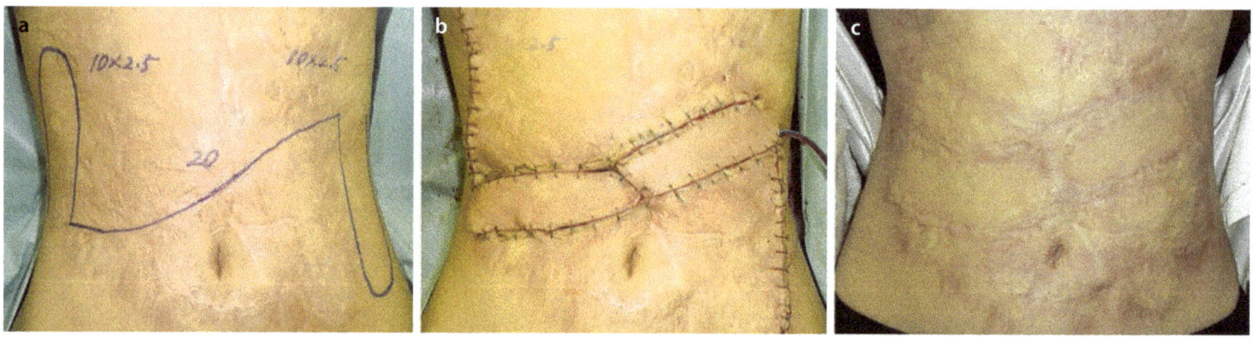

■ **Fig.** Reconstruction of a scar contracture on the abdomen. **a** Preoperative view. **b** View immediately after the operation. **c** One year after the operation. A bilateral transposition flap was designed. The contracture sensation on the abdomen was relieved by the operation

especially useful for reconstructing anterior neck contractures (■ Fig. 35.6).

The Square Flap Method

The square flap method was reported previously by Hyakusoku et al. [5] and is an effective way of elongating the skin, especially for scar contracture release (■ Fig. 35.7). This method consists of a combination of a square flap, one 45° triangular flap, and one 90° triangular flap. The angle of the triangular flaps of Limberg's original method is 30° [6]. However, in the case of scar surgery, the 30° triangular flap can lead to blood flow failure because, in some cases, part of the scar must be included in the flap. Thus, the angles of the triangular flaps in the square flap method should be wider: the combination of a 45° triangular flap and a 90° triangular flap is ideal. One option is to design a four-flap z-plasty and a five-flap z-plasty. However, it is safer to include one square flap. Moreover, the biggest advantage of the square flap method is that one of the flaps has a square shape. This square flap can advance downward and can make a suitably large and pliable floor over the joints and web space. Thus, the method results in three-dimensional reconstruction [7]. In addition, the skin pedicle of the square flap can effectively release tension over time after the operation. This method is particularly indicated for scars on the joints, the neck, the axilla, the digital web, and the mouth commissure (■ Figs. 35.8, 35.9, and 35.10). Theoretically, this method increases the original scar length by 2.8-fold [7].

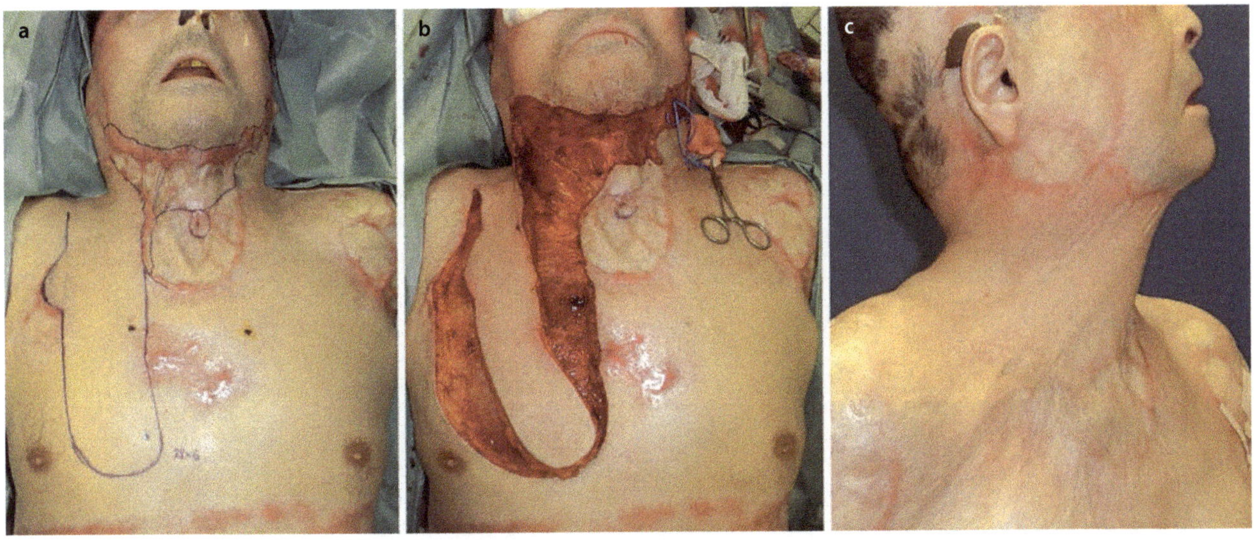

Fig. Reconstruction of a scar contracture on the anterior neck by using a supercharged transposition flap. **a** Preoperative view. **b** Intraoperative view. **c** Two years after the operation. An anterior neck contracture of a 71-year-old man was reconstructed with a supercharged transposition flap. A perforator of the internal mammary artery in the first intercostal space was attached to the flap and anastomosed with the facial artery and vein. The flap allowed full extension of the neck

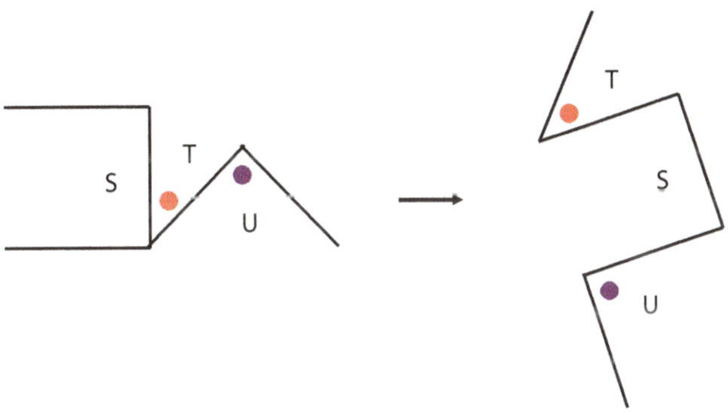

Fig. The square flap method. Theoretically, the method lengthens the original scar length by 2.8-fold

Propeller Flaps

It has been reported that an island flap that can be rotated 90° like a propeller is suitable for the reconstruction of the axilla and cubitus [8] (Fig. 35.11). That was the first time this flap type was described. This original propeller flap was made by using the intact skin in a cubital fossa as a subcutaneous-pedicled island flap to release post-burn linear scar contractures that adjoined the fossa. The subcutaneous pedicle was located in the center of the flap. In the 20 years following this seminal advance, propeller flaps have been refined and modified, and various types of propeller flaps have been reported [9–13]. The most sophisticated of these is the perforator-pedicled propeller (PPP) flap [9]. This type of flap can be harvested from any site on the body that bears a perforator. It employs a skeletonized vascular pedicle that allows the flap to be rotated by up to 180°. Moreover, if the perforator pedicle is located at the edge of the flap, the flap can cover a defect that is a long distance away from the flap donor site. Depending on the case, the flap can be rotated in a clockwise or counterclockwise direction.

The PPP flap is now considered by many plastic surgeons to be a highly viable and particularly sophisticated perforator flap option. This largely reflects the fact that the human body has over 400 perforators whose diameters exceed 0.5 mm. Thus, at least 400 types of propeller flaps can theoretically be harvested. This broad availability means that custom-made PPP flaps can be used to reconstruct defects on many parts of the body. Indeed, PPP flaps are particularly suitable for scars on the trunk and limbs. However, donor site limitations may reduce the suitability of this method for reconstructing the head and neck region.

Since the course and territory of perforators differ for each region, it is advisable to perform a careful preoperative assessment with Doppler ultrasound, color Doppler ultrasonography, or multi-detector low computed tomography (MD-CT). This greatly facilitates the operation, thereby reducing the operative time [14].

It should be noted, however, that propeller flaps have one significant disadvantage: they are always island flaps. Thus, their contracture-releasing effect is lower than that of skin-pedicled flaps. Consequently, propeller flaps are generally only chosen when the available healthy skin adjacent to the defect is limited and a skin-pedicled flap is not possible (Fig. 35.12).

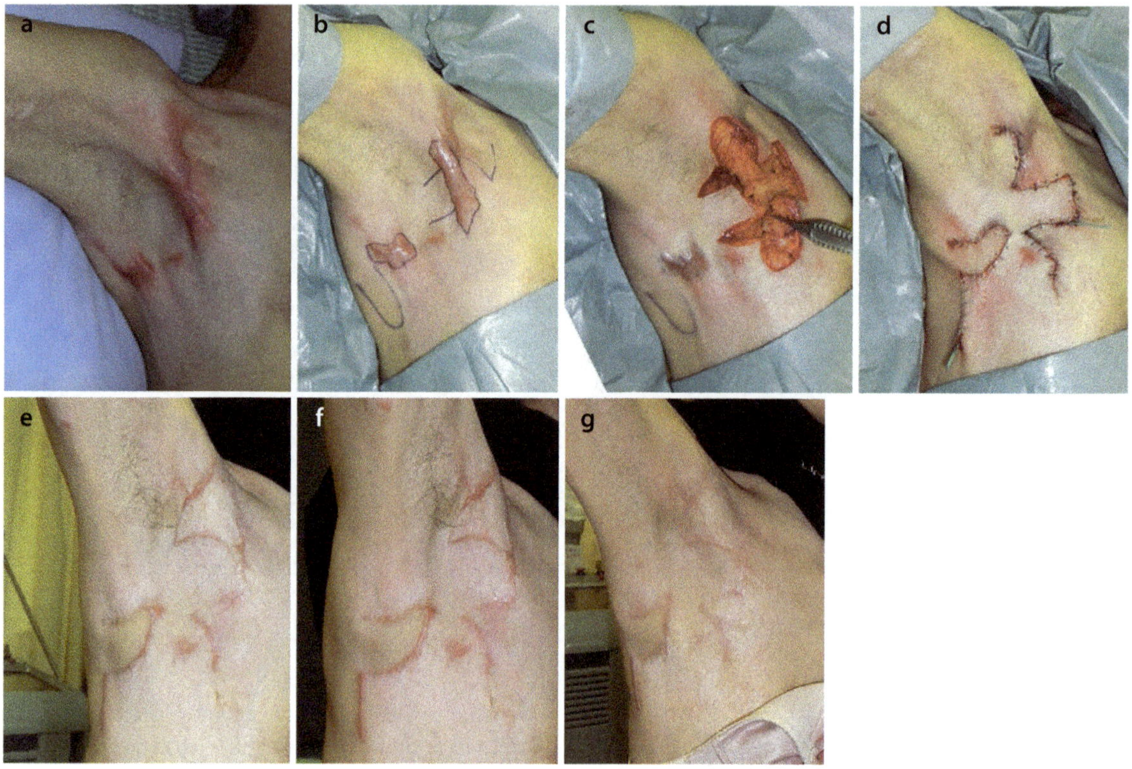

Fig. Reconstruction of a scar contracture on the axilla. **a** Preoperative view. **b** Design of the flap. **c** Intraoperative view. **d** View immediately after the operation. **e** Three months after the operation. **f** Six months after the operation. **g** One year after the operation. The square flap method was used to reconstruct an axillary scar contracture. The square flap gained a triangular shape one year after operation. This indicates that the skin pedicle of the flap extended, thus effectively releasing the tension

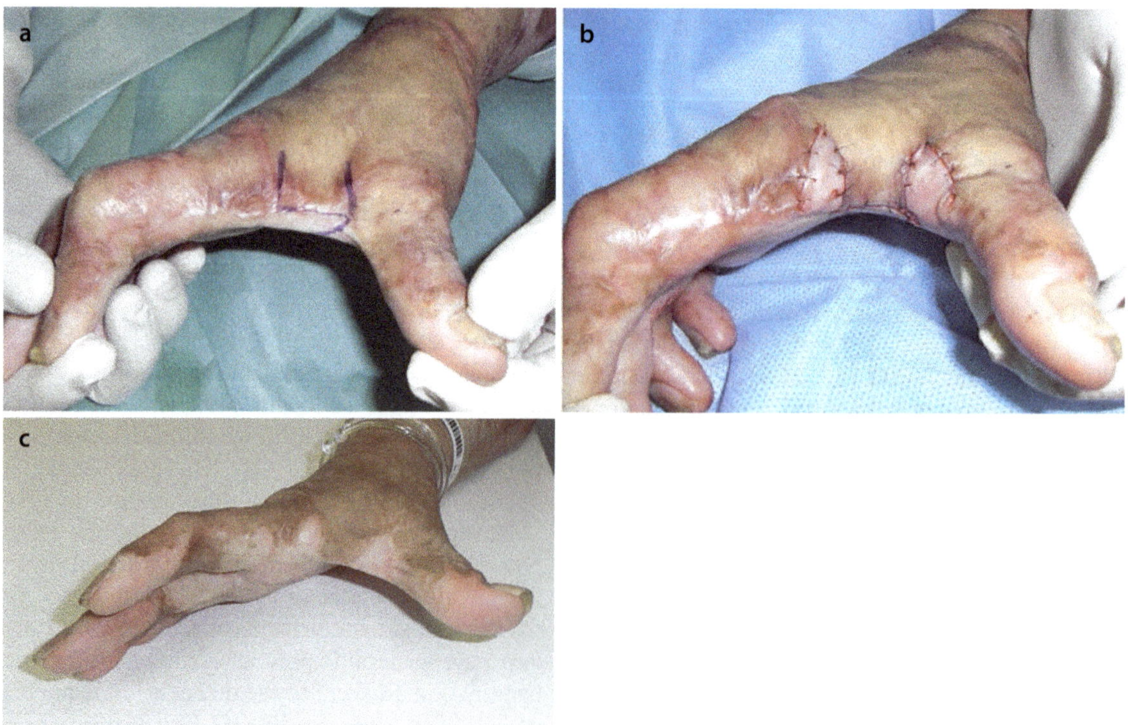

Fig. Reconstruction of a scar contracture on the digital web. **a** Design of the flap. **b** View immediately after the operation. **c** Two years after the operation. The square flap method was used to reconstruct a digital web scar contracture. The skin pedicle of the flap extended, thereby effectively releasing the tension

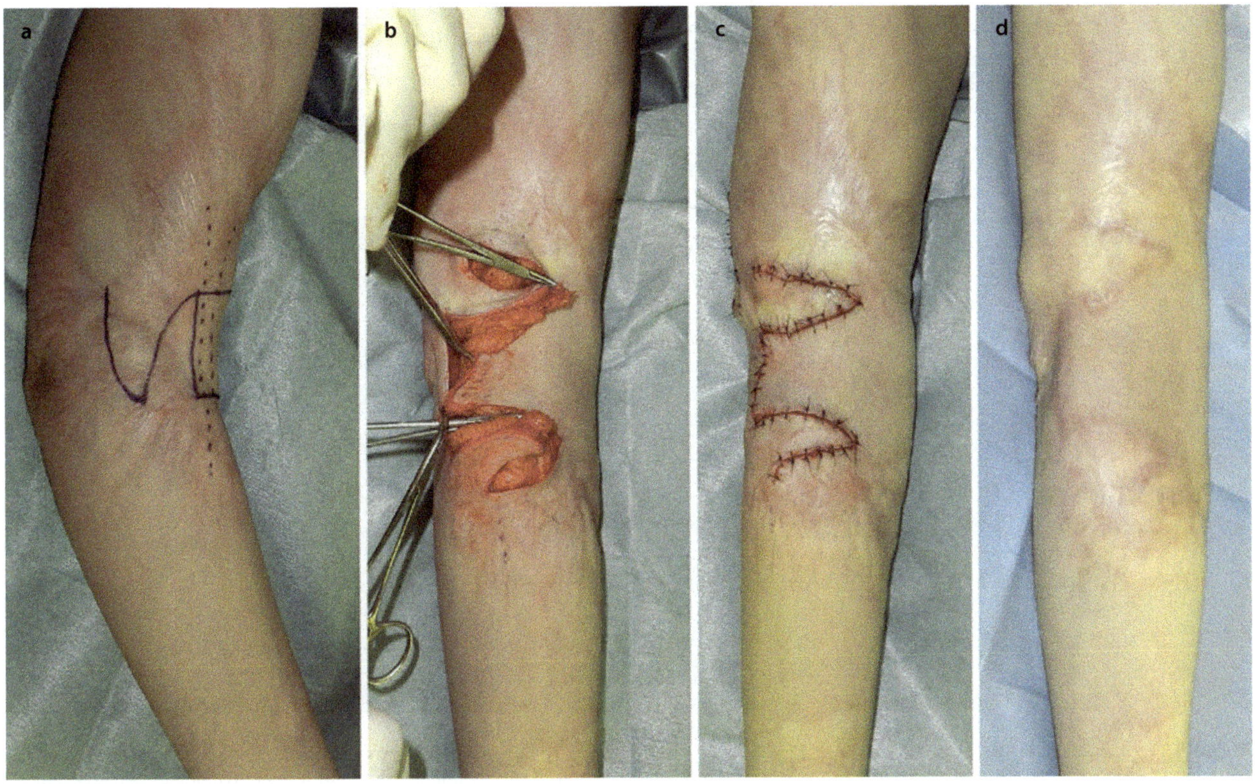

Fig. Reconstruction of a scar contracture on the cubital fossa. **a** Design of the flap. **b** Intraoperative view. **c** View immediately after the operation. **d** Eighteen months after the operation. The square flap method was used to reconstruct a cubital fossa scar contracture. The skin pedicle of the flap extended, thereby effectively releasing the tension

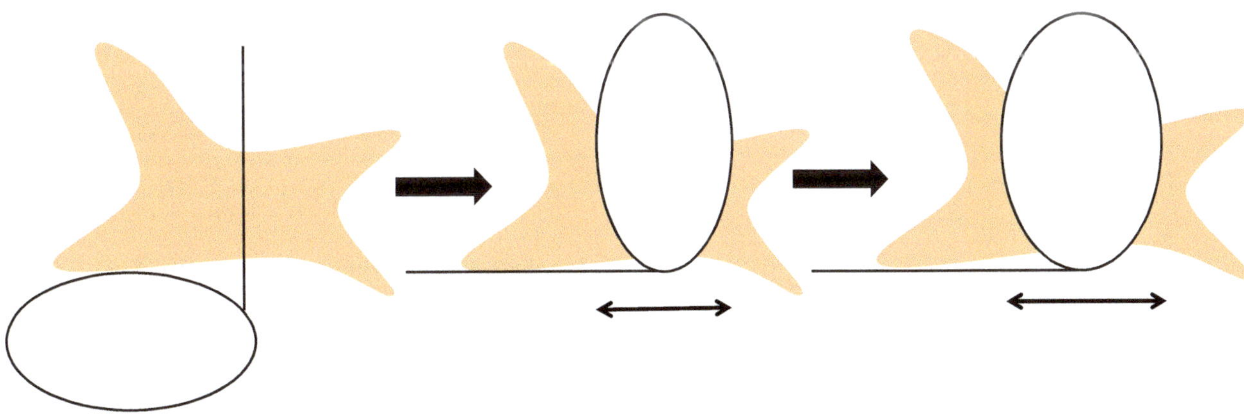

Fig. Propeller flap. The most sophisticated of the propel-ler flaps is the perforator-pedicled propeller (PPP) flap. However, its contracture-releasing effect is lower than that of skin-pedicled flaps. Thus, propeller flaps are most useful when the available healthy skin adjacent to the scar is limited and a skin-pedicled flap cannot be performed

Conclusion

Local flaps generally provide superior functional and aesthetic outcomes. In terms of local flap selection, it is necessary to choose between a skin-pedicled flap and an island flap. It was suggested that skin-pedicled flaps associate with greater scar extension rates than island flaps. Moreover, it should be noted that if the scar is large, it is effective only by dividing the scar with the local flap.

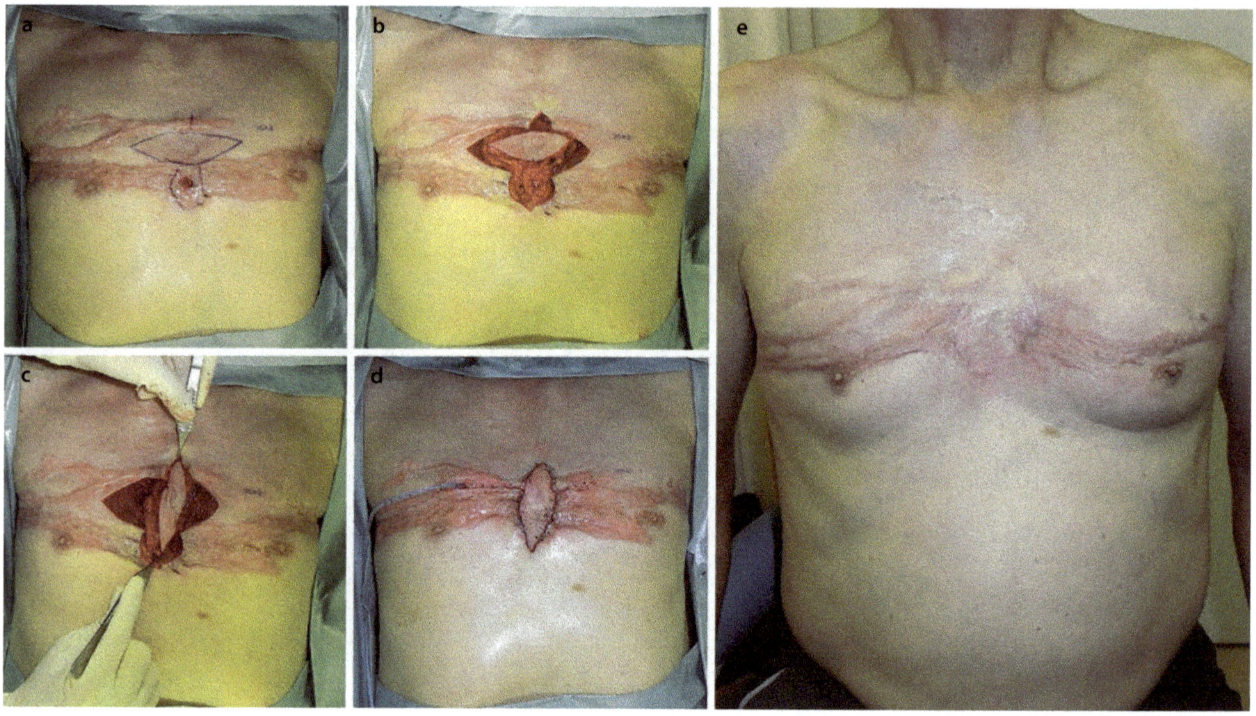

Fig. Reconstruction of a scar contracture on the anterior chest wall. **a** Design of the flap. **b, c** Intraoperative view. **d** View immediately after the operation. **e** Eighteen months after the operation. The propeller flap was designed on the limited space between a scar contracture and an ulcer. Both open wounds were reconstructed by using a 90° rotated propeller flap

Take Home Messages

- Local flaps are superior to skin grafts because the latter can contract, thereby leading to secondary contractures.
- The color and texture match of local flaps is better than that of grafted skin.
- Local flaps, especially skin-pedicled flaps, elongate the scar as effectively as z-plasty.
- It should be noted that if the scar is large, it is effective only by dividing the scar with the local flap.

References

1. Arima J, Dohi T, Kuribayashi S, Akaishi S, Ogawa R. Z-plasty and postoperative radiation therapy for anterior chest wall keloids: an analysis of 141 patients. Plast Reconstr Surg Glob Open. 2019;7(3):e2177.
2. Goutos I, Yousif A, Ogawa R. W plasty techniques in scar revision: geometrical considerations and site-specific technique modifications. Plast Reconstr Surg Glob Open. 2019;7(4):e2179.
3. Yoshino Y, Kubomura K, Ueda H, Tsuge T, Ogawa R. Extension of flaps associated with burn scar reconstruction: a key difference between island and skin-pedicled flaps. Burns. 2018;44(3):683–91.
4. Noda Y, Kuwahara H, Morimoto M, Ogawa R. Reconstruction of anterior neck scar contracture using a perforator-supercharged transposition flap. Plast Reconstr Surg Glob Open. 2018;6(2):e1485.
5. Hyakusoku H, Fumiiri M. The square flap method. Br J Plast Surg. 1987;40(1):40–6.
6. Limberg AA, Wolfe SA. Planning of local plastic operations on the body surface: theory and practice. Lexington: Collamore Press; 1984. p. 382.
7. Huang C, Ogawa R. Three-dimensional reconstruction of scar contracture-bearing axilla and digital webs using the square flap method. Plast Reconstr Surg Glob Open. 2014;2(5):e149.
8. Hyakusoku H, Yamamoto T, Fumiiri M. The propeller flap method. Br J Plast Surg. 1991;44:53–4.
9. Hyakusoku H, Ogawa R, Oki K, Ishii N. The perforator pedicled propeller (PPP) flap method: a report of two cases. J Nippon Med Sch. 2007;74:367–71.
10. Jakubietz RG, Jakubietz MG, Gruenert JG, Kloss DF. The 180-degree perforator-based propeller flap for soft tissue coverage of the distal, lower extremity: a new method to achieve reliable coverage of the distal lower extremity with a local, fasciocutaneous perforator flap. Ann Plast Surg. 2007 Dec;59(6):667–71.
11. Wong CH, Cui F, Tan BK, Liu Z, Lee HP, Lu C, Foo CL, Song C. Nonlinear finite element simulations to elucidate the determinants of perforator patency in propeller flaps. Ann Plast Surg. 2007;59(6):672–8.
12. Pignatti M, Pasqualini M, Governa M, Bruti M, Rigotti G. Propeller flaps for leg reconstruction. J Plast Reconstr Aesthet Surg. 2008;61(7):777–83.
13. Mateev MA, Ogawa R, Trunov L, Moldobaeva N, Hyakusoku H. Shape-modified radial artery perforator flap method: analysis of 112 cases. Plast Reconstr Surg. 2009;123:1533–43.
14. Ono S, Ogawa R, Hayashi H, Takami Y, Kumita SI, Hyakusoku H. Multidetector-row computed tomography (MDCT) analysis of the supra-fascial perforator directionality (SPD) of the occipital artery perforator (OAP). J Plast Reconstr Aesthet Surg. 2010;63(10):1602–7.

6

Specific Attention Areas in Scar Management: Management of Atrophic Scars

Matteo Tretti Clementoni and Ernest Azzopardi

Contents

Background
Common Principles

Atrophic Acne Vulgaris Scarring
Resurfacing and Tightening Techniques
Dermal Lift Techniques
Volume-Imparting Techniques
Isotretinoin Treatment
State-of-the-Art and Combinatorial Approaches

Striae Albae

Burn Atrophic Scars

Conclusion

References

Background

Atrophic scars represent some of the most difficult and insidious pathologies confronting the reconstructive surgeon. Deriving from the ancient Greek "a-trophos" (wasted), the term presents a vivid representation of the clinical picture and an area of scar management particularly worthy of specific attention.

The atrophic scars typically develop as a result of an intracutaneous inflammatory process. Rather than exuberant inflammation, the process results in reduced matrix regeneration and focally reduced collagen production. Focal contraction of the scar tissue will result in uneven soft tissue defects. Clinically, these result in contour defects on the surface of the skin [1].

Several pathologies may result in atrophic scars [2], This chapter is intended for the experienced laser practitioner tackling three clinical conditions presenting to the reconstructive specialties, often as a last resort after exhaustive traditional management: acne, striae albae, and burns. It explores common principles, followed by state-of-the-art management and evaluation of the senior author's experience.

Common Principles

These atrophic conditions wound both tissue and psyche. They tend to be underestimated causes of significant morbidity for the individual patient who often either loses all hope of amelioration or presents with unrealistic expectation. Therefore, its appropriate management entails identification of their concern, their attitude toward the risk/benefit of the management proposed, and setting their expectations at an appropriate and realistic level. It is important to emphasize that current treatment modalities can improve but cannot completely remove atrophic scars. Scarring from acne vulgaris and burns has been associated to a range of mental health issues including depression as well as embarrassment, poor self-esteem, and general social impairment. Early and appropriate involvement of multidisciplinary opinion is key [3, 4].

Appropriate clinical documentation not only helps set the baseline at presentation but also allows the patient to observe progress and build confidence. Both two-dimensional photography and three-dimensional photography are useful adjuncts in management, given reproducible conditions and serial repetition.

Further, an objective grading of the condition is key to identify appropriate therapeutic options in mind. While classification systems are extensively discussed elsewhere, it is our experience that the use of one over the other is not in itself as important as consistency, and familiarity with one system, geared toward a therapeutic solution.

Atrophic Acne Vulgaris Scarring

Atrophic scarring is substantially more common than hypertrophic [5]. Being able to deconstruct the presentation into the component symptoms is crucial. Often the components of the presenting complaint are a mixture of contour and dyschromia, which can be general or specific to particular areas or even single scars. It is important to enquire about the physical consequences which the patient perceives, such as the inability to apply makeup, which are key areas of concern, past treatment regimes, and the frequency of recrudescence. Tendency to hypertrophic, keloid, or poor scarring is asked. Enquiring about postoperative social commitments is important, considering the variation in recovery times with the various treatments while sun exposure without adequate protection may dramatically alter the result and incidence of complications. Examination establishes skin type and excludes residual active inflammation, extent, and grade of disease. Application of the Goodman and Baron classification imparts some degree of objectivity in concluding one's deliberations to focus on the appropriate therapeutic modalities (◘ Table 41.1).

Management of atrophic acne scarring depends on the infrastructure and equipment available to the practitioner; therefore, a critical appraisal of traditional methods is presented first, followed by state-of-the-art methods and our experience thereafter. For ease of reference, these techniques are grouped by their main mode of action into resurfacing and tightening, dermal lifting techniques, and dermal volumization techniques.

Resurfacing and Tightening Techniques

Microdermabrasion

Microdermabrasion is a minimally invasive technique that improves texture but only addresses superficial scars, although its combination with aminolevulinic acid photodynamic therapy (ALA-PDT) is more effective, based on RCT evidence [7]. In principle, subsequent wound remodeling results in neocollagenesis and hence increased dermal thickness. Its main use is for well-defined superficial scars with distinct borders or broad-based scars with indistinct borders. Its main drawbacks are high operator dependence and a suboptimal safety profile. Further adverse effects may include dyschromia and scarring. For these reasons it has been largely replaced by laser.

Table Post-acne scars, qualitative global grading system (Goodman and Baron) [6]

Grade	Disease level	Features and tests
I	Macular	These scars are erythematous, hyper- or hypopigmented macules They do not represent a problem of contour but that of color
II	Mild	Mild atrophic or hypertrophic scars that may not be obvious at social distances of 0.5 m or greater and may be covered adequately by makeup or the normal shadow of shaved beard hair in men or normal body hair if extrafacial
III	Moderate	Moderate atrophic or hypertrophic scarring that is obvious at social distances of 0.5 m or greater and is not covered easily by makeup or the normal shadow of shaved beard hair in men or body hair if extrafacial. Can be flattened by manual stretching of the skin (if atrophic)
IV	Severe	Severe atrophic or hypertrophic scarring that is evident at social distances greater than 0.5 m and is not covered easily by makeup or the normal shadow of shaved beard hair in men or body hair if extrafacial. Cannot be flattened by manual stretching of the skin

Chemical Peels and Microneedling

Chemical peels can improve pigmentation and tone and texture. Bhargava et al. reported that glycolic acid (35%) peels and salicylic (20%) – mandelic acid (10%) peels were more effective for ice-pick than boxcar scars. Twice-weekly stronger strength peels seem to be more effective than daily low-strength creams. Trichloroacetic acid (35%) peels with a short downtime seemed to be particularly effective in darker skin types. Yet others combine needling with TCA peels to good effect. Caution needs to be taken in view of several potential adverse effects including prolonged erythema and post-inflammatory hyperpigmentation. These side effects are more prevalent but by no means limited to deep peels. Paradoxically, very high concentrations of TCA have demonstrated high efficacy in atrophic scars, and boxcar scars in particular, and have been rebranded as chemical reconstruction of skin scars (CROSS). Skin needling is another method, based on the principle of percutaneous induction of collagen, creating dermal microclefts, with collagenesis resulting from the cascade of growth factors unleashed by the wound-healing process. It appears to be more effective on rolling scars, and collagen deposition happens slowly, with the final result taking several repeat sessions and up to a year to be complete. Needling seems to confer added value as a method for transcutaneous drug delivery. Several such applications have been reported, such as combinations with TCA, platelet-rich plasma (PRP), and CROSS. Current best evidence suggests that results are operator-dependent, frequency-dependent, and concentration-dependent and that depth and degree of post-inflammatory hyperpigmentation are unpredictable, requiring experience and expertise; for this reason, the authors have moved away from these techniques toward light and laser therapy.

Dermal Lift Techniques

Punch Excision

Punch excision is a simple and quick technique that converts a discrete atrophic scar into a well-apposed, well-oriented surgical "healthy scar" which is easier to manage by both surgeon and patient. An appropriately sized punch biopsy is used to perform *full-thickness* excision. The wound is then sutured along relaxed skin tension lines (RSTLs). Observing the elongation of the circle into an ellipse with tension allows the practitioner to choose the optimal orientation for closure. It is also useful to avoid closely spaced defects and thus excess traction. Punch excision is replaced by sharp elliptical excision to avoid standing cone formation, when the defect is larger than 3 mm. Once healed, the resulting surgical wounds can be incorporated into laser remodeling.

Punch grafting replaces the punch excision with a similarly sized graft, of better quality in principle, but is laborious and often results in suboptimal color and textural mismatch. Punch elevation is another less commonly practiced technique reserved for boxcar scars with sharp edges and normal bases. The punch biopsy tool is used to excise the scar and its walls down to fat. This is followed by careful tissue elevation for the surface to sit slightly proud of surrounding skin to allow for subsequent retraction. The punched base is then secured. While both techniques are described in the literature, a clear advantage of either compared to punch excision and suturing, or our preferred techniques illustrated hereunder, is not immediately evident.

Subcutaneous Incision

Subcutaneous incision (subcision) frees dermis tethered by fibrous bands causing rolling scars. This technique employs a needle (ideally tribevelled) by severing adherent bands in a subcutaneous plane. Given adequate infiltration with adrenaline-containing local anesthetic, risk of hematoma formation is minimized. The technique does, however, run the risk of subcutaneous nodule formation.

Volume-Imparting Techniques

Filling Techniques

Both autologous (lipotransfer) and alloplast (nonanimal, cross-linked hyaluronic acid, NAHA) have been described to improve the volume underneath atrophic scars. The technique mandates prior release of the tethered scarring, without which the defect may be exaggerated due to volumization surrounding a tethered defect. Additionally, the technique is prone to the same complications of the volumizing agent. There is some evidence that dermal fillers can be used to impart volume which can be useful for soft boxcar or rolling scars [8]. While this produces some improvement of the dermal volume to counter the atrophic nature of the scar itself, the results are dependent on the nature of the dermal filler. Injections of cross-linked hyaluronic acid stimulate collagen formation by dermal fibroblasts and ameliorate skin quality [9]. Several studies claim advantages of different fillers, and this is extensively discussed elsewhere [10]. However, the emerging consensus is that dermal fillers offer very little on their own in the management of atrophic acne scars and work best as combination therapy. Traditionally, fillers care combined with prior subcision [8]. The combination of dermal fillers with high-pressure blast-effect devices is discussed further in this section as part of our current regime.

Dermal and Fat Autografting

Two less common techniques used for correcting volume deficit in atrophic acne scarring are dermal grafting and fat autografting. They are included for completeness, as the practitioner may occasionally encounter patients having been on the receiving end of this technique. In dermal grafting, harvested dermis is processed and implanted into recipient areas. This traditional technique's limitations are that it is limited to atrophic scars at least 4 mm in diameter; necessitates pocket dissection for insetting the graft, which may simultaneously mean subcision; multiple incisions; and inclusion of epidermis may lead to inclusions and dermal cysts.

Lipotransfer involves harvesting, processing, and insetting adipose tissue, which then will be needed to survive by developing a blood supply from surrounding tissues. Evidence regarding its use in atrophic acne scarring is controversial. A combination of fat grafting and condensed nanofat has been successfully used to treat atrophic scars [11]. Other studies claim that this technique may improve atrophic acne scars and texture [12]. Azzam et al. claim that fat grafting proved to be more effective in the treatment of acne scars than ablative fractional CO2 laser treatment. However, it should be pointed out that this study's methodology suffered from limited validity. Follow-up was limited to 3 months after a single lesion of fractional CO_2 laser therapy. Relatively low energies were used as well as a limited number of treatments. Currently, there is no evidence on the long-term success of this modality in the management of atrophic acne scarring [10].

Isotretinoin Treatment

Exposure to isotretinoic acid within 6 months was often cited a contraindication to treatment with a second modality [13], although more recently this view has been challenged. Historically, a few case series reported adverse events (development of keloids and hypertrophic scars, delayed healing) when patients recently completing isotretinoin treatment received dermabrasion and laser. "Spontaneous" keloids were also described in patients on isotretinoin. More recently, literature describes successful treatment of atrophic acne scarring, including fractional laser and dermabrasion; chemical peels in patients on isotretinoin challenge the traditional view of withholding treatment for 6–12 months. Rather, these adverse events result from individual variations in immunologic and inflammatory pathways. Early treatment of acne scars is critical for improved quality of life. The risk/benefit implications of treating the patient early need to be considered in the light of informed consent.

State-of-the-Art and Combinatorial Approaches

Most of the studies published today attempt to perform head-to-head comparison between different treatment modalities, in the attempt to identify the better option. This is understandable from a cost–benefit perspective due to the prohibitive outlay of some therapeutic modalities (◘ Fig. 41.1).

Here we concentrate on combinatorial approach (◘ Table 41.2) for the more taxing Goodman type 3–4 acne scars. There is a clear trend in the literature that favors combination treatments, and trends are now starting to emerge about useful synergies especially for the more severe acne types [2, 14].

Fractional Radiofrequency (FRF)

Fractional radiofrequency (FRF) transmits bipolar currents through contact electrodes or paired microneedles. This results in controlled, loco-temporal thermal dermal injury, inducing a wound-healing response. Clinically, this results in improved texture, tightening, and some improvement of skin clarity. There is consensus in the literature that three to six treatments provide optimal effects, ranging from 25% to 75% improvement and

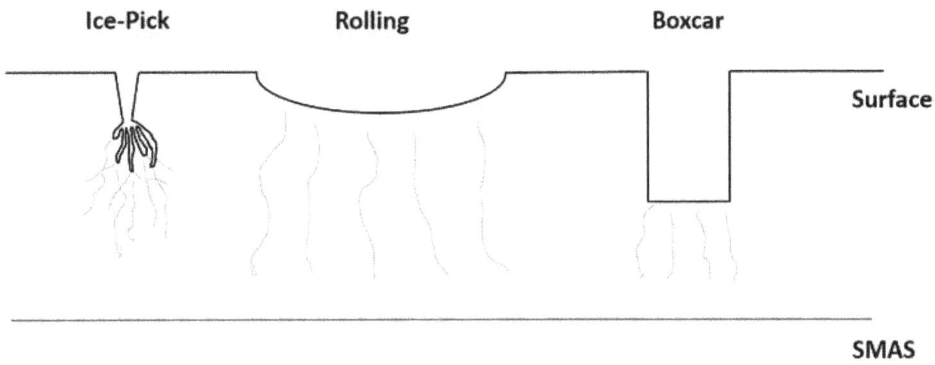

Fig. Morphological classification of post-acne scarring [13]

Table Proposed combinatorial approach and treatment schedule for treatment of atrophic acne scarring

Treatment	Effect	Repeats	Typical interval duration	Typical side effect duration
Bipolar radiofrequency	Regeneration	5	45–60 days	5–7 days
Hyaluronic acid/high pressure	Dermal revolumization	3	45–60 days	1–2 days
Fractional CO_2	Resurfacing/tightening	1/2	9–12 months	5–7 days

Schedule, temporal interval, and side effect duration are based on expert experience, using calibrated and maintained technology. Equipment settings vary between different manufacturers and versions

patient satisfaction. *Radiofrequency with microneedles* (RFM) delivers energy through microneedles (both insulated/non-insulated). The initial, mechanically induced microneedle wound-healing response [15] is followed by controlled thermal energy, up to 3.5 mm deep. This results in focal epidermal ablation, and controlled thermal damage to dermis, and, consequently, neocollagenesis, neoelastogenesis, and ground substance deposition [16]. Clinically, this results in textural amelioration, dermal density, and scar grading, whereas transepidermal water loss and sebum measurements did not change [17]. Some hybrid devices achieve this with a mixture of RF and galvanic energy. Transient posttreatment effects include pain, redness, mild swelling, and some crusting for up to 5 days. Track marks (<6%) and post-inflammatory hyperpigmentation (<3%) have been reported. Lesions arising from ice-pick and hypopigmented acne scars do not respond optimally to this treatment modality from a revolumization perspective, but there may be benefit from resulting skin tightening. Due to the risk of cross-infecting unaffected areas, RFM is contraindicated in patients with any areas of active acne.

Pre- and post-therapeutic regimes are integral to a positive outcome. Makeup removal, and adequate drying of the skin, is essential to avoid short-circuiting and epidermal injury. In contrast to other authors [18], we have achieved acceptability with topical anesthesia only (lignocaine/tetracaine cream 70 mg/g). The patient is advised a rigorous regime of UV protection (≥50%) and emollients to accelerate healing and decrease the risk of PIH.

High-Pressure Dermal Filler Deposition

More recently, low-viscosity NAHA dermal fillers have been employed to replenish volume loss associated to volume loss. Early studies were performed using micro-droplet applicators [19]. Even though these limited studies did report a beneficial effect, with recent improvements in high pressure, needle-less transdermal delivery systems have allowed the development of high-pressure transdermal hyaluronic acid delivery. The latter leads to a controlled “blast effect,” releasing tethered scars while improving delivery of the NAHA to a controlled surface area and depth. The combined physicochemical blast deposition effect is purported to be synergistic and promotes sustained neocollagenesis [19]. Limited level 4 evidence does not allow pooling of data, but consistent beneficial effects have been reported on difficult-to-treat anatomical areas and skin types. Patel et al. used jet volumetric remodeling (JVR) technology to deliver cross-linked hyaluronic acid, using 40–45% pressure vs. levels 4–5 filling, and demonstrated a beneficial effect on ice-pick and boxcar scars. Although level 4 evidence is based on small case series, remarkable results are reported, on

Table Evidence summary for JVR on the face and neck, since 2011, in the literature (English language)

Ref.	Technique	Reported improvement – reduction in Goodman score (%)	Mean age (years)	Follow-up (months)	Area	Skin types (Fitzpatrick)	Areas (*n*)
[21]	JVR/Histo/SP	50	54.7	6	Neck	Korean (II–V)	12
[22]	JVR/SP	27.6 (face)/21.2 (neck)	53.2	3–18	Face/neck	I–IV	34

SP standard photography, *JVR* jet volumetric remodeling, *Histo* histological analysis. Search String "Pneumatic AND Hyaluronic"/limits: English, human since 2010

a cohort of patients which are difficult to manage technically. Benefits include shortened procedure times and minimal downtime for a sustained improvement in the Goodman score. Murine model histological evidence supports the notion that the pneumatic injection of NAHA induces neocollagenesis and dermal thickening [20] (Table 41.3).

Laser

Laser now enjoys a solid evidence base in acne treatment. Traditional ablative laser therapy involved wholesale, partial thickness ablation of diseased dermis. While this produced impressive results, it was associated with significant and prolonged side effects. In our practice this has been entirely overtaken by ablative fractional laser (AFL). Several ablative and non-ablative lasers have been described for the treatment of acne and which are well-described elsewhere [10].

In fractional laser, the laser beam is split into multiple hundred columns, which create noncontiguous zones of thermal injury. These microthermal zones result in noncontiguous columns of epidermal and dermal ablation, resulting in epidermal regeneration and neocollagenesis. There is consensus in the literature that repeat treatment is necessary, when offered in monotherapy, but this may not always be the case when offered as part of a regime intended to address the separate aspects of atrophic acne scarring pathology. Fractional carbon dioxide laser addresses both scar elevation and recontouring (Fig. 41.2).

The skin stretch test of Goodman et al. [6] (Table 41.1) is a good indicator with which to assess the amenability of scars for laser. Scars not correcting with a simple stretch test indicates that it will likely not correct with laser therapy but may require prior treatment with either punch excision or high-pressure injection of hyaluronic acid or, in select cases, subcision.

In a first pass, a narrow size scanning pattern is targeted at the scar base, with the aim of achieving lift (Deep Fx). The second pass targets the edges of sharp-edged scar (such as boxcar scars), contouring it to a smoother scar edge (Deep Fx). In the third pass, active FX is performed to feather out the troughs and crests of the scars. This is typically done at a fixed distance from the skin using a spacer. However, the authors prefer to use a "spray painting" technique, by holding the handpiece still further away from the skin, on increased density, resulting in a more efficient and effective resurfacing (Table 41.4).

Using this technique, substantial improvement has been demonstrated histologically, and efficacy has been maintained for up to 3 years. The results appear to be more significant when compared to non-ablative modalities, albeit at the cost of increased downtime. It is important to advise patients appropriately regarding the importance of pre- and posttreatment regimes (Table 41.5).

Non-ablative laser can also be useful in the correction of acne scarring. This modality trades off minimal downtime, against slower, lower degrees of improvement, compared to ablative laser. Particularly useful is Erbium glass (1565 nm) fractioned laser which may be used to refine dermal texture and contour. In shallow atrophic depressions requiring low energy for adequate penetration, high density may stimulate neocollagenesis, while the corollary settings on elevations may induce flattening.

Picosecond laser may also be used to the same effect with some distinct advantages. Hyperpigmentation may be effectively treated on collimated beam settings, with the picosecond duration resulting in light-reduced inflammatory response. In fractionated mode, picosecond laser results in light-induced optical breakdown (LIOB) which stimulates gentle neocollagenesis.

Striae Albae

Lineae albae present another difficult challenge, especially in darker-skinned individuals. Myriad treatments have been described, none entirely satisfactory. Several eponymous terms are used interchangeably, but we prefer the one proposed by Nardelli's "striae atrophicae," as it embodies the current histopathologic understanding [23].

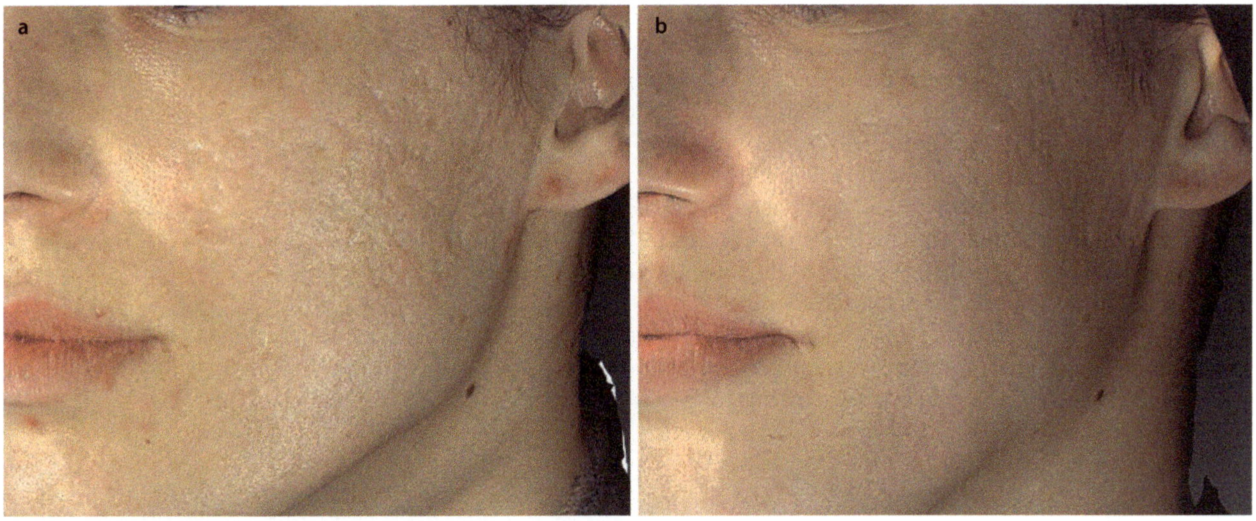

Fig. Figure 1**a** repesents the face before fractional CO_2 procedure and **b** is the patient 6 months later

Table Suggested typical settings for post-acne AFL protocol

Cycle	size	Pulses	Density (%)	Pattern cycle (Hz)	Energy (mJ)	Aim
1 DFX	2	1	5–10	300	15–20	Base of scar
2 AFX	2	1	9	350	40–60	Flange out Boxcar scars, Handpiece at 45°
3 DFX		1	15	300	17.5	Tighten surround[a]
4 AFX		1	3	125	100–	Re surface full face

DFX Deep Fx™, *AFX* Active FX™
[a]For severe scarring (optional)

Table Suggested pre- and posttreatment considerations

Phase	Advice
Pretreatment	
All patients	Back to "normal shade" with complete loss of holiday tan
	SPF 50+ (every 2 h)
Fitzpatrick 3–6	Initiate Kligman regime from 8 weeks pretreatment, stop 2 weeks pre Rx
	tretinoin (0.02%); hydroquinone (4%); vitamin c (3%); hydrocortisone (1%)[a]
Posttreatment	
All patients	Emollients plus SPF 50+ (every 2 h)
	Antivirals PO
	Consider antimicrobials as per local protocols (antifungals, antibiotics)

[a]With particular attention to an airtight container, avoid mucosal, periocular, and perioral areas, and avoid pooling in nasolabial sulcus

Compared to adjacent unaffected skin, striae albae present histologic evidence of attenuated dermal papillae, with the latter nearly entirely substituted with collagen fibers running parallel to the skin.

Trofolastin demonstrates level 2 evidence of positive results for their prophylactic use in SD [24]. Tehranchinia et al. [25] observed some degree of improvement in 80% of patients after two treatment sessions within a 4-week interval. However, 76.7% of patients remained dissatisfied. The authors concluded that this modality resulted in minimal improvement with mild side effects. It also is apparent that Trofolastin's mode of action is related to the deposition of hyaluronic activity [26]. Additionally, it is well established that fractional laser treatments induce long-term clinical and histological improvement of mature atrophic scars [26], including increased architectural reorganization toward normalization, such as collagen structure (from thick surface paralleled hyalinized bundles to uniform dense interwoven fibers with higher vascularization), and decreased inflammation. Unlike Taudorf et al., we do not perform stack pulsing. First as unless there is complete immobility, true stacking is impossible to achieve and, secondly, because stacking does increase risk of excessive thermal damage.

Clinical evidence supports the use of JVR with NAHA promoting sustained neocollagenesis and increased dermal depth, while the blast effect untethers the underlying scarring of lineae alba [27]. The combination of JVR to non-ablative fractional laser gives, in our opinion, a substantial improvement over both techniques used alone. NAFL then provides an effective tool to address dermal recontouring, by stimulating collagen synthesis in troughs and the opposite effect in surrounding areas. While effects of individual treatments appear to be long-lasting, we have also observed that one-off treatments are rarely as effective as repeated cycles spaced 6–8 weeks apart.

Burn Atrophic Scars

Great strides have been registered in acute burn management, resulting in increased burn survival, even with major and previously unsurvivable burns. As a result patients are presenting with increased requirements relating to morbidity and quality of life, arising both from the mechanism of injury and subsequent interventions required to safe life and limb. Atrophic burn scars form an important minority of burn scars. Often interspersed with hypertrophic counterparts, they result in wound instability and breakdown and contribute to poor cosmetic outcomes. The postoperative course of a burn scar is summarized symptomatically in ◘ Table 41.6.

A plethora of lasers have been described in the treatment of atrophic scars (◘ Table 41.7), both non-ablative and ablative with an approximate cutoff of 200 nm. Fractional ablation, first described by Mannstein [28], produces arrays of microscopic thermal damage zones (MTZs) throughout the epidermis and dermis, affecting only a part of the surface area, with consequent remodeling and neocollagenesis for up to 6 months after treatment with permanent results [29]. Less energy is required to achieve the desired depth (≤2 mm) of penetration in atrophic or flat scars, allowing higher fractionated densities to be used, depending on the device, (≤10%).

Non-ablative fractional resurfacing (NAFR), in contrast, leaves the epidermis intact (ad dermis) whilst forming MTZs. A focused dermal injury instigates dermal remodeling and neocollagenesis [28]. The result is a bloodless cylindrical coagulation area within dermis. The clinical advantage is lower risk of infection and pigment alteration, as the epidermis is intact.

Post-procedure discomfort after AFR is surprisingly limited. Patients generally return to normal activity within 1 day, but downtime may be up to 7 days and requires several topical applications which may interfere with clothing and social activity. In contrast, NAFR requires far less downtime, dyschromia, PIH, with lower analgesia requirements, at the expense of more treatment sessions being required. In consideration of these reasons, for flat or atrophic scars, there is

◘ **Table** Therapeutic burn phases

Phase	Typical procedures	Aim
Immediate	Tracheostomy, escharotomy	Life/limb saving
Early	Burn wound excision and grafting	Excise dead tissue Reduce evaporative loss
Intermediate	Periorbital, perioral, address functional gain	Protect special senses Improve ROM deficit arising due to increasing mobility
Late	Incisional/ excisional release	Address functional deficit Improve range of movement Address pain, pruritus

◘ **Table** Wavelengths described from atrophic burn scars

Wavelength (nm)	Lasing medium	Modality	Effect
10,600	CO_2	Fractioned	Lower (×10) water affinity, more coagulation, less bleeding, favorable to LADD
2790	Er, Cr-YSGG	Fractioned	More water affinity, narrower rim of thermal coagulation around MTZs
2940	Er: YAG	Fractioned	
1540,1550,1565	Er: Glass	Fractionated	For scars with a thickness lower than 2 mm

CO_2 carbon dioxide, *Er YAG* erbium-doped yttrium aluminum garnet, *Er,Cr-YSGG* erbium, chromium-doped yttrium scandium-gallium-garnet, *LADD* laser-assisted drug delivery

emerging consensus in the literature that NAFR is the treatment of choice [30]. We also suspect that such wide variety of data exists in part from the prohibitive cost of each technology. Having access to the entire range of technologies in our center, we favor the use of NAFR Er:YAG to raise the base of atrophic scars on higher-density settings.

While the optimal timing of fractional laser therapy is not yet determined, current trends in the literature over the past 5 years favor earlier intervention. Scars of any age can be considered for fractional resurfacing. In practice, the contrast between postoperative regimes required by laser and complex burn surgery poses practical limits on how early a laser intervention may be successfully offered. Notwithstanding, younger scars are more susceptible to remodeling, and some studies now suggest that the ideal timeframe may be as early as 4–12 weeks post-injury, repeated every 1–2 months until response plateaus or the therapeutic aims are attained and may help in scar remodeling, reduce contracture rates, and expedite rehabilitation [31].

Vascular Laser Lasers targeting abnormal scar proliferation have the potential to improve scar characteristics. A number of wavelengths are often used for this purpose, including millisecond range potassium titanyl phosphate (KTP) 532 nm, pulse dye laser (PDL) 595 nm, and neodymium:yttrium aluminum garnet (Nd:YAG) 1064 nm. Although the primary target of PDL is hemoglobin, its mechanism of action is not fully understood. After multiple treatments, PDL results in some softening, flattening, and smoothening [32]. However, melanin acts as a potential competitor; therefore, conservative settings need to be used in darker individuals.

Fractioned picosecond modality laser has the potential to produce light-induced optical breakdown, limited to the dermis, which may stimulate dermal inflammation, remodeling, and neocollagenesis. There is still some controversy regarding the timing of appearance and significance of microscopic epidermal necrotic debris (MEND). In one such study, this phenomenon was noted as early as 3 h (post-pico-532 nm) and within 24 h (both 532 and 1064 nm wavelengths) [6].

Burn reconstruction really starts in the immediate postburn period with adequate first aid therapy that limits the zone of stasis and hyperemia and careful, multimodality management including judicious debridement and maximal attention to dermal sparing. Fractional laser resurfacing for atrophic wounds is an integral part of this armamentarium. Additionally, our recent experience suggests that JVR (NAHA) is a useful adjunct in achieving revolumization of selected atrophic burn wound reconstructions. In particular, resurfacing with split thickness skin grafts often leads to a honeycombed appearance, reduced elasticity, and a feeling of tightness, due to the minimal dermal component of a split-thickness skin graft. Our early experience with this technology has produced excellent results when used in tandem with fractional laser, where we have observed synergistic dermal "re-plumping" and substantial improvement of skin texture.

Conclusion

Atrophic scars present a significant challenge to the reconstructive specialist, with acne, linea albae, and burns being topics worthy of special consideration. Optimal treatment is not based on superiority of one particular treatment over another but rather by the specialist's ability to precisely identify the component parts of the presenting complaint and bringing his entire armamentarium to bear. We believe, based on experience and balance of current evidence, that combined, repeat treatment produces the best results and that these must be carefully balanced against the relative costs: physical, social, and economic, in consideration of each patient's individual needs.

Take Home Messages

- Atrophic scarring is the final common pathway resulting from reduced matrix regeneration and focally reduced collagen production.
- Addressing patient concerns, expectations, and attitude to risk/benefit is key.
- Techniques may be considered according to their principal mode of action: resurfacing and tightening, dermal lifting techniques, and dermal volumization techniques.
- Acne scars affect physical, psychological, and social well-being. Involvement of multiprofessional advice is important.
- In appropriately selected patients, combined RFM-JVR-AFL treatment, tailored to individual needs, is more likely to produce appropriate results.
- Repeat treatment is likely to be needed.
- Color laser may lead to substantial improvement in dyschromias.

References

1. Poetschke J, Gauglitz GG. Current options for the treatment of pathological scarring. J Dtsch Dermatol Ges. 2016;14(5):467–77. https://doi.org/10.1111/ddg.13027. [published Online First: 2016/04/28].
2. Zaleski-Larsen LA, Fabi SG, McGraw T, et al. Acne scar treatment: a multimodality approach tailored to scar type. Dermatol Surg. 2016;42:S139–S49.

3. Koo J. The psychosocial impact of acne: patients' perceptions. J Am Acad Dermatol. 1995;32(5):S26–30.
4. Halvorsen JA, Stern RS, Dalgard F, et al. Suicidal ideation, mental health problems, and social impairment are increased in adolescents with acne: a population-based study. J Investig Dermatol. 2011;131(2):363–70.
5. Layton A, Henderson C, Cunliffe W. A clinical evaluation of acne scarring and its incidence. Clin Exp Dermatol. 1994; 19(4):303–8.
6. Balu M, Lentsch G, Korta DZ, et al. In vivo multiphoton-microscopy of picosecond-laser-induced optical breakdown in human skin. Lasers Surg Med. 2017;49(6):555–62.
7. Linkner RV, On SJ, Haddican M, et al. Evaluating the efficacy of photodynamic therapy with 20% aminolevulinic acid and microdermabrasion as a combination treatment regimen for acne scarring: a split-face, randomized, double-blind pilot study. J Clin Aesthet Dermatol. 2014;7(5):32.
8. Lee JW, Kim BJ, Kim MN, et al. Treatment of acne scars using subdermal minimal surgery technology. Dermatol Surg. 2010;36(8):1281–7.
9. Wang F, Garza LA, Kang S, et al. In vivo stimulation of de novo collagen production caused by cross-linked hyaluronic acid dermal filler injections in photodamaged human skin. Arch Dermatol. 2007;143(2):155–63.
10. Bhargava S, Cunha PR, Lee J, et al. Acne scarring management: systematic review and evaluation of the evidence. Am J Clin Dermatol. 2018;19(4):459–77.
11. Gu Z, Li Y, Li H. Use of condensed nanofat combined with fat grafts to treat atrophic scars. JAMA Facial Plast Surg. 2018;20(2):128–35.
12. Azzam O, Atta A, Sobhi R, et al. Fractional CO(2) laser treatment vs autologous fat transfer in the treatment of acne scars: a comparative study. J Drugs Dermatol. 2013;12(1):e7–e13.
13. Jacob CI, Dover JS, Kaminer MS. Acne scarring: a classification system and review of treatment options. J Am Acad Dermatol. 2001;45(1):109–17.
14. Goodman GJ. Treating scars: addressing surface, volume, and movement to expedite optimal results. Part 2: more-severe grades of scarring. Dermatol Surg. 2012;38(8):1310–21.
15. Doddaballapur S. Microneedling with dermaroller. J Cutan Aesthet Surg. 2009;2(2):110–1. https://doi.org/10.4103/0974-2077.58529.
16. Tanaka Y. Long-term three-dimensional volumetric assessment of skin tightening using a sharply tapered non-insulated microneedle radiofrequency applicator with novel fractionated pulse mode in asians. Lasers Surg Med. 2015;47(8):626–33. https://doi.org/10.1002/lsm.22401.
17. Cho SI, Chung BY, Choi MG, et al. Evaluation of the clinical efficacy of fractional radiofrequency microneedle treatment in acne scars and large facial pores. Dermatol Surg. 2012;38(7 pt1):1017–24. https://doi.org/10.1111/j.1524-4725.2012.02402.x.
18. Ibrahim O, Munavalli GS, Dover JS. Radiofrequency with microneedling. Adv Cosmet Surg. 2018;1(1):109–15. https://doi.org/10.1016/j.yacs.2018.03.001.
19. Halachmi S, Ben DA, Lapidoth M. Treatment of acne scars with hyaluronic acid: an improved approach. J Drugs Dermatol. 2013;12(7):e121–3.
20. Kwon T-R, Seok J, Jang J-H, et al. Needle-free jet injection of hyaluronic acid improves skin remodeling in a mouse model. Eur J Pharm Biopharm. 2016;105:69–74. https://doi.org/10.1016/j.ejpb.2016.05.014.
21. Han TY, Lee JW, Lee JHK, et al. Subdermal minimal surgery with hyaluronic acid as an effective treatment for neck wrinkles. Dermatol Surg. 2011;37(9):1291–6.
22. Levenberg A, Halachmi S, Arad-Cohen A, et al. Clinical results of skin remodeling using a novel pneumatic technology. Int J Dermatol. 2010;49(12):1432–9.
23. Nardelli L. Importanza semiologica delle "striae cutis atrophicae". Boll Sez Region Soc Ital Dermatol. 1936;1:46.
24. Ud-Din S, McGeorge D, Bayat A. Topical management of striae distensae (stretch marks): prevention and therapy of striae rubrae and albae. J Eur Acad Dermatol Venereol. 2016;30(2):211–22. https://doi.org/10.1111/jdv.13223. [published Online First: 10/20].
25. Tehranchinia Z, Mahboubianfar A, Rahimi H, et al. Fractionated CO(2) laser in the treatment of striae alba in darker skinned patients – a prospective study. J Lasers Med Sci. 2018;9(1):15–8. https://doi.org/10.15171/jlms.2018.04. [published Online First: 12/26].
26. Ash K, Lord J, Zukowskl M, et al. Comparison of topical therapy for striae alba (20% glycolic acid/0.05% tretinoin versus 20% glycolic acid/10% L-ascorbic acid). Dermatol Surg. 1998; 24(8):849–56.
27. Cassuto D. Case report: effective treatment of striae distensae using pneumatic injection of hyaluronic acid. Available online on elogioasia.com.
28. Manstein D, Herron GS, Sink RK, et al. Fractional photothermolysis: a new concept for cutaneous remodeling using microscopic patterns of thermal injury. Lasers Surg Med. 2004;34(5):426–38.
29. Stewart N, Lim AC, Lowe PM, et al. Lasers and laser-like devices: part one. Australas J Dermatol. 2013;54(3):173–83.
30. Carniol PJ, Hamilton MM, Carniol ET. Current status of fractional laser resurfacing. JAMA Facial Plast Surg. 2015;17(5): 360–6.
31. Waibel JS, Rudnick A. Current trends and future considerations in scar treatment. Seminars in cutaneous medicine and surgery. Semin Cutan Med Surg. 2015;34(1):13–6.
32. Alster TS, Williams CM. Treatment of keloid sternotomy scars with 585 nm flashlamp-pumped pulsed-dye laser. Lancet. 1995;345(8959):1198–200.

7

Emerging Technologies in Scar Management: The Role of Allogeneic Cells

Clarisse Ganier and Sonia Gaucher

Contents

Background

Allogenic Cell Therapy Studied in Scar Management Field

Human Allogeneic Epidermal Sheets

Cellular Dermal Substitutes and Human Dermal Fibroblasts Therapy

Human Skin Equivalent

Bioprinting of Skin

Injections of Mesenchymal Stromal Cells (MSCs) for Skin Regeneration

Promising Embryonic(-Like) Stem Cells Therapy for Scar Treatment

Conclusion/Discussion

References

Background

After skin injury, the wound-healing process has to occur as soon as possible to prevent excessive blood loss and/or infection. In chronic wounds, this normal healing process fails, which results in a pathologic cycle of inflammation and protease release, leading to the development of a pathologic scar. Also, in the healing of large and deep wounds, scar formation is evident. Nevertheless, in some natural cases, such as fetal skin, humans and animals are able to heal scarless due to the fast wound-healing process and/or specific fetal characteristics [1].

Scars caused by burns, chronic ulcers from diabetes, infections, skin cancer surgery, and other genetic or somatic disease could require effective treatment to avoid functional and psychological troubles and even in some severe cases to prevent mortality. Most of the current treatments do not prevent scarring. They first aim to reduce local inflammation.

Herein, we will discuss about emerging technologies in scar management using allogeneic cell therapy. Allogeneic cell transplants offer the possibility of large prefabrication, cryopreservation for instantaneous use, and repeated applications. They also allow the use of fetal cells that show interesting properties. Furthermore, they are applicable for genetic skin diseases inducing severe scars such as dystrophic epidermolysis bullosa. Current research exploring allogeneic cell therapies for scar treatment show that they are mostly locally delivered by grafting and/or by intradermal injections.

Allogenic Cell Therapy Studied in Scar Management Field

Allogeneic cell therapies combined with scaffolding biomaterials have been employed in tissue engineering approaches for wound care and scar management. We will describe here the cells and their scaffold used in scar management. The common cell types used for scar treatments are fibroblasts and keratinocytes as commercial products for skin regeneration (◘ Table 51.1). The emergence of three-dimensional (3D) printing is gaining commercial interest for large-scale production. Research works on mesenchymal stromal cells (MSCs) therapy for scar management are also increasing and show very promising results.

◘ **Table** Human allogenic cell types used in skin regeneration

Source	Commercial products and their applications	Type of allogeneic cells
Skin	Apligraf® – Venous leg ulcers – Diabetic foot ulcers OrCel® – Partial-thickness burns Clinical trials	Living fibroblasts and keratinocytes
	TheraSkin® – Diabetic foot – Venous leg ulcers Cryoskin® – Chronic nonhealing – Neuropathic diabetic ulcers	Keratinocytes
Neonatal foreskin	TransCyte® – Full-thickness and deep partial-thickness burns – Partial-thickness burns	Dead fibroblasts
	Dermagraft® – Full-thickness diabetic foot ulcers	Living fibroblasts
	Lyphoderm® – Chronic venous ulcer – Partial-thickness burns	Keratinocytes
Fetus	Studied in animal models or involved in clinical trials	Fibroblasts and/or keratinocytes
Bone marrow	Studied in animal models or involved in clinical trials	Mesenchymal stromal cells
Umbilical cord	Studied in animal models or involved in clinical trials	
Adipose tissue	Studied in animal models or involved in clinical trials	

Human Allogeneic Epidermal Sheets

Epidermal sheets consist of human keratinocytes that are differentiated *in vitro* to give rise to a stratified epidermal layer. They can be combined with other biocompatible substrates (bovine collagen, hyaluronic acid), acellular natural human or porcine materials, or nylon or polyglactin meshes. An example of one product using allogeneic keratinocytes is Cryoskin® that is available from frozen cells on a carrier dressing [2]. A single blind study shows the efficacy of this cell therapy for the acceleration of healing of chronic nonhealing neuropathic diabetic ulcers. In general, the clinical outcome of the epidermal sheet grafts is usually not satisfying because of the nonpermanent character, ultimate rejection, and absence of a dermal component.

Cellular Dermal Substitutes and Human Dermal Fibroblasts Therapy

In contrast to epidermal sheets, the dermal substitutes are composed either of autologous or of allogeneic dermal fibroblasts. The scaffold for the cells consists mostly of biomaterials, like benzyl-esterified derivatives of hyaluronic acid (Hyaff-11), polyglycolic acid, or polyglactin. TransCyte® is a comparable product containing a nylon mesh coated with porcine dermal collagen that is seeded with neonatal fibroblasts and fixed to an outer silicone membrane.

The major indication of application consists in transient wound cover after surgery. One of the most successfully bioengineered products is Dermagraft®, an allogeneic cell culture using neonatal dermal fibroblast grown on a biodegradable scaffold. This product showed the capacity to secrete several growth factors, to stimulate angiogenesis, and re-epithelialization from the wound edge, even after cryopreservation and thawing. In diabetic foot ulcers, its efficacy and its safety were demonstrated [2].

In addition, some other clinical trials are ongoing using a medicinal product comprised of viable allogeneic dermal fibroblasts suspended in HypoThermosol®-FRS for remodeling scar contractures from burn patients and from dystrophic epidermolysis bullosa patients. Fibroblasts are from neonatal foreskin, cryopreserved, thawed, and expanded in culture under good manufacturing practice at Intercytex Ltd., UK (▶ ClinicalTrials.gov, Identifier: NCT01564407 [burn patients], ISRCTN67757229 [recessive dystrophic epidermolysis bullosa patients]).

Human Skin Equivalent

Skin equivalent is only composed of a culture of keratinocytes growing on dermal substitutes containing fibroblasts. An example of an allogeneic skin equivalent product is Apligraf® consisting of cultured keratinocytes on a dermal layer of fibroblasts within a bovine type 1 collagen matrix (▶ http://www.apligraf.com/professional/). Apligraf® obtained its Food and Drug Administration (FDA) approval for diabetic foot ulcers and venous leg ulcers applications. This product has been well tolerated in over 150,000 patient applications.

Clinical trials showed that the healing rate of the venous ulcers treated with Apligraf® as well as the healing time was improved. Healing occurs with less fibrosis, which might be because of the construction of the graft itself containing neonatal cells and growth factors/cytokines, stimulating a more fetal-like scarless wound healing. Another product used in clinical trials for the treatment of venous ulcers is OrCel®, a bilayered cellular matrix containing adult epidermal keratinocytes and dermal fibroblasts. Donor dermal fibroblasts are cultured within the porous Type I bovine collagen sponge while keratinocytes, from the same donor, are cultured on the coated, nonporous side of the collagen matrix.

Recently, OrCel® obtained its first FDA approvals for treatment of acute surgical excisions, such as contracture release sites in patients suffering from dystrophic epidermolysis bullosa undergoing hand reconstruction surgery (▶ https://www.accessdata.fda.gov/cdrh_docs/pdf/p010016b.pdf) and also in burn patients undergoing excision and grafting [2]. *In vitro* skin cells used to make OrCel® skin equivalent are extensively expanded that give rise to a low human leukocyte antigen class II (HLA-II) level of the allogeneic cells. Therefore, OrCel® skin equivalent is well tolerated by the recipient after grafting into wound bed. The company reported in both clinical trial and commercial experience no clinical signs of tissue rejection using the cryopreserved OrCel® product. Resorption appears to take place gradually, with no remnants of the donor cells or matrix being detectable by 2 weeks of posttreatment. Their working hypothesis is that extracellular secretion of cytokines and growth factors by the living cells in OrCel® is the major factor for accelerating wound healing.

Bioprinting of Skin

The use of three-dimensional (3D) bioprinting has emerged as a flexible tool in regenerative medicine to bioengineer skin substitutes. There are many kinds of bioprinting technologies, but the four more commonly used are inkjet-based printing, extrusion-based printing, laser-assisted printing, and digital light processing (DLP)-based printing—dynamic optical projection stereolithography (DOPsL). Cell viability can be affected by several factors, including bioprinting technique used.

Jorcano laboratory has developed one bioprinter prototype able to print skin cells, soluble factors, and biomaterials in a desired pattern with the help of high-precision Cartesian robots. The printing skin mimics the structural and molecular structure of the human skin [3]. It is the first functional printer to be introduced to the marketplace. To date, there is no allogeneic 3D printed skin used in patients, but this technology raised great hopes for the treatment of scar in the future.

Injections of Mesenchymal Stromal Cells (MSCs) for Skin Regeneration

MSCs were known to contribute to skin regeneration and to accelerate cutaneous wound healing. MSCs were first isolated from bone marrow in the 1970s by their ability to adhere, proliferate, and develop on a plastic surface, displaying fibroblastic morphology. MSCs are multipotent adult progenitor cells that can differentiate to lineages of mesenchymal cells, including osteoblasts, chondroblasts, and adipocytes. These can be isolated from various adult or perinatal tissues such as adipose tissue or umbilical cord. MSCs have shown positive therapeutic effects in many tissue repair situations through the secretion of trophic factors. In addition, allogeneic MSCs are well tolerated after injections due to their immune-modulating effects [4].

Many studies have demonstrated that MSCs exhibit a number of trophic functions to enhance skin regeneration, such as promoting angiogenesis, modulating the inflammatory response, and limiting tissue fibrosis [5]. In *in vivo* studies, these cells have been used successfully to limit scar formation. Transplanted allogeneic or xenogeneic MSCs transiently survive in the implantation site; their therapeutic potential in wound healing is associated with their secretion of trophic effects on resident cells. One of these *in vivo* studies using a rabbit model showed that intradermal injection of MSCs can regulate inflammation and prevent the formation of hypertrophic scars. The MSCs underwent apoptosis rapidly in the injected site, between 24 and 72 hours postinjection. They demonstrated that apoptosis has an important role in the activation of the inflammatory regulatory abilities of MSCs through TNF-alpha stimulated protein 6 (TSG-6) [6].

An *in vivo* study showed the efficacy of MSCs and dermal fibroblasts combined to minimize skin hypertrophic scarring [7]. They showed that transplanted xenogeneic MSCs influenced positively fibroblast proliferation, migration, and extracellular matrix deposition and reduced inflammation following wounding. This effect was superior to MSC or fibroblast transplantation alone. This study suggests that MSCs, even if eventually rejected quickly after injection, transplanted with fibroblasts normalize matrix regeneration during wound healing. This promising study provides insight into allogeneic cell therapies as a viable method for antifibrotic treatment and demonstrates that even transiently engrafted cells can have a long-term impact via matrix modulation and effect on other tissue cells.

One of the first randomized, controlled clinical trial will study the safety and efficacy of MSCs in skin scar for the treatment of Cesarean section [8]. Eligible patients received transdermal hydrogel MSCs once a day for six consecutive days. Their outcomes should be available soon (► ClinicalTrials.gov, NCT02772289).

Promising Embryonic(-Like) Stem Cells Therapy for Scar Treatment

Embryonic stem cells (ESCs) and induced pluripotent stem cells (iPSCs) are defined as pluripotent cells able to self-renew. In the field of skin, those stem cells showed some promising results regarding fibrosis care.

Many *in vitro* and/or *in vivo* studies are ongoing on embryonic stem cells and induced pluripotent stem cells (iPSC) as potentially promising in scar management [9]. As fetal cells, ESCs are thought to possess antifibrotic ability. An *in vitro* study showed the capacity of ESC-derived macrophages to secrete scarless-like secretome to regulate the altered keloid niche and reverse the profibrotic phenotype of keloid fibroblasts [10]. Because iPSCs are similar to ESCs in many features, they have been evaluated in scar tissue repair. An *in vitro* recent study documented that iPSC-conditioned medium may efficiently suppress hypertrophic scar fibroblast activation [11].

Conclusion/Discussion

The allogeneic cell therapy for scar management shows many advantages: large prefabrication, cryopreservation for instant use, and repeated applications. They also allow the use of fetal cells such as embryonic stem cells. Furthermore, they are applicable for genetic skin disease inducing wound healing without genetic modifications.

Most of current and emerging therapeutics for scar management are using allogeneic fibroblasts and keratinocytes as epidermal sheet, dermal substitute, or skin equivalent. The immune rejection of these adult cells is commonly reported, mostly shown for allogeneic keratinocytes due to different HLA expression and cytokine production. Fetal cells are of particular interest for skin repair due to the high expansion ability, low immunogenicity, and intense secretion of bioactive factors. However, the main cellular effect seems in promoting wound healing through secretion of endogenous and exogenous factors rather than cell survival.

Regarding the viability of allogeneic cells, most of the studies on the literature agree on the fact that allogeneic cells do not survive for a long time after transplantation. But most of their therapeutic potential seems to be based on their secretion of trophic factors such as growth factors, cytokines, and extracellular vesicles at least for MSC therapy and also for dermal fibroblasts therapy. Extracellular vesicles (exosomes, microvesicles, and apoptotic bodies) are secreted by most cells of the organism. These extracellular vesicles are of growing interest among investigators, specially from MSCs across multiple fields, including dermatology as a drug [12]. As MSCs or stem cells, extracellular vesicles demonstrate immunomodulatory properties, accelerate skin cell migration and proliferation, control wound scarring, and improve angiogenesis. Several clinical trials should appear in the future years testing the safety and the efficacy of stem cells and derived products for skin scar treatment.

References

1. Marshall CD, Hu MS, Leavitt T, Barnes LA, Lorenz HP, Longaker MT. Cutaneous scarring: basic science, current treatments, and future directions. Adv Wound Care. 2016;7(2):29–45.
2. Shpichka A, Butnaru D, Bezrukov EA, Sukhanov RB, Atala A, Burdukovskii V, et al. Skin tissue regeneration for burn injury. Stem Cell Res Ther. 2019;10(1):1–16.
3. Cubo N, Velasco D, Jorcano JL, Garcia M, del Cañizo JF. 3D bioprinting of functional human skin: production and in vivo analysis. Biofabrication. 2016;9(1):015006.
4. Najar M, Raicevic G, Fayyad-Kazan H, Bron D, Toungouz M, Lagneaux L. Mesenchymal stromal cells and immunomodulation: a gathering of regulatory immune cells. Cytotherapy [Internet]. 2016;18(2):160–71.. Available from: https://doi.org/10.1016/j.jcyt.2015.10.011
5. Jackson WM, Nesti LJ, Tuan RS. Mesenchymal stem cell therapy for attenuation of scar formation during wound healing. Stem Cell Res Ther. 2012;3(3):20.
6. Liu S, Jiang L, Li H, Shi H, Luo H, Zhang Y, et al. Mesenchymal stem cells prevent hypertrophic scar formation via inflammatory regulation when undergoing apoptosis. J Invest Dermatol [Internet]. 2014;134(10):2648–57.. Available from: https://doi.org/10.1038/jid.2014.169
7. Yates CC, Rodrigues M, Nuschke A, Johnson ZI, Whaley D, Stolz D, et al. Multipotent stromal cells/mesenchymal stem cells and fibroblasts combine to minimize skin hypertrophic scarring. Stem Cell Res Ther. 2017;8(1):1–13.
8. Fan D, Xia Q, Wu S, Ye S, Liu L, Wang W, et al. Mesenchymal stem cells in the treatment of cesarean section skin scars: study protocol for a randomized, controlled trial. Trials. 2018;19(1):4–11.
9. Li Q, Zhang C, Fu X. Will stem cells bring hope to pathological skin scar treatment? Cytotherapy [Internet]. 2016;18(8):943–56.. Available from: https://doi.org/10.1016/j.jcyt.2016.05.008
10. Dreymueller D, Denecke B, Ludwig A, Jahnen-Dechent W. Embryonic stem cell-derived M2-like macrophages delay cutaneous wound healing. Wound Repair Regen. 2013;21(1):44–54.
11. Ren Y, Deng CL, Wan WD, Zheng JH, Mao GY, Yang SL. Suppressive effects of induced pluripotent stem cell-conditioned medium on in vitro hypertrophic scarring fibroblast activation. Mol Med Rep. 2015;11(4):2471–6.
12. Ferreira ADF, Gomes DA. Stem cell extracellular vesicles in skin repair. Bioengineering. 2018;6(1):4.

8

Specific Attention Areas in Scar Management: Specific Scar Management Depending on Anatomical Features (Face, Hair, Breast, Hand, Joints, Foot)

Julian Poetschke and Gerd G. Gauglitz

Contents

Scar Treatment Options for Different Anatomical Localizations
Face
Hair
Hands
Feet
Joints

Conclusion

References

Background

Scarring can have a variety of different detrimental effects on the affected patients. While small scars are often little more than an aesthetically unpleasing blemish, scarring has the potential to drastically affect patients' lives.

Ultimately, not only the scar type but also the dimension of the affected areas and their location play a large role regarding the impairments they might cause.

Different aspects come into play when certain areas of the body are affected by severe scarring, and they should be taken into consideration when planning the treatment.

Severe facial scarring causes a multitude of issues. It is incredibly stigmatizing for affected patients and will likely cause significant psychological suffering. This oftentimes has detrimental effects on the patients' social life leading to isolation and thus further psychological problems. Facial scarring can have a variety of functional impairments, too. It can cause impaired closure of the eyelids leading to lagophthalmos or leading to ectropium or entropium, all of which can endanger the patients' vision and result in pain and unease.

Microstomia is another common consequence of facial scarring, leading to a reduction of the mouth opening, thus greatly impairing the intake of food and beverages as well as hindering speech or oral hygiene all the while causing significant discomfort.

On the head, scarring can lead to hair loss or cicatricial alopecia which, while problematic in men, too, can be downright devastating in women, where hair loss and baldness remain stigmatizing.

The chest is another aesthetically important area where scarring can lead to a significant psychosocial burden, especially in women.

While scarring of the hands can be aesthetically unpleasing, too, its most problematic consequence is the functional impairment it can cause. Especially in burn patients, the functional consequences of the scarring can be so severe that not only the patients' ability to work but to maintain their self-reliance throughout their daily lives is also at risk. Even with immediate physiotherapy and occupational therapy after surgical treatment, functional impairments often remain and are exacerbated by the incipient process of scarring thus leading to a lasting need for further treatment.

Similar problems arise with scarring on the feet. Since walking around throughout the day places a great load on the scars which are often less durable than healthy skin, instable scarring is a common problem around the feet. Scars can lead to deformities of the toes, too, like mallet, hammer, or claw toes which can lead to progressive joint damage and painful clavus.

In general, scarring around functionally important areas of the body like the hands, feet, and joints can cause dire impairments throughout the demands of the patient's everyday life. Problematically, if left untreated, joint damage, a permanent reduction of one's range of movement, and thus progressive worsening of the patient's condition long after the initial trauma are potential consequences.

Therefore, physicians need to make sure that their proposed treatment not only improves the scarring but that it is also suitable to reduce the risk of secondary damage.

In this chapter, we aim to provide an overview of therapeutical options for the treatment of scarring in different anatomical localizations.

Scar Treatment Options for Different Anatomical Localizations

Face

When planning treatment for facial scars, physicians need to take all the aspects of the scarring into consideration. If functional impairments like impaired opening or closure of the eyes and mouth are present, the initiation and success of suitable therapeutic options are required more promptly than it would be with merely aesthetic impairments so that permanent damage beyond the scarring itself can be avoided.

If swift therapeutic success is required, surgical intervention remains the gold standard. Common indications for surgical intervention in facial scarring include microstomia, which is often the result of facial burns, acid attacks, or the ingestion of caustic fluids. It hinders sustentation and oral hygiene and impairs speech. Techniques for commissuroplasty to widen the oral opening through the advancement of mucosal flaps after scar excision have been published as early as 1831 by Dieffenbach and have since been modified and refined by Converse in 1959, Friedlander in 1974, and others (◘ Fig. 42.1). Often, commissuroplasty is aided postoperatively by splinting to avoid fresh scar contractures.

Lagophthalmos is another indication for swift surgical intervention. It, too, is often caused by thermal or chemical injuries. If left untreated, corneal ulcers, infections, and pain are common ailments associated with this affliction, and permanent damage to the patient's vision is a large risk.

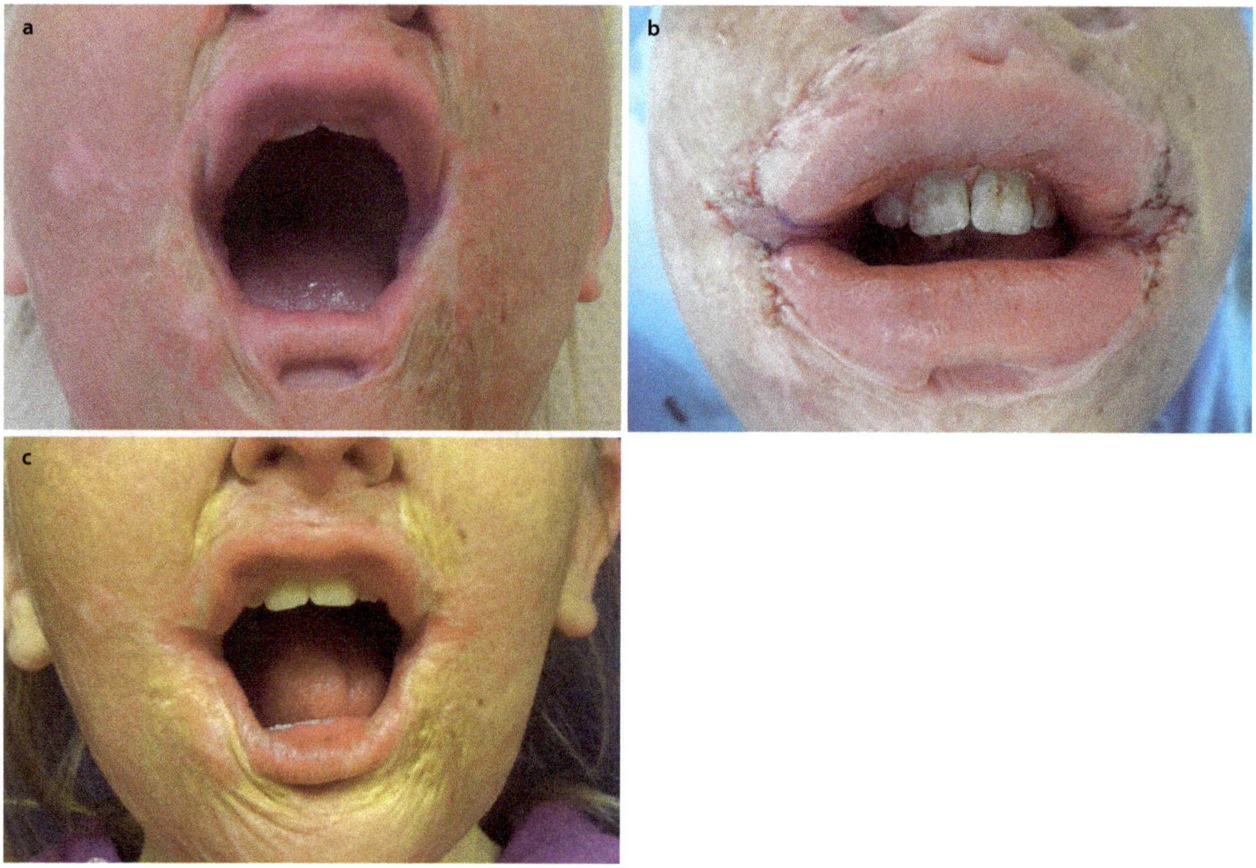

■ **Fig.** A 7-year-old child with severe microstomia due to burn scarring. Scar revision was performed with bilateral commissuroplasty (Converse plasty). Images were taken before **a**, intraoperatively **b**, and 4 weeks after surgery **c**. As a result of the surgery, the teeth are visible again, when the mouth is opened, thus facilitating dental hygiene

Ensuring sufficient closure of the eye is therefore a priority. Consulting an ophthalmologist is important in determining if surgical intervention is necessary and when it is best performed as well as to assess the extent to which reconstructive surgery is necessary.

A variety of treatment options exist for the reconstruction of the eyelids. Where full-thickness defects that affect both the anterior and posterior lamella of the eyelids can require complex reconstructions based on local flaps, oftentimes, only the anterior lamella is affected. Here, reconstruction with full-thickness skin grafts remains the standard (■ Fig. 42.2). In lower eyelid reconstruction, lateral canthopexy is routinely performed to avoid sagging of the lateral corner of the eye, thus leading to ectropion. This technique often results in good function and cosmesis.

Lasers, too, play a vital role in the treatment of facial scarring. Ablative laser treatment has been used for years to treat atrophic acne scars and has proven reliable and effective. Since the advent of fractional lasers, side effects and after-treatment downtimes have been reduced significantly while maintaining a good treatment efficacy. In the treatment of acne scars, the fractional CO_2 laser has proven more effective than its Er:YAG counterpart [1]. Through the radiance of heat into the surrounding tissue, the CO2 laser stimulates heat shock proteins which trigger a cascade of molecular pathways leading to increased levels of scar remodeling factors like transforming growth factor beta 3 (TGF-β3) and matrix metalloproteases. Since treatment with the Er:YAG laser results in almost no heat transfer to the surrounding tissue, those effects are less pronounced.

Widespread hypertrophic scarring as the result of burns, scalds, or chemical agents is becoming a frequent indication for the use of fractional ablative lasers, too. Through its ability to penetrate deep into the scar tissue to stimulate remodeling within the deep dermis all the while being an effective tool for superficial ablation of the irregular, ropelike and tuberose scars that often result from the aforementioned trauma, the CO_2 laser has become an oft-used and reliable tool for facial scar revision. While studies have shown significant improvement of scar texture and firmness after just one session [2], commonly, repeated treatments are necessary to achieve satisfactory results. Furthermore, the scar remodeling stimulated through the treatment continues

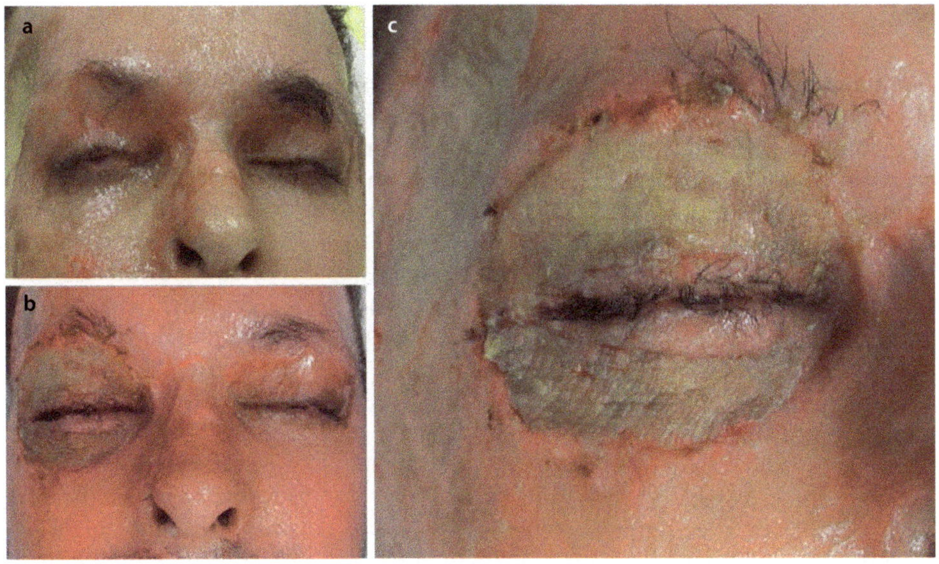

Fig. A patient with pronounced facial scarring and lagophthalmos after sustaining burn injuries. Recurring conjunctivitis and a corneal ulcer led to the indication for surgical revision of the lagophthalmos. The scars were released, and the anterior lamella of the upper and lower eyelid were reconstructed using a full-thickness skin graft from the upper arm of the patient. Image **a** shows the preoperative site, while **b** and **c** show the postoperative results where full closure of the eyelids can be achieved

for months so that final results can only be expected after 6–9 months. Thus, while able to loosen contractures and greatly improve facial scarring, other tools should be chosen where immediate scar relief is required.

Medical needling is another option that aims to improve scarring through percutaneous collagen induction. It has been shown to significantly improve acne and burn scars in connection with a low-risk profile and minimal side effects [3]. Satisfactory scar treatment, however, often requires multiple sessions, and thus far, clinical studies have often relied solely on subjective means of evaluation thus leading to a continued demand for evidence.

Ultimately, it seems best to combine different therapeutic paths. While surgical intervention is paramount for the treatment of severe functional impairments, it is rarely able to improve pliability and texture of scars thus normalizing the look and feel of scarred skin. Here, the combination of surgical intervention with fractional ablative laser treatment might provide a more holistic approach to the treatment of severe facial scarring resulting in improved overall results and lasting patient comfort and satisfaction.

Hair

Scarring in areas of hairy skin will often result in hair loss. This is particularly problematic in widespread scarring. While small scars can easily be excised even on the immobile parts of the scalp, larger scars resulting in pronounced hair loss are often difficult to treat.

On the scalp, the scarred, hairless tissue is excised and replaced by healthy surrounding skin. Ideally, local flaps from the scalp can cover the wound defect after excision; sometimes though, pre-expansion through skin expanders is necessary to provide the required tissue. Side effects of this course of treatment are frequent and include expander malfunction, infection, and dehiscence or "breaking" of the skin over the expanders. If successful, however, the scarred tissue can be excised completely, and permanent hair loss of the scarred areas can be revised.

If neither local flaps, skin grafting, nor tissue expansion are an option after scar excision, free-flap reconstruction can be considered. Here, fasciocutaneous flaps should be considered since the healthy skin architecture seems preferable for receiving a hair transplant as opposed to muscle flaps that have been covered with split-thickness skin grafts. After successful reconstruction and consolidation, fasciocutaneous flaps can easily be thinned to provide a natural contour and integrate well into the surrounding tissue, and consequently, hair transplantation can be attempted to restore a natural appearance. Hair transplantation can also be performed on scars or skin grafts; however, this will require both sufficient thickness of the subcutaneous tissue and adequate tissue perfusion so that the hair grafts are likely to take.

Hair transplantation is the standard therapy for alopecia of the eyebrows or eyelashes, too. While surgical techniques for reconstruction of the eyebrows are available, too, local flaps or composite grafts from the scalp will look different than natural eyebrows. Furthermore, in composite grafts, less so in pedicled flaps, the risk of reduced perfusion might lead to renewed hair loss, thus compromising results. Overall, for this indication, hair transplantation might lead to more natural results.

If hair transplantation is considered, patients should be aware that multiple sessions are required to achieve a satisfactory hair density. Furthermore, it is paramount that sufficient donor sites are available [4].

Hands

Normalizing function in scarred hands is paramount to avoid lasting impairments. Scarring of the hands is common in burns and scalds and often leads to widespread scarring, either through the trauma itself or through the resultant surgical treatment and skin grafting. Oftentimes such scarring will lead to contractures of the web spaces, thus greatly affecting thumb or finger abduction and diminishing grip strength. Closure of the fist is commonly impaired, too, as contractures of the dorsum of the hand and fingers inhibit full flexion.

Such problems are often addressed surgically to allow for swift improvement of the functional impairments and to allow for early mobilization through physiotherapy and occupational therapy.

Loosening of contractures of the web spaces has been described through many different techniques such as single or multiple Z-plasty, butterfly, or jumping man flaps as described by Shaw or Trident flap plasty according to Glicenstein or Hirshowitz (◘ Fig. 42.3). Many other techniques have been described as well, but their common goal is to loosen the contracted linear scar and deepen the affected web space.

It is important when planning web space scar revision that adjacent web spaces are never treated at the same time, to avoid perfusion problems to the finger in between, should one of the neurovascular bundles get damaged during surgery. Therefore, when planning to operate on multiple web spaces on one hand, pairings of web space 1 and 3, 2 and 4, or 1 and 4 are possible, while other combinations should be avoided.

Postoperative regimens vary, but commonly, load-free assisted exercising can be started shortly after surgery. Ideally, compression gloves with silicone spreaders for the affected web spaces are prescribed for overnight use for a year after surgery.

Volar flexion contractures are often treated through multiple Z-pasties, thus lengthening the scar and resolving the contracture.

Especially in widespread dorsal contractures, treatment remains difficult. Ensuring full closure of the fist is central to ensure good hand function; however, scarring is often rigid and restrictive.

To ameliorate these impairments, different techniques should be considered. One option is to replace the scarred tissue. After scar resection, full-thickness skin grafts or dermal substitutes like Integra® in combination with split-thickness skin grafts can be used to create a thicker, more flexible, and pliable skin in commonly stressed areas like the dorsum of the hand. Studies have shown that this might lead to improved pliability and functional results, both in acute and secondary burn reconstruction [5]. This, however, requires adequate coverage of functional structures like neurovascular bundles or tendons so that the grafts will take reliably. Otherwise, local or more likely free-flap coverage will be required. That course of action will, however, likely lead to multiple surgical revisions as flaps are often bulky and require subsequent thinning and contouring.

Laser therapy should be considered when improving the skin quality and rigidity is required. Fractional ablative CO_2 laser treatment has proven effective in releasing contractures and improving scar firmness, and different authors have described swift improvements in range of motion and scar quality in patients with burned hands [6, 7].

After scar revision on the hands, dedicated hand therapy is imperative to achieve lasting improvements regarding hand function and strength. After severe

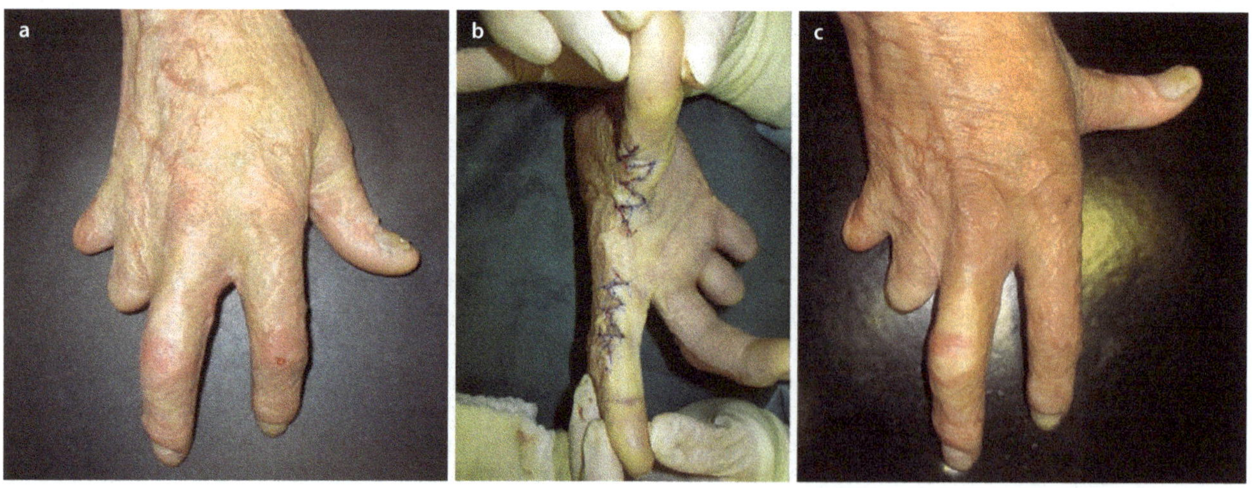

◘ **Fig.** A patient with severe impairment of the abduction of the thumb following burn injuries to the right hand with consecutive scarring of the first web space **a**. After double opposing Z-plasty in the first web space and serial Z-plasty along the radial side of the index finger **b**, abduction of the thumb is drastically improved **c**

trauma and scarring, patients often require months of therapy to reach satisfactory results and to enable self-reliance throughout their daily lives.

The ideal time for scar revision should be carefully weighed, too. Especially in the pediatric patient population, where scar contractures might inhibit physical and functional development, timely intervention is indicated to avoid lasting damages that can be hard or even impossible to reverse.

In general, if possible, the conservative treatment of scarring through compression gloves, silicone finger spreaders, and hand-therapy should be exhausted, especially throughout the phase of scar maturation to avoid unnecessary surgery or even exacerbation of the scarring through stimulation of the scarring process.

Feet

Severe scarring of the feet can lead to a variety of problems for the affected patients. Common causes of scarring located on the feet include burns and scalds but also complex physical trauma.

Oftentimes such injuries cause contractures of the toes that will lead to painful malposition and toe deformities that can greatly impair walking.

Unstable scarring around the feet is a frequent problem, too, and chronic wounds and tears open under the daily stress those scars are exposed to.

These common problems results in a high urgency for scar therapy regarding the feet. The goal is to provide stable skin that is flexible and resistant to the daily strain the feet are exposed to.

Scars resulting from burns or scalds are commonly located on the dorsum of the foot, and resultant contractures of the toes can often be released through excision and Z-plasty or other local flaps, not unlike contractures on the dorsum of the hand. Similarly, though, more severe scarring or unstable scars might require excision of larger scarred areas and then skin grafts or a combination of a dermal substitute (like Integra® or Matriderm®) and skin grafts. Full-thickness scars that require excision onto the extensor tendons might even require free flaps for successful defect reconstruction.

Severely contracted joints might require capsulotomy for release, and sometimes, temporary Kirschner wire transfixation is indicated to achieve lasting rehabilitation of the affected joints [8].

The data on laser treatment for severe scarring of the feet is scarce. In light of the capabilities of fractional ablative lasers, however, it seems prudent to consider this line of therapy as an adjunct in more severe cases or as a primary therapy option in mild to moderate cases where its capabilities to loosen contractures and to soften the scarred skin might yield promising results or at least ease subsequent surgery.

Complications of surgery around the foot include hyperkeratosis, which is especially common around the load-bearing areas like the heel or the ball of the foot, where scarring can often result in this cumbersome problem, which is associated with significant pain, thus hindering walking and resulting in severe discomfort. Authors have noted that hyperkeratosis oftentimes forms protectively around a scarred area to minimize pressure on said area. Especially early on during the wound healing phase after local or free flaps to the heel or the sole of the foot, hyperkeratosis can often hinder the healing process by overgrowing the wound margins and thus inhibiting complete fusion of the wound margins. Therefore, after surgical treatment of the foot, medical foot care presents an important adjunct, not only to ensure patient comfort but also to facilitate wound healing and to minimize complications.

As with treating scarred hands, surgical or laser-based interventions should always go along with conservative means like compression garments, scar massages, and physiotherapy to optimize treatment results. This should be continued until the scar activity has subsided.

Joints

Scarring over joints can be particularly cumbersome to deal with. The constant tension that the healing tissue is exposed through the movement of the respective limb will encourage scar hypertrophy after trauma but also after scar revision. This should be taken into consideration when planning the treatment of scars that run over joints.

Plenty of treatment options are available, but ideally, a combination is chosen to avoid recidivism of problematic scarring.

Linear hypertrophic scarring can be released through Z-plasty or other comparable techniques relying on local flaps. While hypertrophic scars commonly show a great tendency for regress without treatment after an initial phase of growth activity and a consecutive constant phase so that invasive treatments are not considered a first-line treatment option, an exception can be made if hypertrophic scars are under constant tension.

As this stress can be considered a major cause of the scar hypertrophy, resolving it through surgery or fractional ablative laser treatment can result in subsiding hypertrophy and symptoms thus constituting a causal therapy.

Supportive measures that should be considered to avoid renewed hypertrophy include intralesional triamcinolone acetonide or 5-fluorouracil injections, silicone gel or sheets, and pressure therapy.

Widespread scarring can be treated through serial excision. Here, the scar is excised in two to three consecutive operations every 3–4 months. This allows the remaining skin to stretch thus facilitating complete scar removal that would not have been possible in one single step. To avoid stretching of the scar, wound closure should be performed in a layered fashion. The subcutaneous and corium sutures should provide large tensile strength that remains over an extended period. Many studies, most recently by Gupta et al., have shown that superior scar appearance results can be achieved by using intradermal polydioxanone (PDS) sutures when compared to polyglactin 910 (Vicryl) sutures [9].

Alternatively like in other problematic areas, fractional ablative lasers have shown great potential to ameliorate scar contractures and should be considered a treatment option and be discussed with patients [10]. Successful treatment, however, will likely require repeated treatment sessions.

Conclusion

When treating pathological scarring, taking the anatomic location of the scar into account is imperative when choosing the right form of treatment.

Facial scarring can be extremely disfiguring and beyond the aesthetic implications often results in severe functional impairments like microstomia and lagophthalmos, among others. Treatment should be initiated quickly to avoid secondary damage to the affected organs. Commonly, surgical intervention remains the gold standard. Contractures are loosened through local flaps (e.g., Z-plasty), and skin defects after scar excision can be treated through split- or full-thickness skin grafting. Fractional laser treatment as an adjunct has become an important factor in improving facial scarring as they are able to improve scar firmness and smoothen their irregular surface. Similar effects are sought through the use of medical needling, though objective clinical data on its efficacy are largely lacking. Alopecia is a problem when scars affect the scalp. Often, the healthy skin is expanded through skin expanders over several weeks so that the scar can then be excised with the expanded skin now covering the defect. However, such treatment is often difficult because of expander malfunction and infections. Other options include free-flap reconstruction after scar excision, followed by hair transplantation. Especially in hair loss of the eyebrows and lashes, hair transplantation remains the gold standard, and achieving a near natural result in the hands of an experienced surgeon is often possible. Scarring of the hands can result in the loss of self-reliance in affected patients. Oftentimes, the web spaces are contracted thus limiting abduction of the thumb or spreading of the fingers. This can be addressed through deepening of the web spaces, for example, through double opposing Z-plasty. Afterward, compression gloves with silicone spreaders are fitted to ensure permanence of the achieved results and to inhibit renewed contractures. If contractures on the dorsum of the hand inhibit closure of the fist, complex reconstructions can become necessary if larger areas of scarred tissues need to be replaced. Laser treatment can assist in improving scar quality. Overall, a combination of treatment options should be considered. Physiotherapy and occupational therapy as well as compression garment therapy should be included into the treatment algorithm to improve functional results and to inhibit renewed pathological scarring. On the feet, scars often lead to toe deformities which impair walking and make wearing regular shoes uncomfortable or impossible. Here, surgical intervention is indicated. Since the feet are exposed to a lot of strain throughout the day, scars are often unstable and repeatedly crack and tear, leading to chronic wounds and strong patient discomfort. Here, excision and skin replacement through skin grafts, often together with dermal substitutes or even free flap reconstruction, can become necessary.

Overall, it is important to remember that scarring is a multifaceted problem. Through their firmness and contraction, they cause functional problems, their irregular appearance and color can be aesthetically displeasing, and all of these effects can put an enormous strain on the quality of life of the affected patients. Treating such scarring, especially in exposed areas or where function is greatly impaired, should therefore address the complexity of this problem. This is oftentimes only possible by combining surgical, laser-based, and conservative treatment paradigms into an individual treatment plan for the affected patients. This ensures not only immediate but also long-term improvements and inhibits renewed scarring.

Take-Home Messages

- Common functional impairments after scarring of the face include microstomia and lagophthalmos that require swift surgical attention to avoid secondary damage to the affected organs.
- While surgery remains the standard for severe functionally impairing scars of the face, fractional lasers have become a staple in improving scar firmness and surface irregularities and should be used in combination with surgery to improve overall results.
- Hair loss in scarred areas can be addressed in a variety of ways. Expanding healthy, surrounding tissue can help create enough tissue so that the scar can be excised in its entirety and the resultant defect can be covered with the expanded skin.
- If this is not possible, the scarred tissue can be replaced by fasciocutaneous free flaps, and these flaps can then be contoured afterward and receive hair transplants.
- Hair transplants are the gold standard for hair loss of the eyebrows and eyelashes.
- Improving function in scarred hands is imperative to maintain self-reliance in affected patients. Contractures of the web spaces can easily be treated through local flaps to deepen the web space, and results are commonly good when assisted by compression garment therapy afterward.
- Scarring of the feet can be severely impairing for affected patients. Contractures that result in toe malposition or deformities should be addressed to ensure that the patients can walk and wear shoes comfortably.

References

1. Reinholz M, Schwaiger H, Heppt MV, Poetschke J, Tietze J, Epple A, et al. Comparison of two kinds of lasers in the treatment of acne scars. Facial Plast Surg. 2015;31(5):523–31.
2. Poetschke J, Dornseifer U, Clementoni MT, Reinholz M, Schwaiger H, Steckmeier S, et al. Ultrapulsed fractional ablative carbon dioxide laser treatment of hypertrophic burn scars: evaluation of an in-patient controlled, standardized treatment approach. Lasers Med Sci. 2017;32(5):1031–40.
3. Aust MC, Knobloch K, Reimers K, Redeker J, Ipaktchi R, Altintas MA, et al. Percutaneous collagen induction therapy: an alternative treatment for burn scars. Burns. 2010;36(6):836–43.
4. Farjo B, Farjo N, Williams G. Hair transplantation in burn scar alopecia. Scars Burns Heal. 2015;1:2059513115607764.
5. Cuadra A, Correa G, Roa R, Pineros JL, Norambuena H, Searle S, et al. Functional results of burned hands treated with Integra(R). J Plast Reconstr Aesthet Surg. 2012;65(2):228–34.
6. Krakowski AC, Goldenberg A, Eichenfield LF, Murray JP, Shumaker PR. Ablative fractional laser resurfacing helps treat restrictive pediatric scar contractures. Pediatrics. 2014;134(6):e1700–5.
7. Sorkin M, Cholok D, Levi B. Scar management of the burned hand. Hand Clin. 2017;33(2):305–15.
8. Chang JB, Kung TA, Levi B, Irwin T, Kadakia A, Cederna PS. Surgical management of burn flexion and extension contractures of the toes. J Burn Care Res. 2014;35(1):93–101.
9. Gupta D, Sharma U, Chauhan S, Sahu SA. Improved outcomes of scar revision with the use of polydioxanone suture in comparison to polyglactin 910: a randomized controlled trial. J Plast Reconstr Aesthet Surg. 2018;71(8):1159–63.
10. Willows BM, Ilyas M, Sharma A. Laser in the management of burn scars. Burns. 2017;43(7):1379–89.

9

Management of Scars in Skin of Color

Huidi Tchero

Contents

Background

How Scars Evolve Differently in Skin of Color?

Management of Scars in the Skin of Color
Nonsurgical
Surgical
Response Rates and Side Effects in Skin of Color
Recurrence Rate

Management of Scars in Asian Skin

Conclusions

References

Background

Scars are a normal process of dermal healing following laceration, skin incision, or tissue loss. Frequently, they are associated with burns, penetrating wounds, or surgical cuts. Morphologically, they appear erythematous and firm with elevated fibrous masses that are evolving within the margins of the wound and might revert later. They can cause cosmetic disfigurement, functional impairment, and psychological negative outcomes, affecting the patients' quality of life. These patients often seek medical advice to recover the color, texture, pliability, and relief of the associated pain [1]. In this chapter, we discussed how scars evolve differently in the skin of color, explored the available treatment modalities, and recommended planned treatment modalities in keloid management based on the published evidence.

How Scars Evolve Differently in Skin of Color?

Injury to the tissue could significantly produce inflammation, which is in turn associated with infiltration of neutrophils, monocytes, and macrophages, and release of pro-inflammatory cytokines, which induce fibroblast migration and proliferation, resulting in disproportionate extracellular matrix (ECM) deposition besides collagen accumulation [2]. This process is exaggerated when it affects the deep dermis, which would be complicated by the formation of a permanent scar. The scope of scar types varies from atrophic, flat, to raised dermal scars [3].

The pathogenesis of hypertrophic scars might be returned to atypical ECM metabolism following an odd and exaggerated fibroblastic stimulation. Histologically, it exhibits organized overexpression of types I and III collagen, deposition of fibronectin, and overexpression of pro-inflammatory interleukins (IL), such as IL-4, IL-6, IL-13, and IL-21, as well as downregulation of IL-12 and interferon (IFN)-γ expression [2]. The incidence of hypertrophic scars associated with a burn is up to 78%. The risk factor for hypertrophic scar includes dark skin, neck or upper limb age (younger), site, female gender, healing time, the severity of the injury, and the increase in a number of operations.

Keloids are different from hypertrophic scars in a variety of ways: they propagate outside the margins of the wound zone and invade the adjacent skin with no regression, conversely to hypertrophic scars that develop within the edges of the original wound and frequently regress in months. Keloids are a common fibroproliferative disorder that could happen due to abnormal healing process succeeding cutaneous injury. Keloids could evolve in any race; however, persons with more pigmented color (Fitzpatrick IV, V, and VI) are more vulnerable. In Hispanics, African-Americans, and Asians, keloids develop in up to 6–16% of those populations. The tendency for keloid expansion was also observed in patients suffering from dermatological diseases which lead to a protracted inflammatory reaction [1].

The presentation of keloid and hypertrophic scars can vary in patients with skin of color. Scars can be hyperpigmented or very large in patients with darker skin. Although keloid and hypertrophic scars appear usually within 1 year after trauma or surgery, few cases of people with skin of color who developed spontaneous keloid scars were reported within the literature as well.

Under the microscope, keloids appear as a twirling nodular arrangement of collagen fibers, characteristically with hyalinized, coarsened collagen bundles. Moreover, they have an acellular collagen center with adjoining hyper-proliferative fibroblasts. Their center covers dense fibers of immature collagen that are feebly supplied by blood vessels without lymphatic or elastin.

Several mechanisms have been hypothesized for the development of keloids, for example, deviant collagen production, abnormal growth factor regulation, and genetic vulnerability. Elevated levels of *transforming growth factor* beta (TGF-β) are suggested to be involved in keloid development; nonetheless, several other mediators are tending to be elaborated. Still, there is a lack of confirmed hypothesis that could elucidate keloid pathogenesis. Immune cells were also suggested to be involved in keloid scar formation.

Inherited genes increase predisposition for keloid tissue development; however, still, exact genes involved have not been acknowledged. Remarkably, keloid is exclusive to humans, and the animal model of keloid scars is absent. A large Japanese genome-wide association study (GWAS) discovered four single-nucleotide polymorphisms (SNPs) in three chromosomal segments in patients with keloid scars. These SNPs include rs8032158, situated in intron 5 of chromosome 15 that downregulates NEDD4 gene, which chiefly affects keloid severity. A study of admixture mapping recognized potentially mutual genetic regions between a group of Black, Chinese, and Japanese patients on chromosome 15q21.2–22.3, within which NEDD4 inhabits.

In analogous studies among relatives, one on *chromosome 2q23* and the other on *chromosome 7p11* were recognized in Japanese patients and African-American patients, respectively. Notwithstanding evidence of familial keloid formation, there was a changeability in phenotypic presentations and scar severity between families; hence, polygenic inheritance pattern is mostly included in keloid inheritance [4].

Although there are no clear evidence regarding the influence of inherited genes on the higher frequency or severity of scar among patients with skin of color, it was previously observed that the ethnicity of families with multiple affected members is mainly African-American and Indian. Variations in the age of onset, severity of the scars, and response to treatment in the same ethnic group may highlight the role of multiple gene mutations in the pathogenesis of the scar. Nevertheless, the pattern of gene involvements in scar pathogenesis is an area of further research.

Management of Scars in the Skin of Color

The prevention of scars can be achieved by proper cleaning and debridement of wounds, avoidance of unnecessary invasive procedures in high-risk population, and prophylactic measure. Modalities that prevent wound stretch – such as silicone gel sheets or tapes – and intralesional corticosteroids exhibited promising results inn scars prevention; however, the evidence is still weak.

To identify the most suitable management strategy, a thorough clinical examination should be done. This assessment must contain a full medical history, a detailed keloid scar history, any family history of keloids, and a psychosocial assessment. Moreover, a detailed examination should be conducted, including location, color, contour, size, pliability, and symptoms, i.e., pain and itching. Keloid is an untreatable disease, but nonetheless, physicians might be able to manage the manifestations of keloid, counting reducing scar size and redness and mitigating inflammation; this might reduce the recurrence rate of such lesions and may even yield complete extinction of lesions. Deterrence of signs and symptoms' exacerbation and impediment of recurrence after therapy are the main treatment goals of keloids.

Clinically, it is challenging to forecast if a scar will progress into either a hypertrophic scar or keloid. Increasing skin tension in specific locations and orientations while closing the wound and the existence of infections and foreign bodies may amplify the chance of keloid development. The more susceptible sites on the body for keloids include the earlobes, mandibular angle, posterior neck, shoulders, upper arms, upper back, and anterior chest. Bleeding, ulcerative, or firmly attached scars should undergo histopathologic investigation as a differential diagnosis of keloids. The possible differential lesions might be keloidal scleroderma, scar sarcoidosis, dermatofibroma, dermatofibrosarcoma protuberans, morphoeic basal cell carcinoma, and metastatic skin nodules.

Several therapeutic modalities are used in the management of keloid; though, due to unknown resolution rates and high recurrence rates, it is challenging to support any specific therapy. While several strategies exist, owing to the absence of level I evidence, none of them is universally demarcated as the standard. Presently, the treatments used have at best inadequate or indefinite effectiveness, with possible adverse drug reactions. Furthermore, many of these treatments require long treatment durations, might worsen the lesions, or could not prevent recurrence [3]. Multiple treatments for keloid, with varying efficacies, have been stated to date. Traditionally, a number of treatment regimens, for example, cryotherapy, interferon, and verapamil, have been applied for treating keloid, with unreliable success levels. Though, more novel treatments such as intralesional steroid injections, imiquimod, silicone gel, radiotherapy, lasers, electrical stimulation (ES), bleomycin, 5-fluorouracil (FU), surgery, and photodynamic therapy (PDT) have also been tested, not all have revealed efficacy in ethnic pigmented skin. These treatment modalities were reviewed in detail (◘ Fig. 43.1). However, due to the lack of studies on ethnic skin, some included studies presented data on pigmented, as well as nonpigmented keloid skin.

Nonsurgical

Intralesional Steroid Injections

Intralesional injection of corticosteroid (alone or with other agents) is one of the commonest treatment methods for hypertrophic scars and keloids. They are injected each 4–6 weeks as insoluble triamcinolone acetonide (0–40 mg/mL) until pain, scar, and pruritis subside. The response of patients to the treatment ranges from 50% to 100%, while the recurrence rate ranges from 9% to 50%. However, 63% presents with complications like localized ulceration, dermal atrophy, and telangiectasia or hypopigmentation. Noteworthy, pain might be managed through applying a local anesthetic. Corticosteroids alone represent the most efficient for young keloids, while older keloids are further resistant [2].

Silicone Gel/Sheet

Using silicone gel/sheets is assumed to diminish mobility and decrease the scar tension. How silicone gel works is uncertain; however, it may serve as an impermeable membrane to preserve hydration of the skin. A former RCT with 21 patients compared silicone gel with no therapy. Gold et al. found a reduction in hypertrophic scarring and keloid incidence following silicone gel use. However, the limitations of this trial were short follow-up period (only 12 weeks), and the blinding and techniques of randomization were not stated.

In another RCT by De Oliveira and colleagues, 26 patients suffering from keloids or hypertrophic scars had a mixture of silicone gel sheeting and non-silicone gel sheeting, while the control group received no treatment. They found no statistically significant difference

Fig. Treatment modali-ties for a scar in colored skin

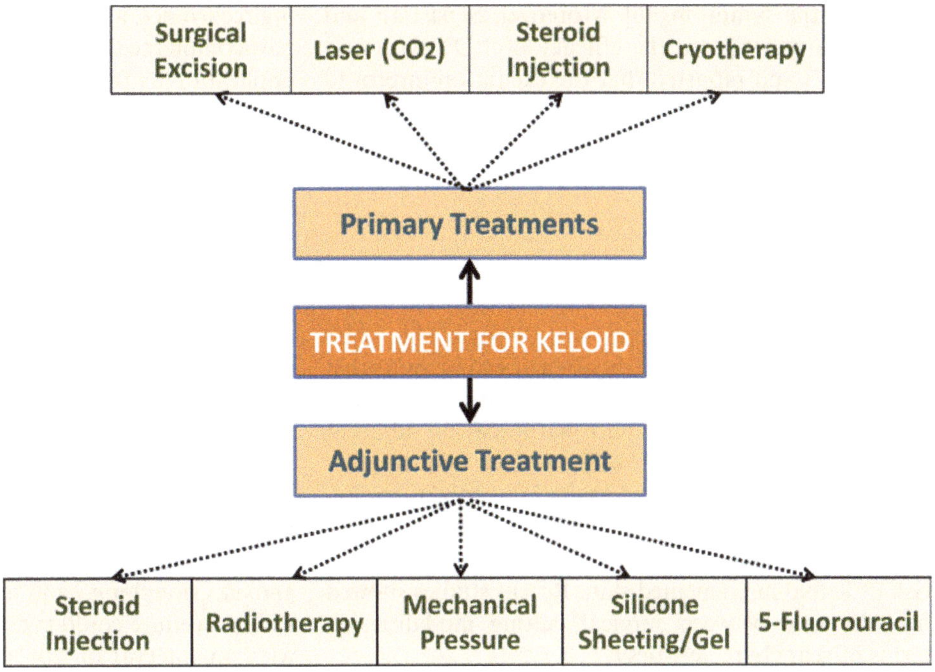

in the symptoms or size of scar by taking any of the treatments; however, both scar types were combined in their analysis, and the follow-up period was <6 months. These findings were in parallel with the results of O'Brien and Pandit study that was carried out among 13 trials including 559 subjects, observing the efficacy of silicone gel in the management of abnormal scarring in vulnerable groups. These studies collectively highlighted the demand for further controlled trials to approve the safety and efficacy of silicone gel sheeting.

Radiotherapy

Radiotherapy is preferred in elder adults who failed to respond to other treatments. It is used only in elderly patients because of the theoretical risk, however, there is a low risk of carcinogenesis. In resistant keloids, we could use ionizing radiation with intralesional excision. It acts via inhibiting collagen synthesis and inducing apoptosis of proliferating cells, which might rebuild a balance between keloid degeneration and collagen synthesis. It is given in doses of 15–30 Gy, ranging from 3 to 40 Gy among the studies, along six periods with accurate dosimetry and proper protection in the postoperative duration [2].

Doornbos et al. retrospectively analyzed 203 patients with keloid lesions using radiotherapy postsurgical excision. They elucidated the correlation between dose and response, with bigger doses decreasing the recurrence rate more efficiently. Conversely, Klumpar et al. found no significant dose–response correlation. Moreover, some investigators as Ragoowansi et al. and Maarouf et al. have supported the use of immediate postoperative radiotherapy [3]. Large-scale clinical trials are required to investigate a dose–response correlation among different races. Using radiotherapy as an adjuvant has revealed good scar resolution rates from 67% up to 98%. Yet, the retrospective study design, different follow-up intervals, and lacking universal clinical evaluation have weakened this success rate.

Photodynamic Therapy (PDT)

The cytotoxic effects of PDT (with methyl-amino levulinate and amino levulinic acid) were investigated in different keloid lesional sites. One study concluded that the success of PDT depends on the photosensitizer precursor, the location, and the number of fibroblasts at the lesion site. A beneficial effect of topical application of methyl-amino levulinate PDT was initially observed in a patient with resistant keloid. There is a case series with 20 keloid patients who were examined for the effect of PDT. The results showed that PDT reduced pain and pruritus scores, reduced flow of blood, improved pliability and reduced levels of collagen in keloid, and resulted in a decrease of volume of keloid without recurrence over the follow-up period (9 months) [5]. These findings direct potential utility of PDT in the management of keloid and necessitate a further high-quality clinical trial to confirm the safety and efficacy of photodynamic therapy.

Electrical Stimulation

Electrical stimulation (ES) was investigated in relieving the keloid symptoms, such as pruritis and pain. Lately, a new in vitro system examined the efficacy of various ES types on collagen expression in keloid fibroblasts and revealed that ES could inhibit formation of collagen I in keloid. Two case series confirmed the efficacy of degraded wave ES in few patients with painful keloids, and the regimen exhibited significant amelioration of the symptoms [6]. Moreover, Sebastian and colleagues investigated the efficacy of PDT with and without ES and reported that the excitation improved the cytotoxic effects of PDT. Large-scale studies are needed to confirm the effectiveness of PDT-ES combination therapy.

Surgical

Surgery is needed in patients with hypertrophic scars with contractures, particularly when affecting joints that result in function loss. Hypertrophic scars may impede movement when they do abnormal forces on adjacent tissues or cross the joints. The elbow, knee, and shoulder are most commonly affected joints by contractures following burn injury. Surgery must be approached with caution as surgical scars may themselves increase the risk of keloid in pigmented skin. Recent studies showed no difference between surgical cutting modalities in terms of scar characteristics [7].

Surgical excision of keloids must be executed with substantial precaution, owing to the high recurrence risk. Excision could result in a bigger lesion and increased possibility of recurrence. The link between scarring and mechanical stress scarring is due to keloid scars occurring primarily in sites of excessive stress and mobility, for example, the shoulder, scapular region, and sternum. Therefore, it has been encouraged that cases subjected to surgery in these specific locations must have a long time of local skin support and splintage.

Surgical Excision and Adjuvant Therapy

The essential method in keloid treatment is surgical removal and primary closure, then injection of local steroid. Initial surgical excision followed by postoperative injection of steroid and silicone sheeting showed a 15% recurrence rate. Other modalities, for example, wearing a body corset or supportive bra, can furthermore decrease the risk of keloid in the mid-sternal region or upper trunk. Precautions to be considered while performing the first keloid surgery include not putting tension on the adjacent skin while closing the lesion. All possible causes of residual inflammation, i.e., entrapped hair follicles or dermal sinus tracts, should be excised to avoid recurrence. In case of large-sized keloid, serial excision would be well thought out to diminish skin tension. The injection of corticosteroid may be performed with surgery, then once every month for about 4–6 months. Surgeons should avoid local Z-plasties, W-plasties, and skin flaps beyond the defect to avert recurrence of bigger keloid. Of note, the use of silicone as a prophylactic method has so far been recommended in many studies except for Niessen et al.'s study. Topical steroid tape has also exhibited effectiveness in preventing recurrence, although it has the potential for unfortunate compliance because it is dependent on its continuous application by the patient [1].

Cryosurgery

Smaller keloid lesions have been treated by cryosurgery; however, substantial pain and occasionally prolonged healing times posttreatment limit its usage. The hypothesized mechanism of action is through ischemic damage that results in cellular anoxia producing necrosis of tissue. Furthermore, it modifies collagen synthesis and stimulates differentiation of keloid fibroblast near normal phenotype, thereby reducing keloid scar size [8].

Intralesional cryosurgery is a technique advanced from simple cryosurgery, which was first announced, by Shepard and Dawber. A simple cryosurgery, including pray technique or liquid nitrogen contact, etc., might produce vascular injury causing necrosis of tissue, anoxia, sloughing, and consequently scar flattening. This procedure could take two to ten treatment sessions with an interval of 20–30 days between each session. The success rate was reported ranging from 32% to 74% following two or more therapies, with superior response rates among hypertrophic scars over keloids. There are complications such as pain and immediate blistering with long-term risk of dermal atrophy that could be hyper- or hypopigmented. Conversely, intralesional cryosurgery includes introducing a recent intralesional cryoneedle (Cryoshape™) inside the scar over the long axis. This probe is formed of an elongated uninsulated needle having double lumen with a safety vent and a sealed, cutting, distal tip prepared to augment the penetration of firm, dense scar. The probe proximal end is linked with liquid nitrogen that is pressurized to circulate within the needle that results in an ice ball forming around the cryoneedle leaving the adjoining scar tissue totally frozen, thus resulting in an apparently normal collagen regarding its structure and organization with a decrease in myofibroblasts and mast cells in the scar. This technique was first described in 1993 by Weshahy and later popularized by Har-Shai et al. and has revealed superior efficacy over simple cryosurgery, with a reported clinical effect ranging from 20% to 75% reduction in the scar volume. The main complications are peritreatment edema and epidermolysis, temporary hypopigmentation, and pain (while this pain is lower than simple cryotherapy). The main advantage of intralesional over simple cryotherapy was melanocyte sparing feature that accounts for a lower incidence of dyschromia as the temperature of skin surface is less influenced in intralesional cryotherapy [2].

A hospital-based clinical trial was performed on 30 patients with keloid using cryotherapy. The findings demonstrated that cryosurgery was an essential treatment regimen for recent keloid, chiefly in smaller lesions. Also, they found that both thicknesses and duration of keloid were the main agents in defining treatment outcome by cryosurgery. These findings were supported by Tziotzios and colleagues who recommended cryosurgery for reduction of scar size. Recently, a case study investigated the efficacy of cryosurgery plus surgical excision combination in 12 participants with keloid after 12 months. They demonstrated that shaving linked to cryosurgery was beneficial in the management of bulky keloid lesions because all cases showed improvement signs. Yet, it is arduous to follow this treatment modality owing to the small sample size [3].

Response Rates and Side Effects in Skin of Color

It is well-recognized that skin type significantly affects scar response to various modalities of treatment. Previous reports have shown that African-American patients had lower vascular response to topical corticosteroid than Caucasian patients. Relatively low response to bleomycin was reported among patients with skin of color. Patients with skin types IV–VI showed low response rates to different types of laser as well.

In terms of safety concerns, patients with skin of color are more reliable to higher incidence of adverse events than patients with lighter skin types. The risk of hypopigmentation after cryotherapy is more prominent in patients with darker skin due to cold sensitivity of melanocytes. While excessive melanin in patients with skin of color can absorb more laser and lead to hyperpigmentation, the high prevalence of melasma among patients with darker skin may contribute to post-laser hyperpigmentation as well. Hereditary hemolytic diseases are more prevalent among African-American, and they may impair healing after laser excision of the scars.

Recurrence Rate

Keloid scars are associated with high rate of recurrence, especially when treated with surgical excision alone. However, there are no current published data that address the effect of skin type on the rate of recurrence after scars treatment.

Management of Scars in Asian Skin

Recent guidelines on the management of scars in Asian patients recommended that scar prevention should be initiated in the immediate postoperative period owing to the high risk of developing poor scars. The recommended first-line therapy was silicone-based products (silicone gel and silicone gel sheets) based on their easy administration and strong supporting evidence. Several second-line therapies were recommended in case of failure of the first-line treatment, including intralesional steroid or 5-flourouracil injections, as well as radiotherapy. Despite lack of strong evidence, laser treatments have been increasingly accepted in these patients; however, further studies are needed to confirm its efficacy and determine the optimal wavelength and amount of energy required. Surgery is generally considered a last resort in resistant keloids. It can be combined with radiotherapy "sandwich technique," which has shown relatively low recurrence rates in Japanese patients [9].

Conclusions

Keloids are considered a challenging medical condition for both patients and medical health professionals owing to its high recurrence rate. The existing body of evidence has tried to investigate the pathophysiology and molecular basis involved in scar development using a reliable and reproducible model of a keloid. These endeavors would optimize the treatment and improve the outcomes of the disease. Currently, it is crucial to robust the published evidence, merged with clinical outcome, to deliver patients with the best therapeutic regimens for scars. Moreover, additional large-scale, long-term, and high-quality RCTs are indispensable to conclude the safety and efficacy of these treatment options further, and also comparative studies are compulsory to identify the best treatment modality for scars in the pigmented skin. Finally, standard guidelines and protocols are mandatory to standardize the progress of such promising treatment modalities on a global scale.

The current body of evidence has emphasized the requirement for additional long-term clinical trials with larger sample size to assess the efficacy of the aforementioned treatments strongly. Several studies were short-term clinical trials with small numbers of patients included, and the others were case series. Besides, lacking stratification of patients into categories according to the type of lesion, i.e., keloid or hypertrophic scars, location, a degree of severity, or ethnicity of the patients, was present in some of these studies. The different types of scars are diverse at the molecular level and morphologically. Furthermore, the difference in skin color, site, number, and size of the scar could respond differently to the same modality of treatment. Therefore, this variability ought to be taken into consideration when designing those studies. Likewise, the measures used to assess scar characteristic and response to treatment were variable among the studies. Therefore, it is a compulsory requirement to use universal tool for assessment and implantation of measures to monitor cellular and metabolic activities in the tissue of keloid which, in turn, would support tailoring specific modality of treatment with each category of patients to ensure the best response of disease to treatment.

Keloid is unique for human tissue. This esoteric nature made keloids' preclinical studies scramble owing to the absence of animal models. Nonetheless, the advent of an in vitro organ culture model of keloid was fundamental in facilitating the study of disease molecular biology, pathophysiology, and the response among variable therapeutic modalities. This model was found to be a valuable tool for investigating new treatments and optimizing the treatment that would exhibit the optimum safety and efficacy in a diminution of the keloid scar mass size. Hence, it is considered as a prospective approach for new therapies assessment.

Take-Home Messages

- Pigmented skin has a higher chance of developing hypertrophic and keloid scars following wounds.
- Thorough history taking and clinical examination are essential for accurate assessment and management of abnormal scars in pigmented skin.
- Several therapeutic modalities for keloid management are available; however, there is lack of evidence to identify one strategy as the gold standard.
- Nonsurgical modalities for keloid management include intralesional steroid injections, radiotherapy, photodynamic therapy, and electrical stimulation.
- Surgery is needed in patients with hypertrophic scars with contractures, particularly when affecting joints that result in function loss.
- Combination therapies of surgical and nonsurgical modalities have shown some promising results; however, further research is needed.
- Large-scale clinical trials and clinical practice guidelines are needed to direct the development of effective treatments for keloid management.

References

1. Visscher MO, Bailey JK, Hom DB. Scar treatment variations by skin type. Facial Plast Surge Clin. 2014;22(3):453–62.
2. McGoldrick RB, Theodorakopoulou E, Azzopardi EA, Murison M. Lasers and ancillary treatments for scar management Part 2: keloid, hypertrophic, pigmented and acne scars. Scars Burns Heal. 2017;3:2059513116689805.
3. Ud-Din S, Bayat A. Strategic management of keloid disease in ethnic skin: a structured approach supported by the emerging literature. Br J Dermatol. 2013;169:71–81.
4. Andrews JP, Marttala J, Macarak E, Rosenbloom J, Uitto J. Keloids: the paradigm of skin fibrosis—pathomechanisms and treatment. Matrix Biol. 2016;51:37–46.
5. Ud-Din S, Thomas G, Morris J, Bayat A. Photodynamic therapy: an innovative approach to the treatment of keloid disease evaluated using subjective and objective non-invasive tools. Arch Dermatol Res. 2013;305(3):205–14.
6. Ud-Din S, Giddings PD, Colthurst J, Whiteside S, Morris J, Bayat A. Significant reduction of symptoms of scarring with electrical stimulation: evaluated with subjective and objective assessment tools in a prospective noncontrolled case series. Wounds. 2013;25(8):212–24.
7. Ismail A, Abushouk AI, Elmaraezy A, Menshawy A, Menshawy E, Ismail M, et al. Cutting electrocautery versus scalpel for surgical incisions: a systematic review and meta-analysis. J Surg Res. 2017;220:147–63.
8. Durani P, Bayat A. Levels of evidence for the treatment of keloid disease. J Plast Reconstr Aesthet Surg. 2008;61(1):4–17.
9. Kim S, Choi TH, Liu W, Ogawa R, Suh JS, Mustoe TA. Update on scar management: guidelines for treating Asian patients. Plast Reconstr Surg. 2013;132(6):1580–9.

10

Additional Invasive Techniques in Scar Management

E. de Bakker, M. C. E. van Leeuwen, O. W. M. Meijer, and F. B. Niessen

Contents

Background

Introduction

Types of Radiation Therapy
External Beam Radiation Therapy (EBRT)
Brachytherapy (Internal Radiation)

Excision and Radiation Type

Recurrence
Complications

Safety Concerns

Additional Thoughts on the Biomechanisms of Radiotherapy in Keloid Treatment

Conclusions

References

Background

Soon after the discovery of radiation, radiotherapy was recognized as a treatment technique for tissue overgrowth. Also, hypertrophic scars and keloid disorder were treated both therapeutically and for prevention of recurrent growth following surgery.

Both patients and care providers might hesitate about radiation treatment considering the associated ominous reputation and tissue burden. While radiation treatment represents a significant burden, for the patient as well as financially and logistically, it is also safe and characterized by low recurrence rates, high patient satisfaction, and, in combination with excision, excellent aesthetic results. Therefore, when other techniques fail in preventing keloid disorder recurrence, radiation treatment is a valid option and should be considered.

This chapter will provide an overview of the history of radiation treatment for keloid disorder. The available techniques and suggested dosages, as well as the authors' experiences and vision on indications and biological working mechanisms, are described.

Introduction

Soon after the discovery of X-ray technology, radiation was recognized as a possible treatment modality for excessive tissue growth. Like malignant tumors, aberrant scars are proliferative tissue overgrowths and were therefore also considered valid targets for treatment with radiation. L. Freund first described the positive effect of roentgen treatment on a hypertrophic scar in 1898. Harris then described the same effect on a keloid disorder in 1901, whereas Wickham recommended radium for the treatment of keloid scars. Already in 1909, Freund combined surgical excision of the keloid with postoperative radiation, where he left the wound open and waited 2–3 days before starting radiation treatment [1]. In the following period, various treatment protocols were described using external radiation with relatively good results. Folke Jacobsson described in 1948 that in 625 cases treated, a total regression of 73.6% was achieved, most of which with radiation alone (*The Treatment of Keloids at Radiumhemmet*, 1921–1941).

External beam radiation therapy uses a radiation source which emits energy onto the target area. The disadvantage of this technique is that it gives a relatively high dose to the adjacent healthy tissue due to the large distance between the radiation source and the target.

Brachytherapy, where the radiation source is placed inside or adjacent to the area requiring treatment, was pioneered in medicine soon after the discovery of radioactivity in 1896 and was widely used in the 1930s to treat various sorts of tumors. The benefit of brachytherapy over external radiation therapy is the ability to deliver radiation as very localized and enabling a higher dose with fewer side effects and fewer treatments needed for the same effect. Brachytherapy for the treatment of keloid scars is nowadays always combined with excision.

After an enthusiastic start, the usage of brachytherapy declined due to the problematic radiation exposure for staff and patients while handling the radioactive materials. The advent of novel radiation delivery methods and the use of new radioactive sources in the 1950s and 1960s caused a renewed interest in brachytherapy. Current remote afterloading devices provide safety by manually placing a hollow catheter (◘ Fig. 40.1b) first and then loading the radioactive source later through the catheter. It was not until 1976 that Malaker et al. introduced this technique for keloid treatment. Current methods focus on excision of the lesion followed by adjuvant radiation therapy. Although this method offers total scar eradication with an optimal aesthetic and low recurrence rates (mean, 10.5%), its use is limited due to significantly higher costs in comparison with other treatment options, as well as availability of the technique in the hospital and the need for more advanced specialist care (e.g., plastic surgeon/dermatologist/radiation oncologist with interest in keloid scar treatment).

Types of Radiation Therapy

External Beam Radiation Therapy (EBRT)

The classic form of radiation therapy uses a radiation source which emits energy onto the target area. Regular X-ray radiation is probably the most widely available and least expensive radiation option. It does not penetrate too deep, so underlying structures remain undamaged. Due to the inaccuracy of the technique, however, more skin side effects are seen. In superficial radiation therapy (SRT), low-energy X-rays (the same range as diagnostic X-rays) emit photons at 20–150 kV reaching an effective depth of 3.5–16 mm. At higher energy of 200–500 kV, an effective depth of 2 cm is reached (orthovoltage radiation). Electron beam radiotherapy uses a linear accelerator to create β-rays. It reaches a depth of 2–6 cm and can be more accurately delivered.

Brachytherapy (Internal Radiation)

In brachytherapy, a hollow catheter is placed either interstitially during closure or superficially on the desired target area (see ◘ Fig. 40.1a–c). After this procedure,

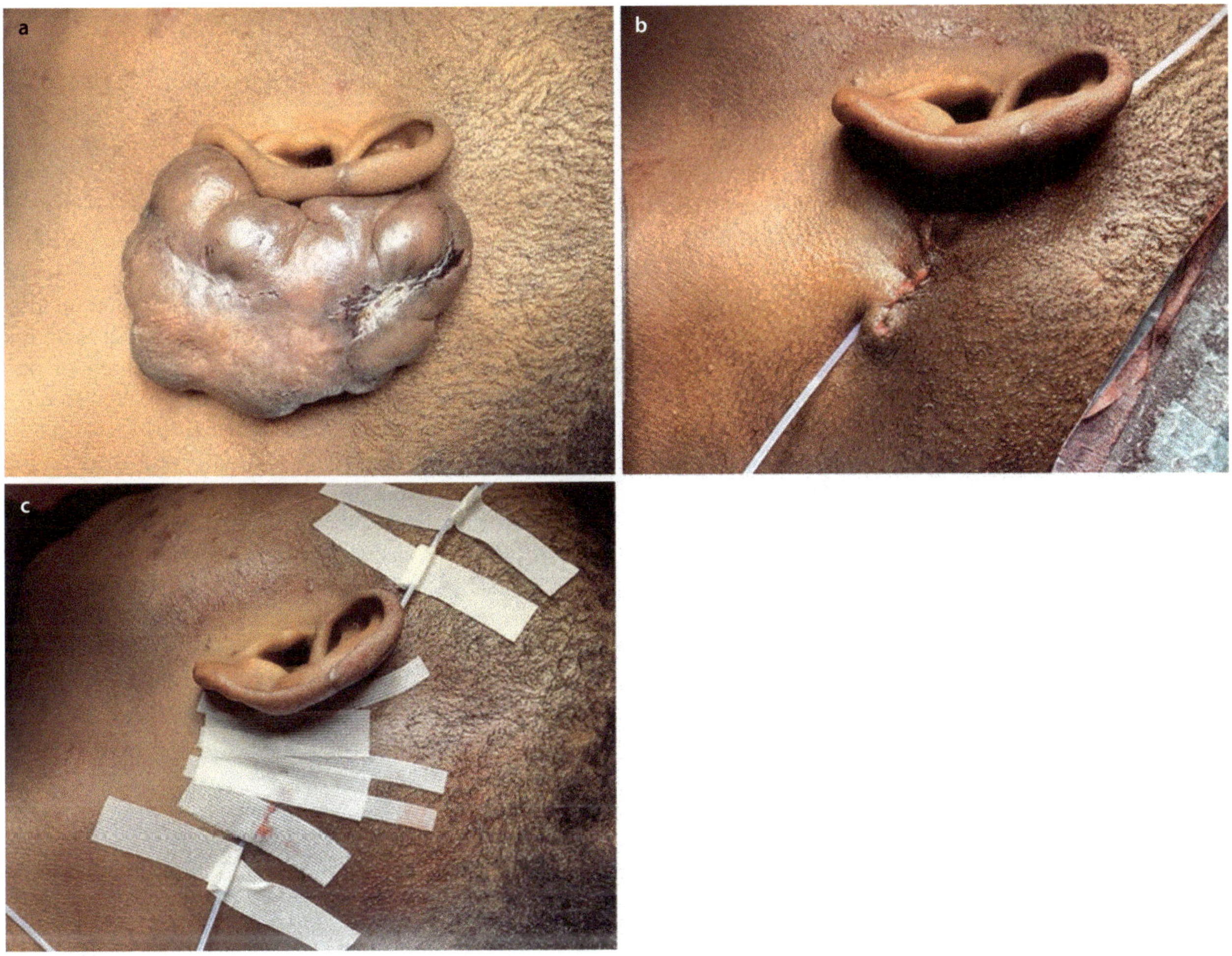

Fig. a Keloid of the earlobe. After excision, a hollow catheter is placed before closing the wound **b**. The catheter is fixed into place to ensure precise radiotherapy delivery **c**

the catheter is loaded with a radioactive source. The treatment regimen can either be low-dose rate (LDR) or high-dose rate (HDR). In LDR a low-dose-rate radioactive source is used to treat for a longer time frame (20–72 hours). It requires hospitalization in a lightly shielded chamber. In HDR the patient is transferred to a shielded chamber after the excision. Here, a high-dose-rate radioactive source is loaded into the catheter remotely by personnel in a separate area for a short exposure (5–10 minutes). Because of the short treatment duration, HDR can effectively be used as an outpatient treatment option and is therefore preferred over LDR. The main advantage of brachytherapy to external beam radiotherapy is the diminished exposure of surrounding tissue, which also provides the possibility to administer a higher dose in a shorter time frame. Additionally, because the applicator can be shaped to fit the desired area, uneven surfaces will receive the same dose, and deeper structures can be avoided. The most commonly used radioactive source is Iridium-192 which emits γ-rays.

Excision and Radiation Type

Radiotherapy should be reserved for recurrent keloid scars because of its invasive characteristic and significant cost. It should be noted that both excision-only and radiation-only have higher recurrence rates compared to excision followed by radiation [2]. The keloid is preferably excised in an extralesional fashion [2] and closed primarily. If this is not an option due to the size of the scar or high tension on the wound edges, skin grafts can be used, or excision of the core of the keloid can be performed.

Close cooperation with the local radiotherapy department is necessary to facilitate radiation therapy for keloids. Radiation equipment usually represents a significant cost to any hospital, and keloid treatment with radiation therapy will most likely only be performed in a small fraction of treatments. This means physicians will probably be bound to techniques that are already available in their hospital. Usually, a form of external radiation will be available, while brachytherapy may be more common in larger medical centers in developed countries.

When planning the procedure, two main considerations should be timing and adequate dosage of the radiation therapy. The first dose should be administered as soon as possible after excision. A clear decrease in recurrence rate was seen in external radiation if treated within 7 hours as opposed to the first 24 hours. HDR brachytherapy should be administered in the first 24 hours after surgery and is also likely more effective in the first 7 hours [3]. Many protocols, therefore, opt to transfer the patient to the radiation department immediately after excision [2]. Choosing the right dosage is important and there is no "gold standard" (yet). The concept of biological effective dose (BED) is important in the radiation regimen to be formed. BED is the measure used to quantitatively indicate the biological effect of any radiotherapy treatment. Because it corrects for the dose per fraction given and the fraction number, it will allow comparison of all kinds of treatments and modalities. In keloid treatment, it would appear that administering less than a BED of 10–12 Gy is correlated with a higher recurrence rate [2]. Literature suggests there seems to be a strict threshold because doses of less than 10 Gy repeatedly report higher recurrence rates. This would also mean that a single fraction could be enough, possibly preventing an overnight stay and/or additional hospital visits. At present, there are not enough studies yet in support of this, and a recent study even found a higher recurrence rate in a 13 Gy single-faction protocol [4]. In a multicenter comparison of HDR brachytherapy, 2 × 6 Gy (BED of 19) treatment gave an equally low recurrence and lower complication rates than using 2 × 9 and 3 × 6 Gy [4]. Administering more than a BED of 20 Gy seems unnecessary in HDR brachytherapy [4]. In the treatment of earlobe keloids with EBRT, a BED of 15–22.5 over two fractions (2 × 10 Gy) was found to be sufficient [5]. In a recent systematic review, HDR brachytherapy achieved the lowest mean recurrence rate, followed by LDR brachytherapy and external radiation therapy (HDR, 10.5 ± 15%; range, 0–44; LDR, 21.3 ± 2.1%; range, 19.4–23.6; external, 22.2 ± 16%; range, 0–72) [2].

Recurrence

When reviewing the literature, it should be kept in mind that recurrence is often defined differently. It can be described as any regrowth of tissue, mild or total relapse, or even regrowth extending beyond the borders of the original lesion. Symptoms like pain or itching or any other complaint in the operated area not related to radiation may be counted as recurrence. With respect to radiation therapy, recurrence is usually correlated to the administered BED; the higher the BED, the lower the recurrence and vice versa. Since the opposite can be said of complications, a balanced approach should be made toward BED. Recurrence rate is also influenced by location; in a recent meta-analysis, Mankowski et al. found the chest and trunk to have higher recurrence rates (34%) as opposed to the ears (12%) [5]. Furthermore, to properly assess recurrence, a follow-up of at least 1 or 2 years posttreatment should be considered to avoid bias by missing recurrences.

Complications

Complications following radiotherapy of the skin are scored with the toxicity criteria of the Radiation Therapy Oncology Group (RTOG) and the European Organisation for Research and Treatment of Cancer (EORTC) [6]; see ◘ Table 40.1. Since radiotherapy influences wound healing, wound-related complications like wound dehiscence, infection, and the failure of the wound to close (chronic wound) are additional entities to consider. The most commonly seen complications are erythema, temporary and permanent pigmentation disturbances, and telangiectasia. Wound-related complications are rarely seen when administering doses as

◘ **Table** Toxicity criteria of the Radiation Therapy Oncology Group (RTOG) and the European Organisation for Research and Treatment of Cancer (EORTC) [6]

Grade	1	2	3	4
Acute	Follicular, faint or dull erythema/epilation/dry desquamation/decreased sweating	Tender or bright erythema, patchy moist desquamation/moderate edema	Confluent, moist desquamation other than skin folds, pitting edema	Ulceration, hemorrhage, necrosis
Late	Slight atrophy; pigmentation change; some hair loss	Patch atrophy; moderate telangiectasia; total hair loss	Marked atrophy; gross telangiectasia	Ulceration

discussed earlier. Reported recurrence and complication rates vary. A recent retrospective study comparing 2 × 9 Gy, 3 × 6 Gy, and 2 × 6 Gy reported minor complications in 57%, 40%, and 33.7%, respectively, and 18.6%, 13.8%, and 3.3% major complications, respectively. Recurrence was the same for all groups (25%) [4]. Pigmentation complications are more commonly seen in people with a darker skin (Fitzpatrick V–VI) who seem to benefit from brachytherapy in which the irradiated area is greatly reduced [7]. It should be noted that pigmentation differences are less prevalent in brachytherapy in comparison with cryotherapy [8]. Furthermore, HDR brachytherapy yields good results in patient-reported outcomes such as the Patient and Observer Scar Assessment Scale [7].

Safety Concerns

When administering radiotherapy for benign diseases, concerns will arise about the risk of inducing secondary malignancy in the treated area. As of now, only a few cases have been described in external radiotherapy, and Ogawa et al. found the risk to be very low, with an estimated incidence of 0.1–0.0335% [3]. No cases of late malignancy have been described while using brachytherapy. Of course, the possibility should be mentioned when discussing therapeutic options with the patient [3].

Additional Thoughts on the Biomechanisms of Radiotherapy in Keloid Treatment

The working mechanism of radiation therapy to prevent the recurrence of the keloid scar is still the subject of research. Initially, the application was based on the principle that radiation inhibits tissue growth, and since both keloid disorder and hypertrophic scars are considered tissue overgrowth reactions, they were treated as such. Early irradiation, within 7 hours of surgery, has been shown to result in lower recurrence rates as opposed to a later moment [2]. This suggests that interfering in the early stages of wound healing is paramount in preventing recurrence of the disorder. Radiation is especially harmful to dividing cells; the fact that particularly the most proliferative cells are vulnerable explains its effectiveness in treating cell overgrowth.

Fibroblasts have been linked to keloid disorder for a long time, and ionizing radiation has been proven to influence keloid fibroblast proliferation [9]. Current theories consider keloids to be an immunological problem where endothelial cells and neovascularization may play a pivotal role as well [10]. During surgery or trauma, the tissue is damaged, and blood vessels are severed. To provide the upcoming immune cells and fibroblasts with enough nutrients and oxygen, new blood vessels are formed along the wound edges, while the surroundings of the wound show redness as a sign of vasodilation. This process starts during the first hours following wounding [11]. Endothelial dysfunction has been linked to abnormal wound healing [10, 12, 13], so by suppressing endothelial cells and therefore angiogenesis due to radiation, the formation of dysfunctional blood vessels could be prevented and inflammation decreased, ultimately potentially suppressing keloid formation and preventing recurrence [1, 10].

In the classic definition, hypertrophic scarring is confined within the boundaries of the original lesion, whereas a keloid scar grows beyond its boundaries. However, in close visual inspection of hypertrophic scars, we see that they also can extend beyond the borders of the original lesion. The extension beyond the scar borders is less compared to keloid disorder, and the ongoing process of scar formation stops earlier. In the case of keloid disorder, the vascularity is the highest just around the keloid as may be observed clinically during excision (◘ Fig. 40.2).

Conclusions

Radiotherapy is a last resort option for recurrent and therapy-resistant keloids and hypertrophic scars. It represents a significant burden, both financially and logistically as well as to the patient. On the other hand, It is a very efficacious treatment option (in preventing recurrence) while obtaining the most optimal esthetic result. It is a safe procedure and most patients experience no or minor side effects. The therapeutic goal should be to try and excise the entire keloid (extralesionally) and start radiation treatment as soon as possible, preferably within 7 hours. Between external radiation and LDR and HDR brachytherapy, the most preferable option is high-dose-rate (HDR) brachytherapy because of the

- Ability to customize the device per treatment area, therefore only radiating the target area while minimizing radiation damage to the healthy surrounding tissue
- Lower total BED compared to external radiation to achieve the same effect
- Ability to deliver the desired BED in a short period of time, allowing an outpatient setting

The optimal dose appears to be around a BED of 20–30 Gy; however, more research works are needed to determine treatment protocols. Physicians should adjust their therapies on the merit of experience and existing

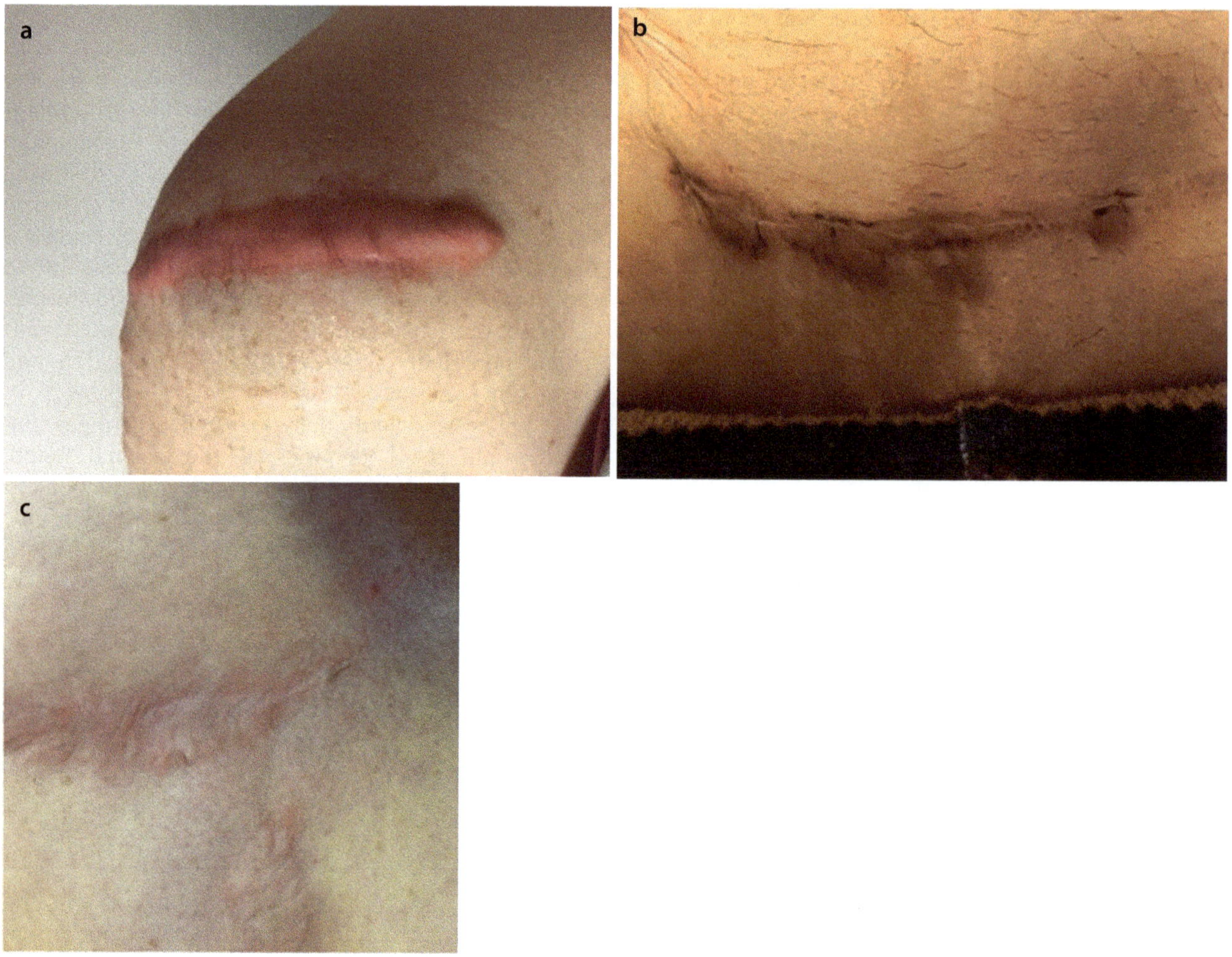

◘ **Fig.** **a** Hypertrophic scar on the shoulder (age 18 months) with apparent vascular involvement. **b** Hypertrophic scar after cesar-ean section (age 5 years) extending beyond its borders. **c** Hypertrophic scar after breast reduction surgery (age 2 years) extending beyond its borders

literature in collaboration with the local radiotherapy department and in accordance with the wishes of the patient.

Take Home Message

- Consider excision and radiotherapy as a last resort for therapy-resistant keloids.
- HDR brachytherapy started <7 hours after surgery and a BED of ±20 is recommended.
- The chance of secondary malignancy seems very low.

References

1. Ogawa R, Yoshitatsu S, Yoshida K, Miyashita T. Is radiation therapy for keloids acceptable? The risk of radiation-induced carcinogenesis. Plast Reconstr Surg. 2009;124(4):1196–201. https://doi.org/10.1097/PRS.0b013e3181b5a3ae.
2. van Leeuwen MCE, Stokmans SC, Bulstra AEJ, et al. Surgical excision with adjuvant irradiation for treatment of keloid scars: a systematic review. Plast Reconstr surgery Glob open. 2015;3(7):e440. https://doi.org/10.1097/GOX.0000000000000357.
3. Goutos I, Ogawa R. Brachytherapy in the adjuvant management of keloid scars: literature review. Scars, Burn Heal. 2017;3:2059513117735483. https://doi.org/10.1177/2059513117735483.
4. Bijlard E, Verduijn GM, Harmeling JX, et al. Optimal high-dose-rate brachytherapy fractionation scheme after keloid excision: a retrospective multicenter comparison of recurrence rates

and complications. Int J Radiat Oncol Biol Phys. 2017;100(3): 679–86.
5. Mankowski P, Kanevsky J, Tomlinson J, Dyachenko A, Luc M. Optimizing radiotherapy for keloids: a meta-analysis systematic review comparing recurrence rates between different radiation modalities. Annals of Plastic Surgery. 2017;78(4):403–11. https://doi.org/10.1097/SAP.0000000000000989.
6. Cox JD, Stetz J. Toxicity criteria of the radiation therapy oncology group (RTOG) and the European organization for research and treatment of cancer (EORTC). Int J Radiat Oncol Biol Phys. 1995;31(5):1341–6.
7. Van Leeuwen MCE, Stokmans SC, Bulstra AEJ, Meijer OWM, Van Leeuwen PAM, Niessen FB. High-dose-rate brachytherapy for the treatment of recalcitrant keloids: a unique, effective treatment protocol. Plast Reconstr Surg. 2014;134(3):527–34. https://doi.org/10.1097/PRS.0000000000000415.
8. Bijlard E, Timman R, Verduijn GM, Niessen FB, Hovius SER, Mureau MAM. Intralesional cryotherapy versus excision with corticosteroid injections or brachytherapy for keloid treatment: randomised controlled trials. J Plast Reconstr Aesthetic Surg. 2018;71(6):847–56. https://doi.org/10.1016/j.bjps.2018.01.033.
9. Ji J, Tian Y, Zhu YQ, et al. Ionizing irradiation inhibits keloid fibroblast cell proliferation and induces premature cellular senescence. J Dermatol. 2015;42(1):56–63. https://doi.org/10.1111/1346-8138.12702.
10. Huang C, Liu L, You Z, et al. Endothelial dysfunction and mechanobiology in pathological cutaneous scarring: lessons learned from soft tissue fibrosis. Br J Dermatol. 2017;177(5):1248–55. https://doi.org/10.1111/bjd.15576.
11. Butzelaar L, Schooneman DPM, Soykan EA, et al. Inhibited early immunologic response is associated with hypertrophic scarring. Exp Dermatol. 2016;25(10):797–804. https://doi.org/10.1111/exd.13100.
12. Butzelaar L, Ulrich MMW. Mink van der Molen AB, Niessen FB, Beelen RHJ. Currently known risk factors for hypertrophic skin scarring: a review. J Plast Reconstr Aesthet Surg. 2016;69(2):163–9. https://doi.org/10.1016/j.bjps.2015.11.015.
13. van der Veer WM, Bloemen MCT, Ulrich MMW, et al. Potential cellular and molecular causes of hypertrophic scar formation. Burns. 2009;35(1):15–29. https://doi.org/10.1016/j.burns.2008.06.020.

11

Scar and Scarring in the Elderly

Hester Colboc and Sylvie Meaume

Contents

Introduction

Epidemiology of the Elderly: A Factor to Consider

Definition of Elderly in Medicine: Should We Make Distinctions?

From Skin Aging to Dermatoporosis

Consequences of Age on Wound Healing

Frequent Comorbidities Altering Wound Healing in the Elderly

What Scarring Problems Are Usually Observed in the Elderly?

Conclusion

References

Aims of the Chapter

- To provide demographic data on the elderly and the definition of elderly in medicine
- To bring elements of skin aging and dermatoporosis
- To describe the consequences of age on healing and major comorbidities in elderly that impair healing
- To address the main problems raised by scars in the elderly – these scars are not the hypertrophic scar, the keloids, or the scars due to cosmetic aspects but the recurrence of a wound on a scar, the Marjolin's ulcer, the hyperkeratosis, the unstable scars, and the adhesion to the deep plane of old scars

Introduction

The population is getting older all over the world. This means that more people are living with chronic illnesses, which reduce their independence and force them to take various medications. Healthcare professionals should take this into account when managing scar and scarring problems in older patients. Until now, research works primarily focus on the treatment and prevention of wounds in the elderly – acute (dissecting hematoma, skin tears, etc.) or chronic (pressure ulcers, leg ulcers, diabetic wounds of the foot, etc.) – but too little was done concerning the problem of scarring itself and even less on scars associated with the loss of skin function along the time.

Epidemiology of the Elderly: A Factor to Consider

According to the United Nations' report on the aging of the world population, adults over 60 years will outnumber younger people by 2050 [1], and in Europe alone, more than 20% of the population will be over 65 years in 2025 [2]. As this population ages, many older people will live with chronic conditions, reduced independence, polypathology, and polypharmacy, a situation healthcare professionals should take into consideration when dealing with dermatological, scarring, and scar conditions. While governments encourage the growing trend in Europe to promote an adapted elderly management, the specific wound healing and scarring care provided by surgeons, physicians, and caregivers is increasingly important but scarcely discussed [3].

Definition of Elderly in Medicine: Should We Make Distinctions?

If the WHO defines elderly as over 65 years of age, the increase in life expectancy in good health means that when we talk about elderly people in the medical environment, these are subjects of more than 75–80 years, and the distinction between the healthy elderly and the polypathological elderly becomes important. The state of health of the elderly is multifactorial. It depends on genetic, environmental, social, psychic factors, and the existence of multiple pathologies. It is not necessarily linked to age. For 30 years the concept of fragile old man/woman has been developed [4]. It obeys to several definitions and criteria which vary accordingly to the numerous publications of which it is the subject and makes it a dynamic medical concept. Only 10–20% of the nonagenarians or centenarians are considered fragile. These are the so-called geriatric patients who require specific management. Most people over the age of 75 are not frail and considered "fit" with good functional autonomy and good social integration and few pathologies. Conversely, the frail elderly present functional limitations and a decline in their ability to adapt and anticipate. To distinguish these two types of elderly population, standardized geriatric assessments have been developed using validated scales of autonomy, nutrition, cognition, etc. [5]. This evaluation is not only performed by geriatrician if one wishes exhaustive but can also be realized by nonspecialists and paramedics: nurses, physiotherapists, social workers, dieticians, occupational therapists, and speech therapists. The objective of such assessments is to provide a supportive plan adapted to each patient, a compromise between what is desirable and feasible or reasonable and what is not (◘ Table 44.1).

◘ **Table** Main factors of frailty in the elderly
Age over 85 years
Loss of autonomy for an activity of daily life or more
Impairment of cognitive functions
Reduced nutritional reserves
Inadequate social support (loneliness, poverty)
Sedentary lifestyle, confinement, postural instability
Poorly compensated sensory disturbances
Kidney and liver failure
Depressive symptoms
Polymedication

From Skin Aging to Dermatoporosis

Skin aging leads to alteration of the skin and consequently to the loss of its physiological barrier role. Skin aging leads to alteration of the skin and consequently to the loss of its physiological barrier role. It is the consequence of intrinsic (genetically programmed) and

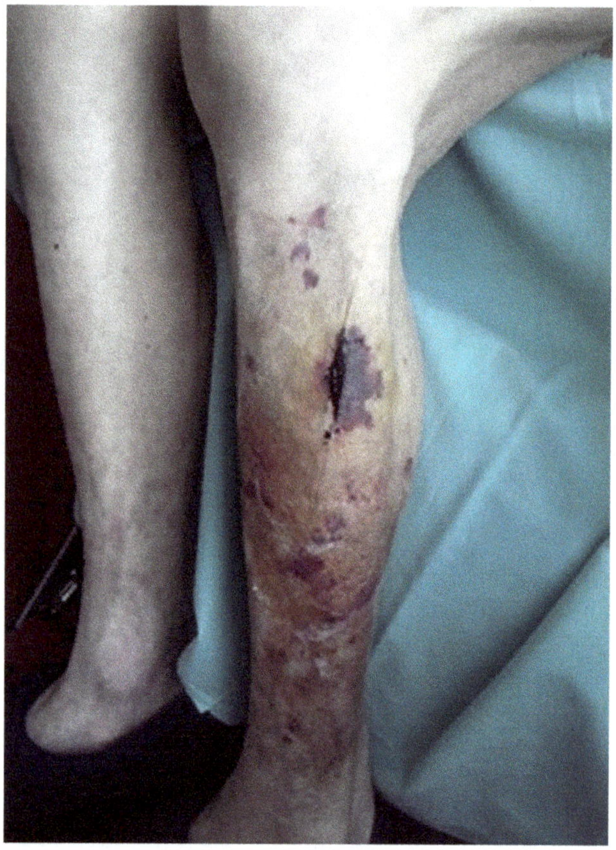

Fig. Dermatoporosis: Bateman purpura, skin tears, hyperpigmentation, and spontaneous stellar pseudo-scars

extrinsic factors. These extrinsic factors are numerous, and include more specifically drugs aggravating the physiological xerosis (hypolipidemic oral, allopurinol, hydroxyurea and cimetidine) [6], deficits in essential fatty acids, in vitamins (B group vitamins, E, PP, C, A), zinc, magnesium as well as malnutrition frequent in the elderly patient and environmental factors such as smoking and exposure to ultraviolet (UV). For some patients, skin aging can become can constitute a real functional organ failure, far from cosmetics considerations. The term "dermatoporosis" was recently proposed by Saurat [7, 8] to cover all the manifestations and implications of this chronic skin syndrome linked to skin fragility and insufficiency.

The clinical manifestations of dermatoporosis (Fig. 44.1) include morphological markers of fragility (skin atrophy, Bateman's purpura, spontaneous stellar pseudo-scars, hyperpigmentation), as well as the functional expression of skin fragility (skin tears, poor healing, dissecting hematoma). The first signs appear around the age of 60, while the disease itself, with its related complications, is observed between the ages of 70 and 90.

On a microscopic scale, skin aging is manifested by a thinning of the dermo-epidermal junction and an extension of the keratinocyte renewal time. In the dermis, there is observed a decrease in the number of fibroblasts and thus the density of fiber collagen and glycosaminoglycans, with thinning of the dermal thickness. Associated with this quantitative drop is a qualitative drop in residual fibers. During aging, a decrease of hydrophilic character of the glycosaminoglycans, responsible for the hydration of the dermis, is observed. This chemical modification can explain the dermal thinning and xerosis seen in the elderly. These changes also affect the microvascularization, with thinning of the vessel wall, which may explain the tendency to hematoma and purpura (Batman's purpura) typically observed in the elderly.

Consequences of Age on Wound Healing

Physiological healing has three main stages, directly impacted by aging: the first stage is hemostasis and inflammation, second stage is cell proliferation, and third stage is tissue remodeling. With age, platelet adhesion to the damaged endothelium is increased, decreasing the healing time. The local inflammatory answer to injury is reduced, following a decrease in the expression of molecules of adhesion. The proliferation phase is also impaired by slowing the renewal keratinocyte evokes above and also a decrease in response to growth factors. Finally, tissue remodeling, the final stage of wound healing, is also impaired in the aging subject due to an imbalance between metalloproteinases and their physiological inhibitors, in favor of metalloproteinases and therefore the destruction of collagen [9]. The different healing phases are therefore altered by these phenomena in the elderly: reduction of the wound contraction, cell proliferation, neovascularization, delay of the inflammatory phase, and slower epithelialization [10].

Apart from these deleterious aspects, elderly healing presents some advantages. Thanks to a decrease in inflammation, pathological scarring such as hypertrophic scars and/or keloids is rarely observed in elderly. After skin excision for tumor, sometimes needing a consistent loss of substance, the aged patient skin laxity generally allows an easy reapproximation of the edges and the suture may be realized without tension, issuing to good scarring. However, suturing itself can be impacted by the increased skin tears risks due to the dermatoporosis.

Frequent Comorbidities Altering Wound Healing in the Elderly

Many comorbidities frequent in the elderly can decrease wound healing. Undernutrition and diabetes can delay all type of wound, while arterial or venous diseases and edema (linked to heart, kidney or liver failure) can delay healing of lower limbs wounds. Elderly patients are also more exposed to treatments that can delay healing, especially systemic corticosteroid therapy and cancer chemotherapy.

What Scarring Problems Are Usually Observed in the Elderly?

Traumatic and surgical acute wound healing is rather good even in very old patients, and *hypertrophic or keloid scars are rare*, at least in the Caucasian population [11].

The poor quality of the scar is usually not a major problem (appearance, color, shape) [12] except in exposed regions (face) or when impacting the function (heel, eyelid, and periorificial areas).

Pruritus and/or pain may appear very lately after the trauma/surgery and occur after 20 or 30 years. They are linked to dermatological problem (dry skin) or neurogenic disorders. These situations may be treated symptomatically with appropriate cosmetics [13]. A few of them need surgery, but war, posttraumatic, and postsurgery scars are not usually reasons to go to see a doctor.

Atrophic and adherent scars can be improved by injecting fat under the scar, a recent technique presenting the advantage of being scarcely invasive when anticoagulation is not needed or should be stopped (◘ Fig. 44.2).

The reappearance of a wound on a scar should be considered differently. The recurrence of a tumor may be at the origin of the scar. A biopsy or the recurrence of a chronic ulcer (arterial or venous, pressure, or diabetic foot ulcers) is needed to diagnose a malignant transformation.

It can also lead to the reassessment of the patient and indication of preventive treatment of compression or discharge (cushion, shoe, soles).

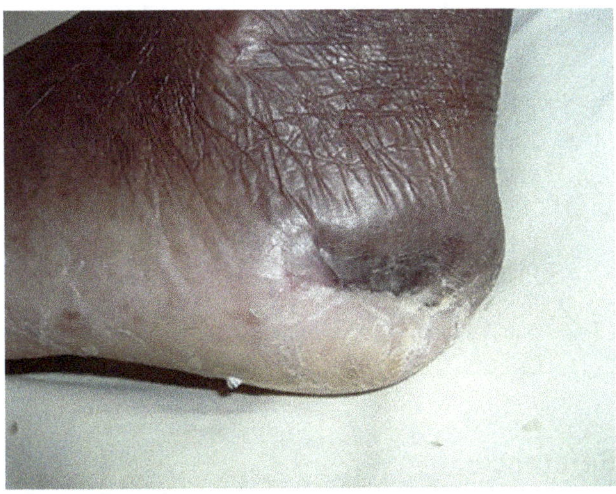

◘ **Fig.** Atrophic scar/defect: In this stage 4 pressure ulcer, the healing process led to a neoskin adherent to the underlying structures like aponeurosis, muscle, tendon, and bone. The possibility to inject adipose tissue under the skin should be discussed

Post-irradiation scars in cancer treatments (breasts for example) pose the problem of radiodermatitis and radionecrosis which evolves and worsens over time, in particular in the elderly who were irradiated at a time when the administered doses were high.

Some scars from childhood linked to operated orthopedic malformations are associated with joint deformations of osteoarthritis because of mechanical forces pressure or friction exerted on those scars or because of underlying medical problems in the region: arterial disease or neuropathy.

Marjolin's ulcer [14], a rare and aggressive skin cancer, develops late on scars from burns (◘ Fig. 44.3) or from delayed wound-healing problems: chronic osteitis, burns, pressure ulcers, lupus scar, skin graft, and radiodermatitis. Squamous cell carcinoma are more frequently observed than basal cell carcinoma, melanoma, or sarcoma. The occurrence of a wound on a scar aged of more than 20 years always requires a biopsy [15].

Hyperkeratosis is common especially on scars on plantar aspect of the foot, the heel, next to the Achilles tendon, or on the toes and the lateral aspects of the foot, due to a thickening of the stratum corneum reaction to friction or to mechanical conflict, especially in case of loss of sensibility (diabetes, nerve damage). Cracks can appear and constitute entry doors exposing to the risk of deep infection (◘ Fig. 44.4).

Unstable scars may appear because of their location, sometimes due to a poor quality of the dermal component (absent or fibrotic) or insufficient preventive measures taken against external agents (shoes, stockings, bandages, prosthesis, etc.).

These wounds finally closed after a succession of closure and multiple reopenings, source of discomfort, and risk of cancer transformation (◘ Fig. 44.5). The treatment of these unstable scars becomes more and more complex due to the underlying diseases and comorbidi-

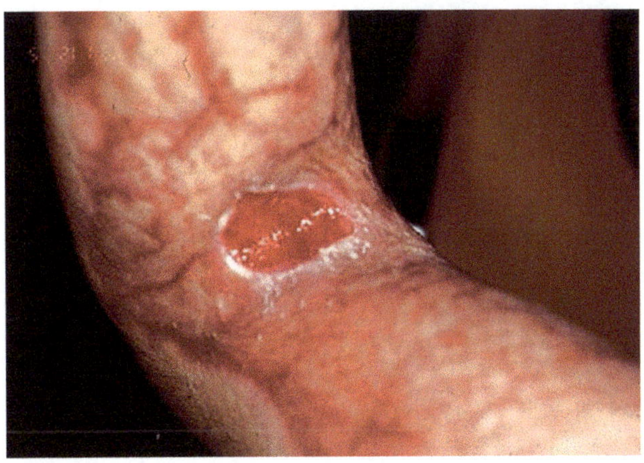

◘ **Fig.** Marjolin's ulcer on an old burn scar

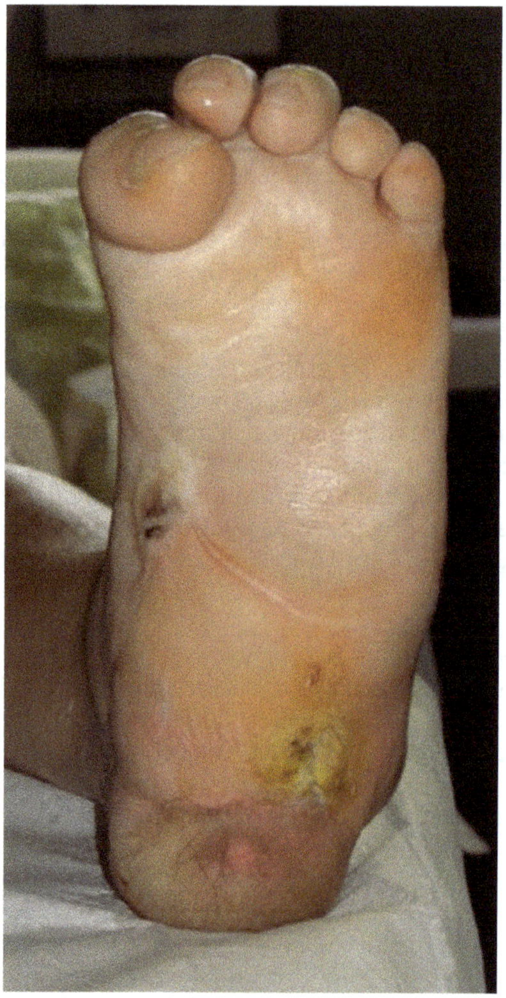

Fig. Scar becoming problematic with the age due to mechanical forces, trauma, pressure over the scar, underlying pathology (osteitis, diabetes, vascular diseases venous or arterial) issuing to hyperkeratosis, and potential neoplasic transformation

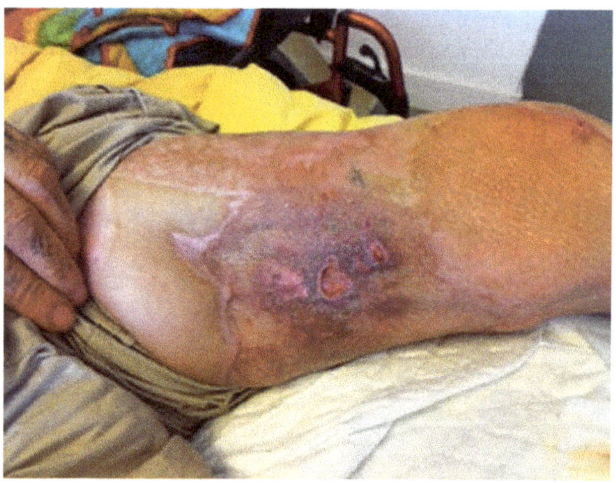

Fig. Scar instability: consequence of poor quality of der-mal component (absent or fibrotic) and poor preventive measures taken against external mechanical agent (shoes, stocking, bandage, prosthesis, etc.). Succession of closure and reopening phases

ties. Biopsies often need to be done to rule out a malignant degenerescence.

Adherence to the depth is a problem that worsens with age. Healing occurring on a wound with loss of deep substance (dermis, fat, gliding capacities) and not correctly repaired (for exemple using negative pressure therapy, skin substitute or flap) may lead to an atrophic scar adherent to the deep plans. These adherent scars can disrupt normal skin movements and mobilisation of the patient, specially when located near an articulation. These adherences are exposed to skin reopening due to the loss of elasticity of age-related skin.

Conclusion

Epidemiological studies are lacking and the literature is poor on the subject. Hypertrophic and keloids do not seem to be a frequent problem in the elderly. The absence of inflammation and tension on the scar is undoubtedly an explanatory factor that perhaps merits more basic research. However, persistent functional problems lead aged patients to consult. Chronic wounds or sites of a long-lasting healing process are associated to an increased risk of malignant transformation, that must be take into consideration by the clinician. Regarding scars, elderly patients are usually less concern by the cosmetic aspects and its impact on the quality of life. The existence of underlying diseases can reopen certain scars or pressure ulcers and therefore the treatment must be adapted according to the comorbidities. The geriatrician sometimes has a role to play in establishing the therapeutic plan.

Take-Home Messages

- The number of elderly people is increasing.
- The tension on the scars is often less because the skin of the elderly is less elastic (modification of the extra cellular matrix).
- Keloid and hypertrophic scars are rare in the elderly.
- Scars problems are more often malignant degenerescence, hyperkeratosis, atrophy, instability, or adherence to the depth.
- A biopsy must be performed if the scar reopens or persists in an elderly patient.

References

1. United Nations. World population ageing: 1950–2050. New York: United Nations; 2001.
2. European Commission. Ageing. Available from: http://ec.europa.eu/health/ageing/policy/index_en.htm. Accessed December 2014.

3. Rechel B, Doyle Y, Grundy E, McKee M. Policy brief 10: how can health systems respond to population ageing? vol. 36. Geneva: World Health Organization; 2009.
4. Buchner DM, Wagner EH. Preventing frail health. Clin Geriatr Med. 1992;8(1):1–17.
5. Dent E, Kowal P, Hoogendijk EO. Frailty measurement in research and clinical practice: a review. Eur J Intern Med. 2016;31:3–10.
6. Greist MC, Epinette WW. Cimetidine-induced xerosis and asteatotic dermatitis. Arch Dermatol. 1982;118:253–4.
7. Saurat JH. Dermatoporosis – the functional side of skin aging. Dermatology. 2007;215:271–2.
8. Kaya G, Saurat JH. Dermatoporosis: a chronic cutaneous insufficiency/fragility syndrome. Clinicopathological features, mechanisms, prevention and potential treatments. Dermatology. 2007;215:284–94.
9. Quan T, Fisher G. Role of age-associated alterations of the dermal extracellular matrix microenvironment in human skin aging: a mini-review. Gerontology. 2015;61(5):427–34.
10. Sgonc R, Gruber J. Age-related aspects of cutaneous wound healing: a mini-review. Gerontology. 2013;59:159–64.
11. Monarca C, Maruccia M, Palumbo F, Parisi P, Scuderi N. A rare case of postauricular spontaneous keloid in an elderly patient. In Vivo. 2012;26(1):173–5.
12. Brands-Appeldoorn A, Maaskant-Braat S, Zwaans W, Dieleman J, Schenk K, Broekhuysen C, Weerdenburg H, Daniel R, Tjan-Heijnen V, Roumen R. Patient-reported outcome measurement compared with professional judgment of cosmetic result afeter breast-conserving therapy. Curr Oncol. 2018;25(6):553–61.
13. Humbert P, Dréno B, Krutmann J, Luger AT, Triller R, Meaume S, Seité S. Recommendations for managing cutaneous disorders associated with advancing age. Clin Interv Aging. 2016;11: 141–8.
14. Cruickshank AH, Gaskele E. Jean-Nicolas Marjolin: destined to be forgotten? Med Hist. 1963;7:383–4.
15. Yu N, Long X, Lujan-Hernandez JR, et al. Marjolin's ulcer: a preventable malignancy arising from scars. World J Surg Oncol. 2013;11:313.

12

Scars After Breast Reconstruction

Wouter B. van der Sluis

Contents

Conclusion

References

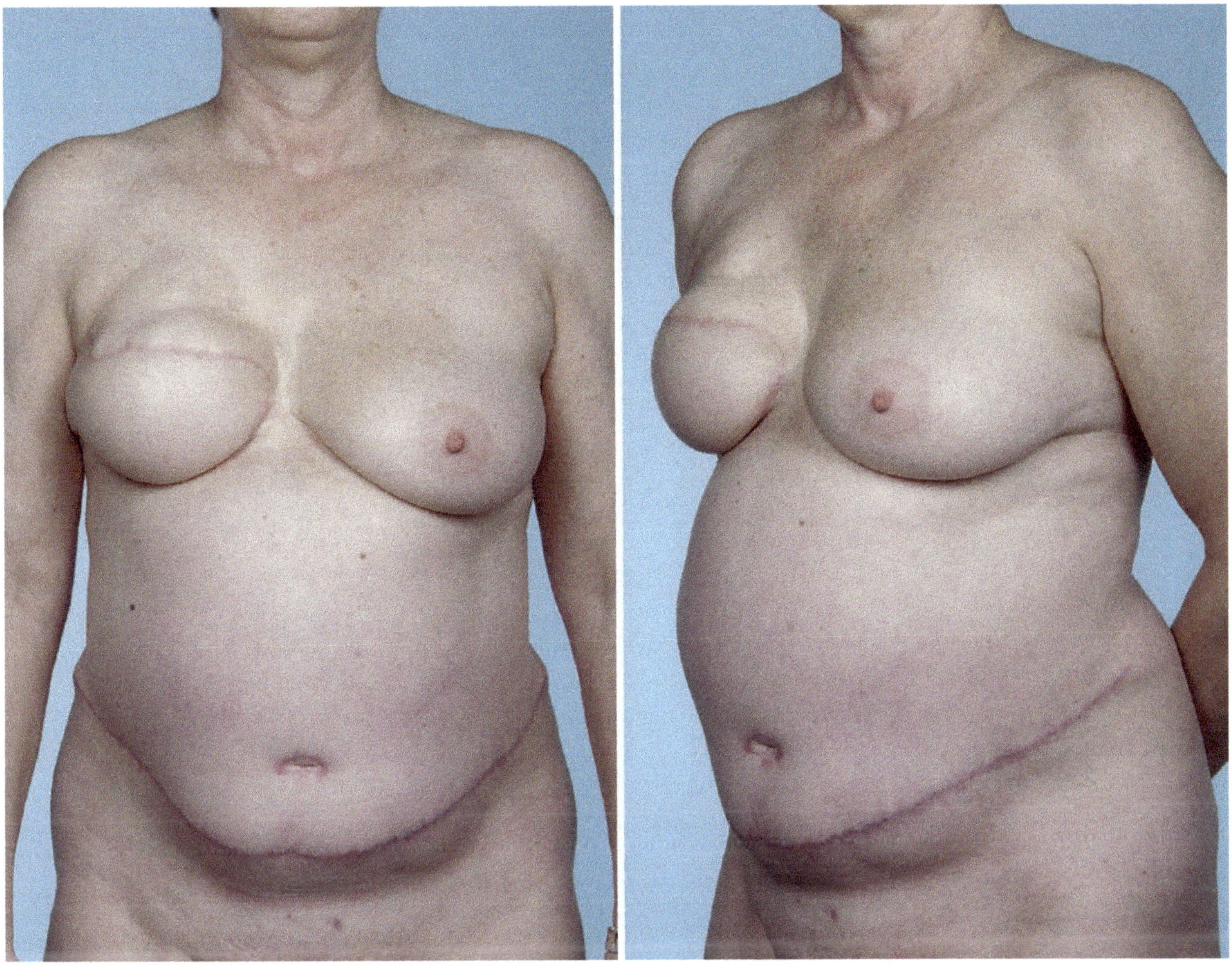

■■ Medical History

A 47-year-old woman visited the outpatient clinic because of a scar on the right breast. She previously underwent deep inferior epigastric perforator (DIEP) flap breast reconstruction after nonskin, non-nipple-sparing mastectomy, chemo- and radiotherapy, because of breast cancer. She had attended her oncological regular check-ups without problems. She now complained of a painful scar on the right breast, which she also found unaesthetic.

? Questions (4 max)

- Q1. Which anatomic areas need to be examined as well during outpatient clinic consultation?
- Q2. Define the problems in terms of anatomy.
- Q3. What could be a (non-)surgical approach of the problem?
- Q4. What should always be checked in postoncological patients before surgery?

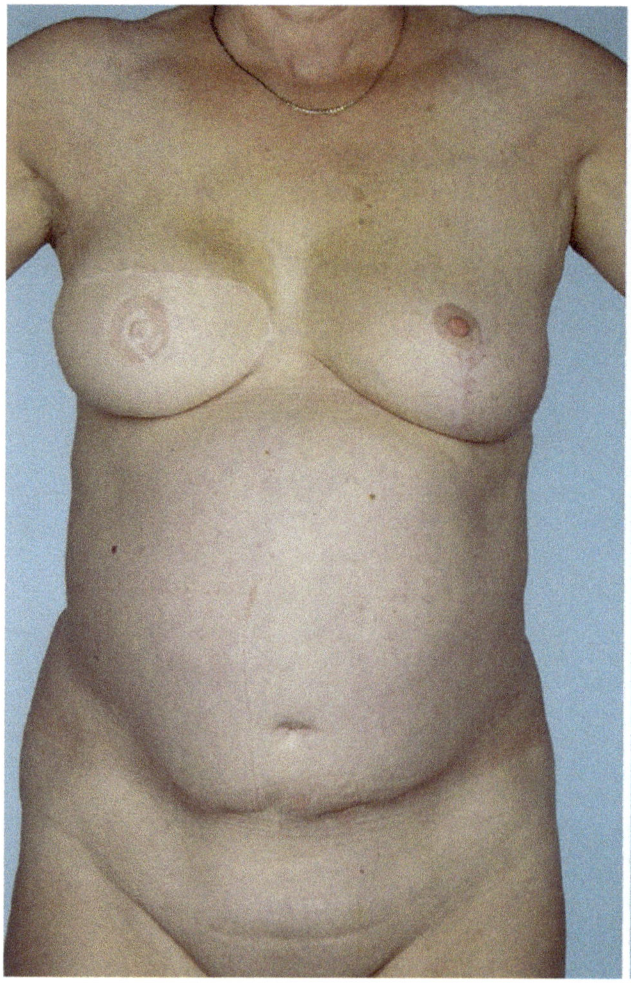

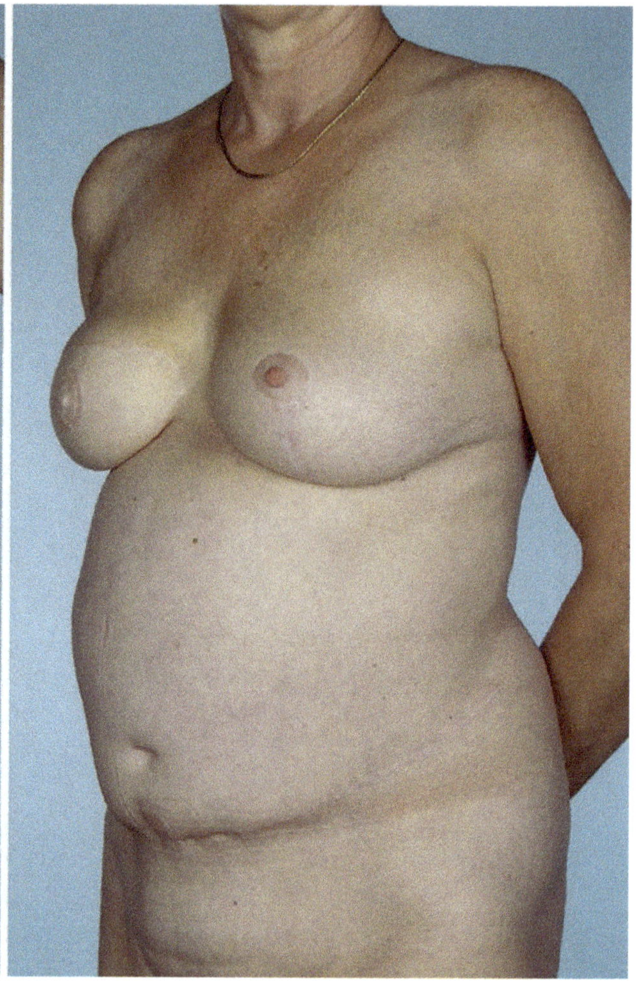

■ **Immediate Postintervention Situation**

In one surgical session, a donor-site dogear correction, scar lipofilling, and contralateral breast reduction were performed. Liposuction was used to correct the excess of fat at the region of the abdominal scar. The same fat was used for lipofilling of the upper pole of the right breast and the right breast scar. Nipple tattooing was performed at the outpatient clinic.

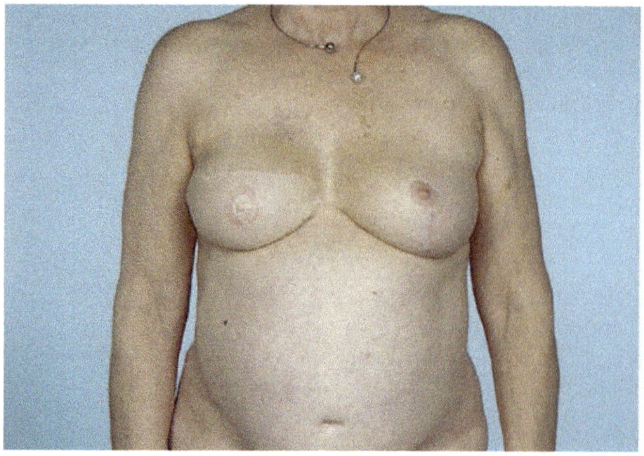

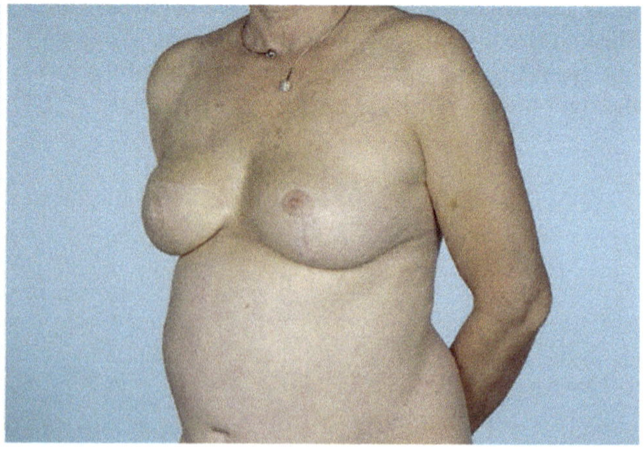

With 24 months of clinical follow-up, the patient was fully satisfied with the end result.

Argumented answers and explanation according to the five references (cited later): 20 lines

- Q1. Which anatomic areas need to be examined as well during outpatient clinic consultation?
- A1. The contralateral breast, the donor-site scar, and possible donor sites for future fat harvesting.

- Q2. Define the problem in terms of anatomy.
- A2. There is volume asymmetry between the left and right breasts. Right breast: lack of nipple, irregularities, and volume deficit of upper pole. Donor site: dogears, scar irregularities, and scar hypertrophy.

- Q3. What could be a nonsurgical approach of the problem?
- A3. Silicone application on all hypertrophic scars.

- Q4. What could be a surgical approach of the problem?
- A4. Donor-site dogear correction, nipple plasty or tattooing, scar lipofilling, contralateral breast reduction, or a combination of these strategies.

- Q5. What should always be checked in postoncological patients before surgery?
- A5. If they have attended routine oncological checkups.

Conclusion

There are different surgical options for breast reconstruction: immediate or delayed prosthesis-based reconstruction, oncoplastic reconstruction, fat grafting, and free or pedicled flap reconstructions [1–4]. Different techniques leave different scars on the breast. Nonsurgical approaches for breast scarring after reconstruction are silicone application and/or corticosteroid injections. Physical examination should always include examination of the contralateral breast, the donor-site scar, and possible donor sites for reconstructive purposes. There is a great role for autologous fat grafting in these reconstructive procedures. Other (minor) corrections can be performed simultaneously.

Take-Home Message

- Scar problems after various types of breast reconstruction are common. Many different corrections can be combined in one or multiple sessions.

References

1. Ho PJ, Hartman M, Young-Afat DA, Gernaat SAM, Lee SC, Verkooijen HM. Determinants of satisfaction with cosmetic outcome in breast cancer survivors: a cross-sectional study. PLoS One. 2018;13:e0193099.
2. Jaspers ME, Brouwer KM, van Trier AJ, Groot ML, Middelkoop E, van Zuijlen PP. Effectiveness of autologous fat grafting in adherent scars: results obtained by a comprehensive scar evaluation protocol. Plast Reconstr Surg. 2017;139:212–9.
3. Mureau MAM, Breast Reconstruction Guideline Working Group. Dutch breast reconstruction guideline. J Plast Reconstr Aesthet Surg. 2018;71:290–304.
4. van Turnhout AA, Fuchs S, Lisabeth-Broné K, Vriens-Nieuwenhuis EJC, van der Sluis WB. Surgical outcome and cosmetic results of autologous fat grafting after breast conserving surgery and radiotherapy for breast cancer: a retrospective cohort study of 222 fat grafting sessions in 109 patients. Aesthet Plast Surg. 2017;41:1334–41.

13

Atrophic Scars: Reinforcing the Flap Mattress Using Adipocyte Transfer in Paraplegic Patients at Risk of Pressure Ulcer Recurrence

Luc Téot

Contents

Medical History

References

Medical History

A 28-year-old man became paraplegic after a car accident 10 years ago. He presented repetitive pressure ulcers on the sacrum and the ischions, with successive surgical procedures (flaps, negative pressure, and skin grafting) on both sides.

He was successfully treated on the left side using a rotation flap for an ischiatic pressure ulcer, allowing to restart verticalization. The seated position was allowed after 2 months, progressively allowing a 12-hour-a-day seated position. The flap was followed every month and a progressive crushing of the fat under the ischial tuberosity was noted for a long time, with transient signs of redness appearing 1 year after surgery (◘ Fig. 63.1) A Coleman technique using 300 cc of fat was proposed.

❓ Questions to Medical History

- What is the rationale of using fat transfer in a patient who seems not to respect the postoperative restrictions?
- How to calculate the volume of fat to inject?

▪▪ Intervention 1:

One year later, a Coleman technique was proposed and administered, using 300 cc of fat obtained from the abdomen by liposuction. The fat was centrifugated 3000 t/min during 3 min, and then the substratum was extracted and used as a filler (◘ Fig. 63.2). The patient was authorized to remain seated 1 hour a day after 2 weeks and then progressively 1 hour more each month, till 12 hours a day.

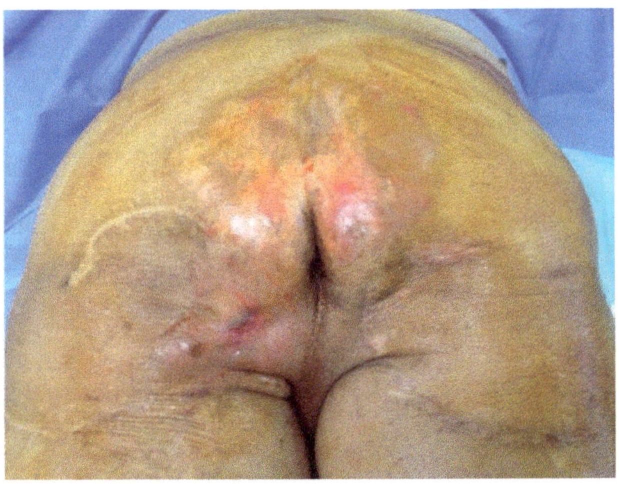

◘ **Fig.** Paraplegic patient operated 1 year before using a rotation ischial flap on the left side. The fat mattress under the flap skin begins to crush, exposing the patient to the risk of recurrence

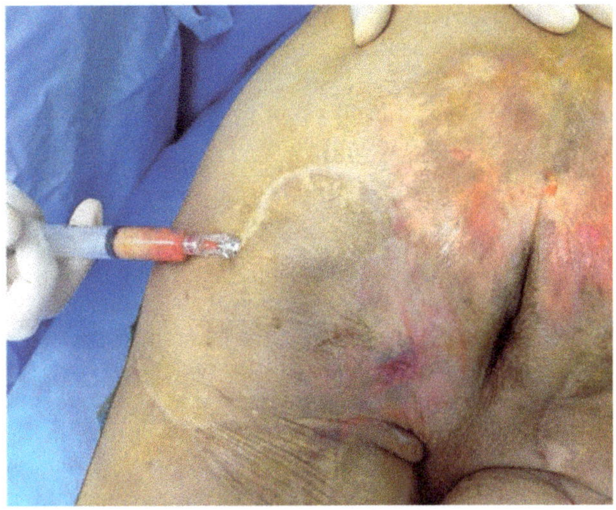

◘ **Fig. 63.2** Fat injection 300 cc, under the flap skin in the most exposed area when the patient is seated

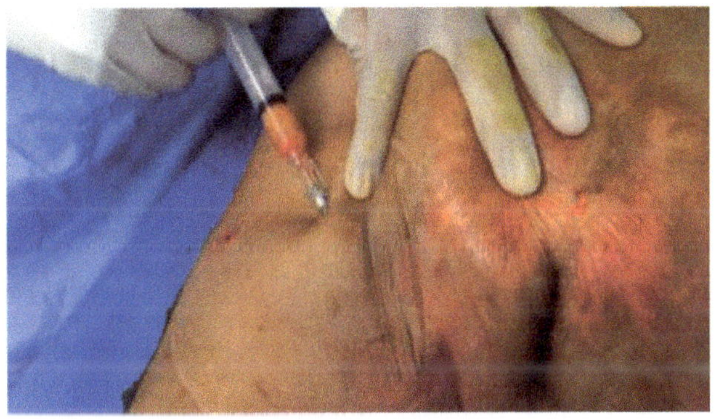

◘ **Fig.** A second 450 fat injection was administered 1 year later

❓ Question Intervention 1

- Is there a risk to inject a large fat volume under a suffering skin?
- Which postoperative protocol is given to the patient in order to prevent the recurrence?

▪▪ Intervention 2:

The patient was followed regularly, and a second injection was done 1 year after the first one (◘ Fig. 63.3), in order to compensate a recurrent diminished fat volume. The injected fat volume was increased to 450 cc. The patient was informed to limit his seated position to a maximum of 6 hours a day and to check every day the ischial area, the cushion was reanalyzed and changed.

The patient did not present any recurrence after 2 years of follow-up.

Question Intervention 2

- Has the patient been informed about the risk of recurrence?
- How to adapt the behavior of the patient during the postoperative period in order to prevent the recurrence?

Answers

Fat transfer has been proposed since a long period of time as a filler [1], and used alone or in combination with PRP [2]. However, the literature suggests that transplanted adipocyte stem cells bring some mechanical properties [3] and help to regenerate the subcutaneous tissues [4], a reason why injections can be administered even under a lightly suffering skin. In this case the postoperative pressure applied over the flap and then over the fat injected area was too high and the patient was not correctly following the protocol. A second chance was given after some alarming signs of suffering on the ischial area had appeared. The volume of injected fat was increased and the therapeutic education provided to the patient was enhanced. The patient was particularly encouraged to limit the daily seating, which he finally accepted, a crucial point to prevent another recurrence.

Take Home Message

Adipocyte stem cells have provided some evidence in scar improvement. This chapter introduces the use of adipocyte derived fillers in scars presenting adherence to the underlying structures or depressions compared to adjacent areas. The use of fat grafting prepared with simple techniques is now considered as a useful adjunctive technique in resurfacing pathological scars.

References

1. Moseley TA, Zhu M, Hedrick MH. Adipose-derived stem and progenitor cells as fillers in plastic and reconstructive surgery. Plast Reconstr Surg. 2006;118(3 Suppl):121S–8S.
2. Alser OH, Goutos I. The evidence behind the use of platelet-rich plasma (PRP) in scar management: a literature review. Scars Burn Heal. 2018;4:2059513118808773. https://doi.org/10.1177/2059513118808773. eCollection 2018 Jan–Dec.
3. Atashroo D, Raphel J, Chung MT, Paik KJ, Parisi-Amon A, McArdle A, Senarath-Yapa K, Zielins ER, Tevlin R, Duldulao C, Walmsley GG, Hu MS, Momeni A, Domecus B, Rimsa JR, Greenberg L, Gurtner GC, Longaker MT, Wan DC. Studies in fat grafting: Part II. Effects of injection mechanics on material properties of fat. Plast Reconstr Surg. 2014;134(1):29–38.
4. Scioli MG, Bielli A, Gentile P, Mazzaglia D, Cervelli V, Orlandi A. The biomolecular basis of adipogenic differentiation of adipose-derived stem cells. Int J Mol Sci. 2014;15(4):6517–26. https://doi.org/10.3390/ijms15046517. Review.

14

Hyperpigmented Scar

Julian Poetschke and Gerd G. Gauglitz

Contents

Medical History

References

Medical History

A 23-year-old healthy Caucasian patient suffered from a deep dermal burn (IIb) 2 years ago due to contact with an open fire. Despite initial professional burn care and aftercare using silicone-based products, the patient developed an elevated hypertrophic scar in an area of 18 × 12 cm with an approximate height of 1 cm on her left lower leg. Repetitive treatments with cryotherapy and intralesional injections with triamcinolone acetonide at the local university hospital did not result in significant improvements; however, as a side effect of the treatment, brownish hyperpigmentations appeared in the treated area. At initial presentation in our clinic, the patient did not complain about any pain except some tension and pruritus but was severely disturbed by the appearance of the scar (◘ Fig. 58.1).

Questions to Medical History

- What is the rationale for the formation of postinflammatory hyperpigmentations after the initial therapy?
- Which therapeutic alternatives exist?
- Are there any medical precautions that should be considered for initiating any additional therapy?

Intervention 1

One pass using a Q-switched ruby 4 mm/4 J (Asclepion) under local anesthesia cream. Aftercare with fusidic acid and a class III steroid containing cream.

Interventions 2–6

Eight weeks later significant improvement of hyperpigmentation and some minor flattening (◘ Fig. 58.2), five additional sessions with fractional CO_2 (Lumenis, UltraPulse, SCAAR FX 60–90 mJ, 1–3%, 300 Hz) under local anesthesia cream, additional 5-fluorouracil (5-FU)

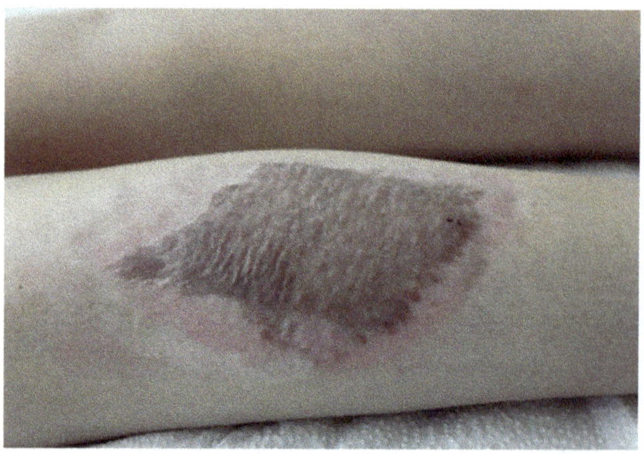

◘ **Fig.** Baseline situation: elevated hypertrophic scar in an area of 18×12 cm with an approximate height of 1 cm on the left lower leg at initial presentation. Surrounding erythema due to mild reaction to the local anesthesia cream applied prior to the laser therapy

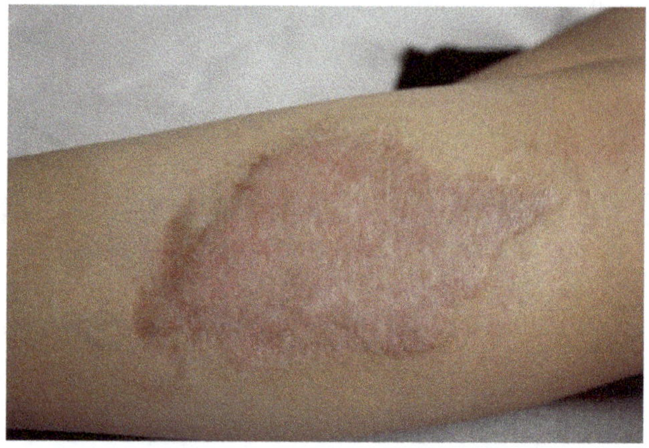

◘ **Fig.** Presentation 8 weeks after initial Q-ruby laser treatment

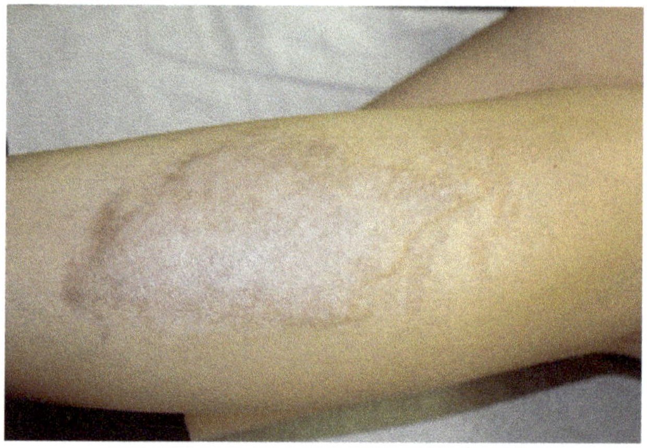

◘ **Fig.** Presentation 12 weeks after last laser treatment

50 mg/cc for drug delivery on the scar surface. Wound dressings with gauze, fusidic acid, and a class III steroid containing cream. Repetitive treatments approximately every 4–6 weeks apart.

Questions Interventions

- Why use the Q-ruby first before initiating therapy with fractional CO_2?
- What is the rationale for the time intervals in between laser sessions?
- Potential risk of laser therapy?
- Why combination with 5-FU?

Intervention 7

Another pass using a Q-switched ruby 4 mm/4 J (Asclepion) under local anesthesia cream. Aftercare with fusidic acid and a class III steroid containing cream. Final results 12 weeks after last treatment shown in ◘ Fig. 58.3.

Discussion

Hyperpigmented scars are relatively common; however, most frequently scar therapy is directed toward reducing possible symptoms like pruritus, pain or tension, and reduction of excess scar tissue through various approaches. Nevertheless, using nanosecond or picosecond lasers with wave lengths of 532, 694, 755, or 1064 nm known from laser tattoo removal or treatment of benign pigmentated skin lesions do have potential to improve appearance of hyperpigmented scars. In our case, treatment using a q-switched Ruby laser has been chosen as initial therapy simply due to the fact that the hyperpigmentation was the main concern of our patient. The hyperpigmentation was most probably a response to previous cryotherapy sessions; however, in darker-skinned patients, hyperpigmentations of scars are frequently seen without any previous therapy. Alternatively, a hydrochinone-containing cream may be used, but they are often less effective compared to respective laser treatments [1]. Caution should be paid to possible melanocytic lesions, which can easily be ruled out through dermatoscopy and should be excluded from laser therapy.

The use of fractional CO_2 lasers for the improvement of hypertrophic scars has been demonstrated in numerous studies. Combining deep fractional ablation with high fluences and a low density to stimulate dermal matrix remodeling with superficial smoothening of the scar through ablation of individual scar strands, followed by extensive fractional surface ablation, has been shown to greatly improve widespread hypertrophic scarring [2–4]. On a molecular basis, the heat radiated into the treated tissue results in the activation of heat-shock proteins, predominantly from the HSP-70 family, as well as the alteration of remodeling factors like matrix-metalloproteases and antifibrotic isotypes from the transforming-growth factor beta family (TGF-β) [5, 6]. Although these processes have not yet been fully elucidated, clinical studies have shown a normalization of the dermal matrix architecture following fractional CO_2-laser treatment [7, 8]. Its combination with triamcinolone acetonide or 5-FU appears to further improve results and, in our experience, seems to minimize the total number of sessions necessary to achieve satisfying results [9, 10]. We usually allow the scar tissue to settle in between laser sessions for 4–8 weeks as scar tissue needs time for remodeling. While hypertrophic scars usually respond very well to fractional lasers, some caution should be paid when treating keloids as here, activation of the keloid with further enlargement is relatively frequently seen.

Take-Home Message

- Different scar types do benefit from combinational therapies. Interestingly, hyperpigmentations of scar do respond relatively well to QS-ruby or picosecond lasers.

References

1. Imhof L, Dummer R, Dreier J, Kolm I, Barysch MJ. A prospective trial comparing q-switched ruby laser and a triple combination skin-lightening cream in the treatment of solar lentigines. Dermatol Surg. 2016;42(7):853–7.
2. Blome-Eberwein S, Gogal C, Weiss MJ, Boorse D, Pagella P. Prospective evaluation of fractional CO2 laser treatment of mature burn scars. J Burn Care Res. 2016;37(6):379–87.
3. Cervelli V, Gentile P, Spallone D, Nicoli F, Verardi S, Petrocelli M, et al. Ultrapulsed fractional CO2 laser for the treatment of post-traumatic and pathological scars. J Drugs Dermatol. 2010;9(11):1328–31.
4. Poetschke J, Dornseifer U, Clementoni MT, Reinholz M, Schwaiger H, Steckmeier S, et al. Ultrapulsed fractional ablative carbon dioxide laser treatment of hypertrophic burn scars: evaluation of an in-patient controlled, standardized treatment approach. Lasers Med Sci. 2017;32(5):1031–40.
5. Paasch U, Sonja G, Haedersdal M. Synergistic skin heat shock protein expression in response to combined laser treatment with a diode laser and ablative fractional lasers. Int J Hyperth. 2014;30(4):245–9.
6. Qu L, Liu A, Zhou L, He C, Grossman PH, Moy RL, et al. Clinical and molecular effects on mature burn scars after treatment with a fractional CO(2) laser. Lasers Surg Med. 2012;44(7):517–24.
7. Orringer JS, Kang S, Johnson TM, Karimipour DJ, Hamilton T, Hammerberg C, et al. Connective tissue remodeling induced by carbon dioxide laser resurfacing of photodamaged human skin. Arch Dermatol. 2004;140(11):1326–32.
8. Ozog DM, Liu A, Chaffins ML, Ormsby AH, Fincher EF, Chipps LK, et al. Evaluation of clinical results, histological architecture, and collagen expression following treatment of mature burn scars with a fractional carbon dioxide laser. JAMA Dermatol. 2013;149(1):50–7.
9. Sabry HH, Abdel Rahman SH, Hussein MS, Sanad RR, Abd El Azez TA. The efficacy of combining fractional carbon dioxide laser with verapamil hydrochloride or 5-fluorouracil in the treatment of hypertrophic scars and keloids: a clinical and immunohistochemical study. Dermatol Surg. 2019;45(4):536–46.
10. Waibel JS, Wulkan AJ, Shumaker PR. Treatment of hypertrophic scars using laser and laser assisted corticosteroid delivery. Lasers Surg Med. 2013;45(3):135–40.

15

Secondary Lip Correction in a Cleft Lip Patient

Wouter B. van der Sluis and Johan P. W. Don Griot

Contents

Suggested Reading

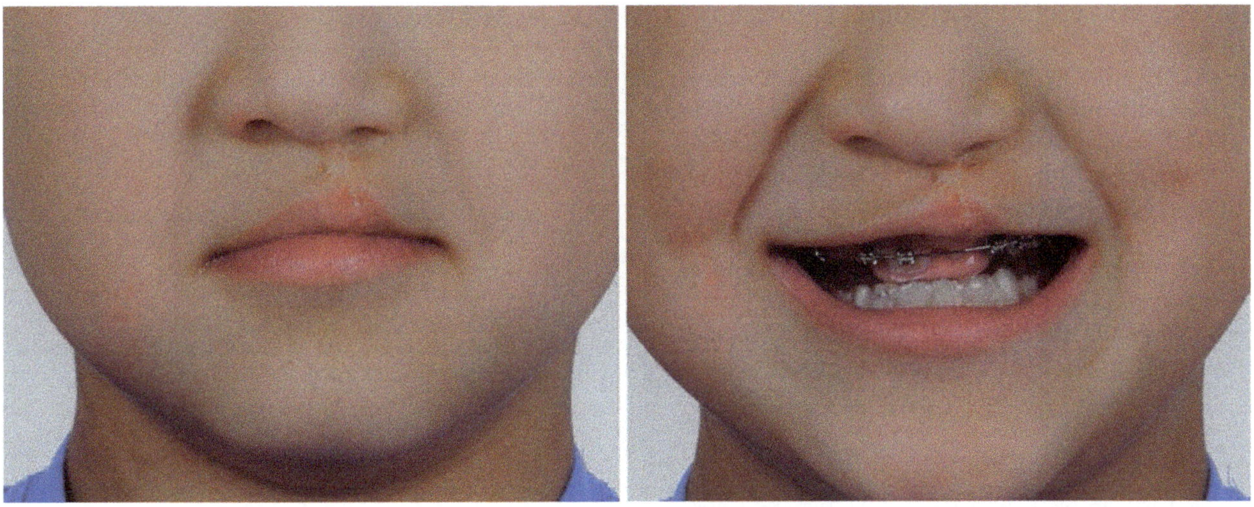

▪▪ Medical History

A 11-year-old male visited the outpatient clinic with his parents because of unpleasing esthetic result after surgical correction of unilateral cleft lip and palate in China. There are no additional operative data available. The cleft palate and lip were not part of a genetic syndrome. There were no other comorbidities.

He stated that he was not pleased with the aesthetic result of the cleft surgery and that the main problem for him was asymmetry of the perioral area. There were no functional complaints in the domains of speech, eating, and/or drinking.

❓ Questions (4 max)

- Q1. Define the problem in terms of anatomy
- Q2. What is the Rose–Thompson effect?
- Q3. What would be the surgical approach to this problem?
- Q4. What (non)surgical methods can be chosen to optimize postoperative scarring?

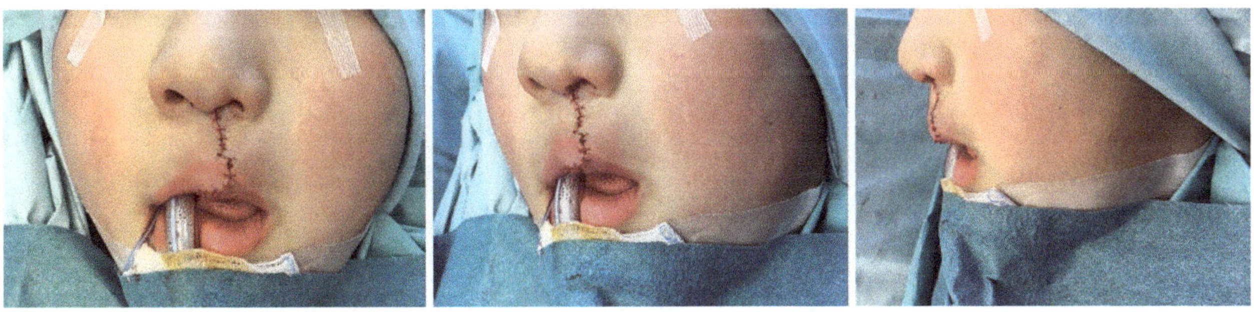

Immediate postintervention situation: Correction of these deformities in children is best performed under general anesthesia. Intubation is performed using an RAE (Ring-Adair-Elwyn) tube, which is a prebent tube that facilitates adequate reach of the operative area. The operative area is marked using skin marker that does not wash away or fade out during sterile exposition and surgery. The operative region is infiltrated with a mix of lidocaine and adrenalin.

The scar was excised using a concave excision pattern, making use of the Rose–Thompson effect. With one additional Z-plasty, adequate scar length was achieved. Reconfiguration of misaligned lip mucosa was achieved in the same session. The subcutaneous plane was closed using resorbable sutures. The skin was closed using skin glue.

Argumented answers and explanation according to the five references (cited later): 20 lines

- Q1. Define the problem in terms of anatomy.
- A1. Postoperative scar contracture of philtral scar with subsequent effect on nose and lip esthetics. Also, misalignment of lip mucosa was observed.

- Q2. What is the Rose–Thomson effect?
- A2. The effect of scar lengthening by using concave excisions of the scar, which is subsequently closed in a straight line

- Q3. What would be the surgical approach to this problem?
- A3. Use of the Rose–Thompson effect in combination with one or multiple Z-plasties or a combination of these strategies. An alternative approach might be using fat grafting of the scar; however, this probably provides a less predictable result.

- Q4. What (non)surgical methods can be chosen to optimize postoperative scarring?
- A4. Injecting the orbicularis oris with botulinum toxin, silicon application in the postoperative phase, using glue instead of sutures for tissue approximation.

Take-Home Messages

- Cleft lip scars influence lip, philtrum, and nose aesthetics.
- In secondary lip correction, cleft surgeons typically make use of the Rose–Thompson effect, one or multiple Z-plasties, or a combination of these strategies.

Suggested Reading

1. Deshmukh M, Vaidya S, Deshpande G, Galinde J, Natarajan S. Comparative evaluation of esthetic outcomes in unilateral cleft lip repair between the Mohler and fisher repair techniques: a prospective, randomized, observer-blind study. J Oral Maxillofac Surg. 2019;77(1):182.e1–8.
2. Farmand M. Secondary lip correction in unilateral clefts. Facial Plast Surg. 2002;18(3):187–95.
3. Mulliken JB, Zhu DR, Sullivan SR. Outcomes of cleft lip repair for internationally adopted children. Plast Reconstr Surg. 2015;135(5):1439–47.
4. Stal S, Hollier L. Correction of secondary cleft lip deformities. Plast Reconstr Surg. 2002;109(5):1672–81.

16

Vacuum Massage in the Treatment of Scars

Peter Moortgat, Jill Meirte, Ulrike Van Daele, Mieke Anthonissen, Tine Vanhullebusch, and Koen Maertens

Contents

Working Mechanism of Vacuum Massage in Relation to Pathological Scarring

The Effects of Vacuum Massage on Scars
General Effects
Physical Effects
Physiological Effects
Mechanical Effects

Conclusion

Bibliography

Background

Vacuum massage is also known as depressomassage, vacuotherapy, or Endermologie®. It is a non-invasive mechanical massage technique performed with a mechanical device that lifts the skin by means of suction, creates a skin fold, and mobilizes that skin fold [1, 2] as displayed in ◘ Figs. 54.1 and 54.2.

Vacuum massage originates from cupping therapy, a traditional Chinese medicine therapy dating back 2000 years or more. A local suction on the skin is created using heat or mechanical forces in order to create vasodilatation. In the late 1970s, Louis-Paul Guitay suffered from severe skin burns after a car accident. During his rehabilitation, he had to endure hours of manual massages every day. This multi-month process was normal practice for burn victims with extensive scar tissue in the late 1970s. Massage sessions typically lasted 3– 4 hours a day and consisted of rigorous routines. The therapist rolled skin and tissue back and forth to regain elasticity. As days grew into weeks, Guitay became dissatisfied with these incessant treatments. They were time-consuming, labor intensive, and he noticed his results varied drastically based on the skills of each individual therapist. Endermologie®, taken from the French term meaning "through the dermis", was Louis-Paul Guitay's way of standardizing massage therapy to maximize the effect of each treatment. He developed a mechanical device to copy the manual massage techniques by means of negative pressure. This method allowed him to perform the massage in a more consistent way and was less time consuming. From then onward, Endermologie® or vacuum massage has been frequently used to treat traumatic or burn scars.

Although vacuum massage was invented to treat burns and scars, very little literature is available on the effects of this intervention. Soon after its development, the device was used extensively in Europe to treat trauma and burn scars [2]. In the course of its use, care providers soon noticed its ability to improve the appearance of cellulite, and consequently most studies mainly focused on lipodystrophy to investigate its working mechanism. The number of studies concerning cellulite is three times higher than those of burns or scars.

The aim of this chapter is to present an overview of the available literature with the physical and physiological effects of vacuum massage. This was done in order to find the underlying working mechanisms of Endermologie® that could benefit the healing of burns and scars. Analyzing the physical and physiological effects of this treatment can increase insights in the influence on the scarring process and may clarify the outcome.

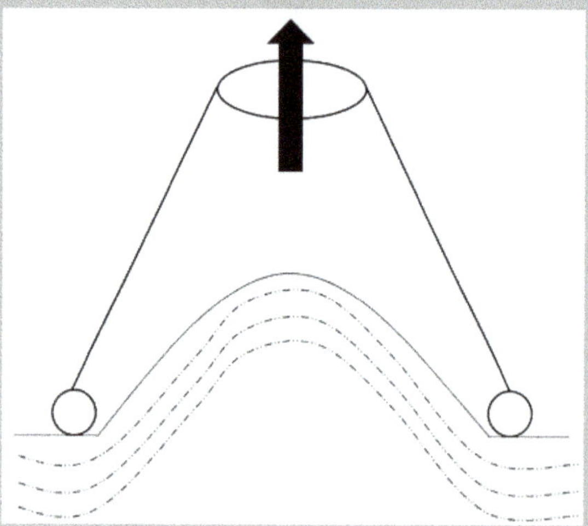

◘ Fig. Vacuum massage creates a skin fold and mobi-lizes that skin fold

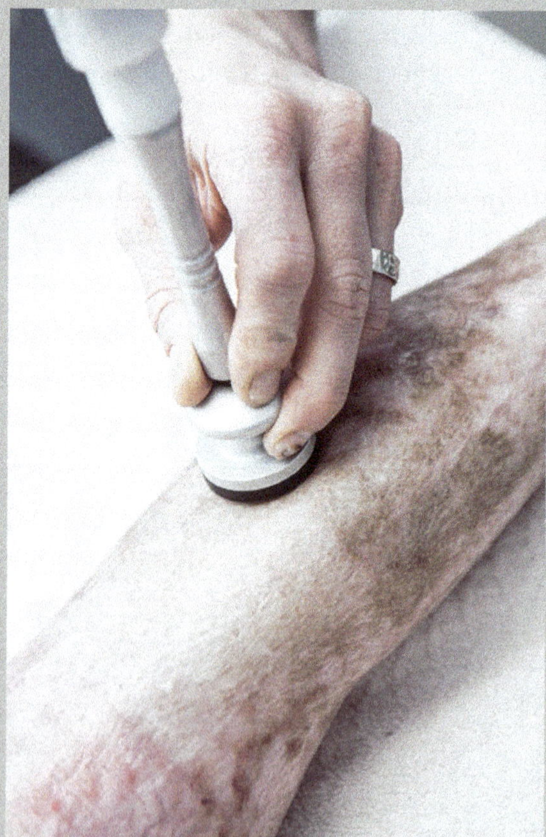

◘ Fig. Vacuum massage on scars

Working Mechanism of Vacuum Massage in Relation to Pathological Scarring

In recent years, there has been an increasing interest in the mechanobiology of scars. The influence of mechanical forces on skin has been examined since 1861 when Langer first reported the existence of lines of tension in cadaver skin [3]. Internal tension in the dermis leads to cell–extracellular matrix (ECM) and cell–cell interactions transferring external mechanical forces into biochemical signals inside the cell [4]. Khan et al. reclaimed the term "mechanotherapy" and presented the current scientific knowledge underpinning how mechanical load may be used therapeutically to stimulate tissue repair and remodeling. It has long been thought that the effectiveness and efficiency of physical therapy would improve if our understanding of the cell biology/biochemistry that participates in mechanics could be improved. Traditional physical therapy focuses primarily on rehabilitation, but recent developments in mechanobiology that illuminated the effects of physical forces on cells and tissues have led to the realization that the old therapy model should be updated. Recent studies showed how mechanotherapies target particular cells, molecules, and tissues. The role of mechanical force in various therapies, including micro-deforming soft tissue techniques, shockwave, vacuum massage, tissue expansion, skin stretching, and tension reduction (tissue targeting) therapies is the subject of numerous ongoing clinical trials [5–7].

All adherent cells including endothelial cells, fibroblasts, and myofibroblasts sense tension originate from the environment. Tension is transmitted via cell–ECM contacts, leading to reorganization of the cytoskeleton and the elicitation of specific signals that modulate gene expression. In skin, alterations of mechanical forces are continuously recognized by cells, and their functions are adapted according to the biological requirements. If mechanical tension is removed, those tissues undergo atrophy, indicating the important role of mechanical signals for maintaining proper functioning of the organism. Obviously, fibroblasts and myofibroblasts are cells implicated in scarring, which is strongly influenced by mechanical tension.

The precise mechanisms by which different cell types transmit mechanical signals are not fully understood. They might involve stretch-activated ion channels, direct interactions between structural and signaling components, or activation of small GTPases. As outlined above, many cooperative interactions exist between integrins and growth factor signaling. In particular, fibroblast to myofibroblast conversion and alpha-smooth muscle actin (α-SMA) expression crucially depend on a combination of mechanical tension and TGF-β. Thus in scarring, generation of tension can induce myofibroblast formation, causing a self-perpetuating loop. A similar autocrine loop is discussed for the induction of collagen synthesis in fibroblasts by mechanical tension. In this case, TGF-β is induced by tension, which in turn activates collagen synthesis via the classic pathways. In addition, fibronectin is induced by the application of cyclic strain to fibroblasts. In parallel, many proteases are downregulated, whereas protease inhibitors are upregulated. As a result of these events, modulation of mechanical tension results in alterations of fibroblast and myofibroblast activity. . Tension directly modifies gene transcription, induces signaling from integrins affecting small GTPases, or induces/inhibits growth factor signaling, which then indirectly affects ECM protein synthesis by fibroblasts/myofibroblasts [8]. By a combination of these mechanisms, mechanical tension induces an activated, contractile fibroblast/myofibroblast phenotype characterized by high levels of synthesis of ECM proteins, low protease activity, and high production of fibrogenic cytokines. Translated into a clinical situation, this means a retractile scar with adhesions between the dermal tissue and the underlying viscera.

The mechanotransduction theories provide possible evidence for several physical non-invasive treatment options. It was suggested that many of the physical scar management methods, including compression therapy, silicone therapy, adhesive tape, and occlusive dressing therapy, are related to mechanotransduction mechanisms. Mechanical compression seems to induce apoptosis and to regulate cytokine release, thus reducing hypertrophic scarring. The effects of mechanical tension on TGF-beta1 and collagen synthesis leads to the hypothesis that brief, moderate stretch of scar tissue seems to downregulate hypertrophy and retraction of scars and could be the best option for splinting, positioning, and postural stretching [9].

The Effects of Vacuum Massage on Scars

General Effects [1 10 12] –

General effects are defined as the effects inherent to the intervention itself or to the individual who performs the treatment. A number of studies mentioned the measured effects were dependent on the number of treatments. The more the treatment, the higher the effect. After this ascertainment, Adcock et al. also discovered that the principal force applied to the tissue during the therapy depended on the particular type of maneuver performed, with the suction and the roller tension being of minor importance. Moreover, they observed a major decrease of tension in thicker tissue.

In four studies performed, the results showed a setback after a follow-up period without treatment, but one study demonstrated the opposite. All these results are shown in ◘ Table 54.1.

Table Basic information available in the literature describing effects of vacuum massage on several skin layers

Literature	Etiology	Study design	Targeted skin layer	No. of patients	Assessment	LESS score
Moortgat et al. [16]	Burn scars	CCT	Epidermis/ dermis	48	POSAS, touch pressure threshold, DermaLab elasticity	18
Anthonissen et al. [15]	Burn scars	CCT	Epidermis/ dermis	47	POSAS, Tristimulus colorimetry, trans-epidermal water loss	18
Adcock et al. [1]	Pig skin	RCT	Dermis/ hypodermis	12	Histology	17
Adcock et al. [12]	Pig skin	RCT	Hypodermis	4	Intra-dermal tonometry	16
Revuz et al. [11]	Aging skin	CCT	Dermis	24	Subjective assessment of skin laxity and skin loosening, stereophogrammetry, cutometer	16
Moseley et al. [18]	Scar like	RCT	Dermis/ hypodermis	10	Likert scale, tonometry	16
Lucassen et al. [19]	Healthy skin	Pre/post	Dermis/ hypodermis	19	High frequency ultrasound	13
Watson et al. [2]	Healthy skin	RCT	Epidermis/ dermis	5	Laser-Doppler imaging, lymphoscintigraphy, venous flowmetry	13
Innocenzi et al. [14]	Lipodystrophy	CCT	Epidermis/ dermis	12	Descriptive histology	11
Innocenzi et al. [20]	Lipodystrophy	CCT	Epidermis/ dermis	15	Quantitative histology	10
Ortonne et al. [21]	Lipodystrophy	RCT	Dermis/ hypodermis	30	High frequency ultrasound, fringe projection, skin fold thickness	13
Bourgeois et al. [13]	Scars	RCT	Epidermis/ dermis	20	Subjective assessment of pain, itch, tightness, erythema and skin smoothening, profilometry	13
Monteux et al. [22]	Lipodystrophy	Pre/post	Dermis/ hypodermis	9	Skin fold thickness	11
Marques et al. [10]	Healthy skin	Pre/post	Hypodermis	12	Gene profiling, micro-array	11
Scuderi et al. [23]	Healthy skin	RCT	Epidermis/ dermis	10	Subjective assessment of skin smoothening and skin tone	10
Majani et al. [24]	Scars	Pre/post	Epidermis/ dermis	26	Subjective assessment of skin smoothness, pain, tenderness, oedema and aesthetic improvement, histology	10
Marquez-Rebollo et al. [25]	Scar like	Pre/post	Epidermis/ dermis	70	Number of indurations	10
Gavroy et al. [26]	Scars	CCT	Details not available	606	Test de glissement	7
Lattarulo et al. [27]	Healthy skin	Pre/post	Epidermis/ dermis	34	Laser-Doppler imaging, $tcpO_2$	7
Worret et al. [28]	Scar like	Pre/post	Dermis	10	Subjective assessment of pain, color and elasticity, quality of life, cutometer	7
Delprat et al. [29]	Scars	Pre/post	Details not available	132	Test de glissement	5

RCT randomized controlled trial, *CCT* controlled clinical trial, $tcpO_2$ transcutaneous oxygen pressure

Physical Effects [13–16]

An improvement of the tissue hardness and the elasticity of the skin were the two most observed effects. However, most of the studies used subjective methods to quantify these effects. Other reported physical effects were decreased skin fold thickness, decreased face volume, improved skin laxity, increased epidermal thickness, and improved skin roughness. Recent studies have shown that elasticity and redness, measured with subjective and objective assessment tools, were significantly improved after 1 year when the scar was treated for 6 months. The results of one study also revealed that the vacuum massage had minimal value as additive treatment to pressure garments and silicone when it concerned redness. For elasticity, on the other hand, vacuum massage + pressure therapy and silicone seemed to perform better than pressure therapy and silicone alone. The results are set out in ◘Table 54.2.

Physiological Effects [2, 10, 13, 15, 17]

An improvement in blood perfusion was noticed in four studies. Fibroblast proliferation was enhanced together with an increase in collagen content. Two studies mentioned an improved venous and lymphatic flow together with increased transcutaneous oxygen pressure. Smoothening of the dermo-hypodermal junction and a decreased dermal interstitial space were also observed. One study mentioned altered gene expression profiles in adipose tissue. In another study, a significant decrease of trans-epidermal water loss (TEWL) was found and indicated a recovery of the skin barrier. After correction for baseline and age of scar, there was evidence for lower mean TEWL values in the vacuum massage group, significant after 3 months ($p = 0.006$). Humbert et al. investigated the histological effects of vacuum massage and discovered an increased migratory ability of fibroblasts together with increased elastin and hyaluronic acid presence which indicated induced remodeling capacity. The upregulation of MMP-9 suggests degradation of the existing damaged ECM to induce remodeling. These findings were somehow confirmed by the study of Meirte et al., where an increased dermal thickness together with a decreased dermal density were already noticed in the first 2 hours after a vacuum massage treatment. These results are shown in ◘Table 54.3.

Mechanical Effects

The suction forces generated by vacuum massage could elicit an array of mechanical forces within the tissues, associated with a relaxation of those mechanical forces. Once stress forces on a wound were relieved, apoptosis of myofibroblasts would occur. This finding implies that vacuum massage may release the mechanical stress associated with scar retraction, and thus induce apoptosis. This can be another plausible theory for its mechanism of action to improve the outcome of (burn) scars.

Conclusion

Although vacuum massage initially had been developed for the treatment of burn scars, literature reveals little evidence for the efficacy of this treatment. Very few studies investigated the effects of vacuum massage on human models with scars. The heterogeneous population and the wide diversity of study designs make it very hard to translate the previously mentioned results toward the burns and scars population in humans. Although the present study contributes additional evidence for the working mechanism of vacuum massage as an anti-scarring agent, the results should be confirmed by studies on human models. Variations in duration, amplitude, or frequency of the treatment have a substantial influence on collagen restructuring and reorientation, thus implying possible beneficial influences on the healing potential by mechanotransduction pathways. Vacuum massage may release the mechanical tension associated with scar retraction, and thus induce apoptosis of myofibroblasts. Suggestions for future research include upscaling the study design, investigating molecular pathways and dose dependency, comparing effects in different stages of repair, including evolutional parameters and the use of more objective assessment tools.

Table Overview of the physical effects of vacuum massage on epidermis/dermis/hypodermis

Paper	Tissue hardness subjective	Tissue hardness objective	Elasticity subjective	Elasticity objective	Skin fold thickness	Scar adhesions	Face volume	Skin laxity	Epidermal thickness	Skin roughness	Color subjective	Color objective
Delprat et al. [29]						Decreased						
Gavroy et al. [26]						Decreased						
Adcock et al. [12]		Decreased										
Revuz et al. [11]				No changes			Decreased	Decreased				
Innocenzi et al. [14]									Increased			
Innocenzi et al. [20]									Increased			
Ortonne et al [21].					Decreased					Decreased		
Worret et al. [28]	Decreased		Increased	Increased							Decreased	
Moseley et al. [18]	Decreased	Decreased	Increased									
Bourgeois et al. [13]	Decreased									Decreased	Decreased	
Monteux et al. [22]					Decreased							
Scuderi et al [23].	Decreased							Decreased				
Marquez-Rebollo et al. [25]	Decreased		Increased									
Majani et al. [24]	Decreased		Increased									
Moortgat et al. [16]			Increased	Increased								
Anthonissen et al. [15]												Decreased

Table Overview of the physiological effects of vacuum massage on epidermis/dermis/hypodermis

Paper	Blood perfusion	Dermo-hypodermal junction	Collagen content	Collagen orientation	TEWL	Lymphatic flow	$tcpO_2$	# fibroblasts	Fibroblast phenotype	Dermal interstitial space	Superficial vascular surface	Pain	Itch	Altered gene profile
Lucassen et al. [19]		Smoothened												
Adcock et al. [1]			Increased	Dense longitudinal bands										
Watson et al. [2]	Increased					Increased								
Lattarulo et al. [27]	Increased						Increased							
Revuz et al. [11]				Dense longitudinal bands										
Innocenzi et al. [14]								Increased	Secreting					
Innocenzi et al. [20]								Increased	Secreting	Decreased	Increased			
Ortonne et al. [21]		Smoothened												
Worret et al. [28]												Decreased		
Bourgeois et al. [13]											Increased	Decreased	Decreased	
Marques et al. [10]														Yes
Majani et al. [24]										Decreased				
Moortgat et al. [16]												Decreased	Decreased	
Anthonissen et al. [15]					Decreased									

$tcpO_2$ transcutaneous oxygen pressure, *TEWL* trans-epidermal water loss

Take-Home Messages

- Vacuum massage is a way of standardizing massage techniques to optimize the treatment.
- Mechanotransduction is the presumed working mechanism behind vacuum massage.
- Improved tissue hardness and elasticity are the two most observed physical effects.
- The effect of vacuum massage is highly dependent on the type of maneuver performed.
- The more treatments are carried out, the higher the effect.
- Fibroblast migratory and proliferative capacities are enhanced by vacuum massage.
- Vacuum massage improves scar elasticity, which will probably lead to amelioration of function.
- Vacuum massage may release the mechanical stress associated with scar retraction.

Bibliography

1. Adcock D, Paulsen S, Davis S, Nanney L, Shack RB. Analysis of the cutaneous and systemic effects of Endermologie in the porcine model. Aesthet Surg J. 1998;18:414–20.
2. Watson J, Fodor P, Cutcliffe B. Physiological effects of Endermologie: a preliminary report. Aesth Surg. 1999;19:39–45.
3. Silver FH, Siperko LM, Seehra GP. Mechanobiology of force transduction in dermal tissue. Skin Res Technol. 2003;9:3–23.
4. Ingber DE. Cellular mechanotransduction: putting all the pieces together again. FASEB J. 2006;20:811–27.
5. Moortgat P, Maertens K. "The science of stretch": clinical implications of Mechanobiology of scars. Middle East Wounds Scar Meet. 2014.
6. Huang C, Holfeld J, Schaden W, Orgill D, Ogawa R. Mechanotherapy: revisiting physical therapy and recruiting mechanobiology for a new era in medicine. Trends Mol Med. 2013;19:555–64.
7. Verhaegen PDHM (2011) On burn scar reconstruction - clinimetric, experimental and clinical studies. ISBN: 978-90-5335-413-1
8. Eckes B, Nischt R, Krieg T. Cell-matrix interactions in dermal repair and scarring. Fibrogenesis Tissue Repair. 2010;3:4.
9. Bouffard NA, Cutroneo KR, Badger GJ, White SL, Buttolph TR, Ehrlich HP, Stevens-Tuttle D, Langevin HM. Tissue stretch decreases soluble TGF-??1 and type-1 procollagen in mouse subcutaneous connective tissue: evidence from ex vivo and in vivo models. J Cell Physiol. 2008;214:389–95.
10. Marques M-A, Combes M, Roussel B, Vidal-Dupont L, Thalamas C, Lafontan M, Viguerie N. Impact of a mechanical massage on gene expression profile and lipid mobilization in female gluteofemoral adipose tissue. Obes Facts. 2011;4:121–9.
11. Revuz J, Adhoute H, Cesarini J, Poli F, Lacarrière C, Emiliozzi C. Clinical and histological effects of the lift device used on facial skin aging. Les Nouv Dermatologiques. 2002;21: 335–42.
12. Adcock D, Paulsen S, Jabour K, Davis S, Nanney LB, Shack RB. Analysis of the effects of deep mechanical massage in the porcine model. Plast Reconstr Surg. 2001;108:233–40.
13. Bourgeois JF, Gourgou S, Kramar A, Lagarde JM, Guillot B. A randomized, prospective study using the LPG technique in treating radiation-induced skin fibrosis: clinical and profilometric analysis. Skin Res Technol. 2008;14:71–6.
14. Innocenzi D, Balzani A, Panetta C. Modifications Morphologiques De La Peau Induites Par La Technique LPG®. DERMOtime settembre 1–4. 2002.
15. Anthonissen M, Meirte J, Moortgat P, Maertens K, Daly D, Fieuws S, Lafaire C, De Cuyper L, Van den Kerckhove E. Influence on clinical parameters of depressomassage (part I): the effects of depressomassage on color and transepidermal water loss rate in burn scars: a pilot comparative controlled study. Burns. 2018;44:877–85.
16. Moortgat P, Lafaire C, Dom Y, Douws P, Van Tichelen J. The effect of prus depressomassage on elasticity and skin fold thickness of burn scars. Burns. 2011;37:S6–7.
17. Fanian F, Humbert P, Lihoreau T, Jeudy A, Elkhyat A, Robin S, Courderot-Masuyer C, Tauzin H, Lafforgue C, Haftek M. Mécano-stimulation of the skin improves sagging score and induces beneficial functional modification of the fibroblasts: clinical, biological, and histological evaluations. Clin Interv Aging. 2015;10:387.
18. Moseley A, Piller N, Douglass J, Esplin M. Comparison of the effectiveness of MLD and LPG technique®. J Lymphoedema 2007;2:2–8.
19. Lucassen GW, Sluys WLN, Herk JJ, Nuijs AM, Wierenga PE, Barel AO, Lambrecht R. The effectiveness of massage treatment on cellulite as monitored by ultrasound imaging. Skin Research and Technology 1997;3(3):154–160
20. Innocenzi D, Balzani A, Montesi G, La Torre G, Tenna S, Scuderi N, et al. Evidence des modifications cutanées induites par la technique LPG via une analyse d'images. DermoCosmetologia 2003:1–7.
21. Ortonne J-P. Treatment of cellulite. Nouv Dermatol 2002;22: 261–269.
22. Monteux C, Lafontan M. Use of the microdialysis technique to assess lipolytic responsiveness of femoral adipose tissue after 12 sessions of mechanical massage technique. Journal of the European Academy of Dermatology and Venereology 2008; 22(12):1465–1470
23. Scuderi N. Randomized clinical trial on patient compliance and the ergonomics of two appliances for mechanical massage. 2008. http://www.icoone.pl/files/scuderi_eng.pdf. Accessed 30/09/2013.
24. Majani UGO, Majani A. Tissue mechanostimulation in the treatment of scars. Acta Medica Mediterr 2013;29:133–134.
25. Márquez-Rebollo C, Vergara-Carrasco L, Díaz-Navarro R, Rubio-Fernández D, Francoli-Martínez P, Sánchez-De la Rosa R. Benefit of Endermology on Indurations and Panniculitis/ Lipoatrophy During Relapsing–Remitting Multiple Sclerosis Long-Term Treatment with Glatiramer Acetate. Advances in Therapy 2014;31(8):904–914
26. Gavroy J.P., et al. LPG and the cutaneous softening of burns. J Plaies Cicatrices 1996;5:76–84.
27. Lattarulo P, Bacci PA, Mancini S. Physiological tissue changes after administration of micronized Diosmin / Hesperidin , individually or in association with Endermologie ®. Int J Aesthetic Cosmet Beauty Surg 2001;1:25–28.
28. Worret W-I, Jessberger B. Effectiveness of LPGR treatment in morphea. Journal of the European Academy of Dermatology and Venereology 2004;18(5):527–530
29. Delprat J, Ehrler S, Gavroy JP, Romain M, Thaury MN, Xenard J. Raideur et Tissus Mous. La Raideur Articul 1995:46–51.

17

Management of Scarring Following Aesthetic Surgery

Alexandra Chambers

Contents

Introduction

Patient Selection for Cosmetic Surgery
Evaluating Medical Risks
Assessment of Constitutional and Genetic Risks
Modification of Lifestyle
Psychological Assessment and Expectations Management

Prophylactic Measures in Cosmetic Surgery to Reduce Excessive Scarring
Choice of Surgical Techniques
Methods to Control Better Healing

Treatment of Scars Following Aesthetic Surgery
Surgical Treatments
Non-surgical Treatments
Long-Term Management of Patients with Scars After Cosmetic Surgery

Conclusion

References

Introduction

> **Aesthetic (Cosmetic) Surgery**
> Aesthetic surgery's principal purpose is to improve physical appearance and self-esteem.

Demand for cosmetic surgery procedures continues to grow at a rapid pace around the world, with a 9% increase in treatments performed in 2017 compared to the previous year. This translated into 20 million more cosmetic surgery procedures [1]. According to the International Society of Aesthetic Plastic Surgery (ISAPS), the USA, Brazil, Japan, Italy, and Mexico account for 41.4% of the world's cosmetic interventions. Breast augmentation, liposuction, eyelid surgery, rhinoplasty, and abdominoplasty were the most popular treatments.

All surgical procedures have inherent risks, and aesthetic surgery is not an exception. One of the risks is poor scarring, and this can occur from postoperative infection, wound dehiscence, tissue necrosis, or simply from abnormal healing tendencies. Unfavorable scarring is not uncommon following cosmetic surgery; the incidence can vary from 5% after breast augmentation to as high as 8% after abdominoplasty [2, 3]. The impact of excessive scarring can be disturbing to a patient and can incite significant morbidity and psychological distress. The experience can also be disheartening for the surgeon, as the patient will likely blame them for scars. For example, in the UK, approximately a quarter of medical malpractice claims after cosmetic surgery are related to poor scarring and, on average, generate roughly £300,000 in awards [4]. The cost of remedial scar treatment can be quite expensive, taking time and resources of both the patient and the surgeon.

Given the risks of poor scarring, it makes sense for cosmetic surgeons to take as many precautions as possible to avoid inferior outcomes. This chapter explores preventative measures to preclude the occurrence of unacceptable scars, as well as treatment strategies for when they nevertheless develop.

Patient Selection for Cosmetic Surgery

All cosmetic procedures are elective, and identifying patients at risk for poor scarring is a key starting step. It is important to develop a selective approach in offering aesthetic treatments to reduce unfavorable outcomes and to mitigate potential problems. Patients must be included in the decision-making process, beginning with providing a clear explanation of the risks for their specific case. The surgeon must take the time to explain and to provide realistic management of patient expectations. Only after clearly describing the risks and answering questions can patients make a valid informed decision.

The scar risk and acceptance matrix (◘ Table 45.1) is an example of a simple clinical tool that can be used to quantify the risks of cicatrix formation. This is a communication tool that can help a patient's understanding and, when used in a clinical practice, only requires a few minutes of consultation time. The parameters taken into account for this calculator are the preexisting medical conditions that might affect healing, life style risks, the patient's constitutional tendencies to poor scarring, and the patient's expectations about scar appearance.

Each row of the matrix can contribute an integer value from 1 to 5 according to the descriptions in each column. Adding the results from each row gives a total score, with low values corresponding to low risk. Patients with medium and high risk should be well counseled before their procedure, and the preventative measures (to be described later in this chapter) should be taken before surgery. A very high-risk score might justify declining treatment. The following subsections describe each row of the calculator in more detail.

Evaluating Medical Risks

Reviewing a patient's medical history is key for identifying patients who might be at risk for the types of complications that can lead to poor scarring. The following examples illustrate some of the issues to consider.

- Individuals with cardiovascular disease and hypertension might be at higher risk of bleeding or inadequate tissue perfusion.
- Chronic lung disease and poor peripheral circulation can cause inadequate oxygenation of skin. This in turn could lead to a potential necrosis at the surgical site.
- Autoimmune and connective tissue diseases can give rise to excessive fibrosis and scar thickening. They can also lead to suboptimal collagen deposition, resulting in atrophic or widened scars.
- Immunosuppressed or diabetic patients will have a greater chance of postoperative infection and a problem healing.
- Allergies to certain medications or substances, like latex or adhesive dressings, might compromise an otherwise successful surgery.
- Some medications and supplements can promote postoperative bleeding or predispose to hyperpigmentation.
- Patients, who have previously developed unsightly scars, might be prone to keloid and hypertrophic or atrophic healing.

Table Scar risk and acceptance matrix

Score	1	2	3	4	5
Medical risks	None	Hypoxic chronic state CVD Hypertension	Suppressed immunity, including steroid use Diabetes	Autoimmune connective tissue diseases Post-bariatric surgery malabsorption	Peripheral Vascular disease Hyper-viscosity states
Fitzpatrick skin type and constitutional tendencies	Skin 1–3 No history of poor scarring Dry skin with low sebaceous activity	Any skin type Red, pigmented or slightly uneven and lumpy scars BMI > 30	Any skin type Multiple stretch marks, very loose skin Atrophic scars present	Skin 4–5 Previous hypertrophic scar Post-inflammatory hyperpigmentation BMI < 18 Thick skin, higher sebaceous activity	Skin 6 Previous keloid scars
Lifestyle	Healthy life style	Sedentary, hectic lifestyle Binge dieting	No sun protection and overuse of sun beds	Alcohol abuse Recreational drugs use	Smoking (any type) Nicotine replacement
Psychological assessment and patient expectations	Expects scarring Accepts possibility of a poor scarring, including keloid	Expects scarring Hopes for no poor scarring	Expects scarring, which can be easily disguised	Expects scarring but only a minimal	Expects no scar at all

A cumulative score of 5 or below is indicative of low risk for unfavorable scarring and low probability of patient distress with a scar. Scores 6–10 indicate medium risk, scores 11–15 predict high risk, and scores 16–20 very high risk

In summary, a good understanding of the patient's medical history and how this could affect the scar formation process is important for the surgeon's treatment plan, which also helps the patient understand their specific risks. A discussion of these issues is an important part of helping the patient to make an informed decision.

Assessment of Constitutional and Genetic Risks

Being either under- or overweight increases surgical risks, and this also has an effect on postoperative recovery [5]. Patients with one of these characteristics may suffer from nutritional or metabolic abnormalities (or both). Accounting for this before proceeding with a cosmetic surgery is strongly advisable.

Also of note is the specific case for patients who have undergone bariatric surgery to control their weight. These patients often develop a condition of malabsorption and a significant metabolic shift.

For some individuals, there will be inherent familial or racial risks that can contribute to excessive scarring. Although, no specific genetic mechanisms have yet been identified, individuals with the skin type 4–6 on the Fitzpatrick scale are at higher risk for more noticeable scars [6]. Both the *MYH9* gene (coding for a non-muscle myosin) and apolipoprotein1 (APOL1) have been implicated in non-diabetic kidney disease and keloid scarring in people of African descent (see Fig. 45.1). There is a hypothesis that a haplotype *MYH9-APOL1* is likely responsible for keloid formation [7]. Brown et al. [8] found a genetic association between *HLA-DRB1*15* status and the risk of developing keloid scarring in individuals with a pale complexion.

In a practical clinical consultation, the surgeon can simply enquire about ethnicity and make an examination of the patient's skin. Pigmentation tendencies and any previous scars or marks (for example from vaccinations or injections) will help estimate risks. Figure 45.2 illustrates a tendency to form a keloid scar following mesotherapy injections for improving fine décolletage lines.

Note that age plays a role in constitutional scarring tendencies. Older patients with thinner and dryer skin have almost no chance of developing keloid scarring, whereas teenagers with higher sebaceous and cellular activity have a higher chance of developing pronounced scars.

As already stated, poor scarring can negate the benefits of the cosmetic surgery. A careful explanation of the risks is essential before embarking on a procedure.

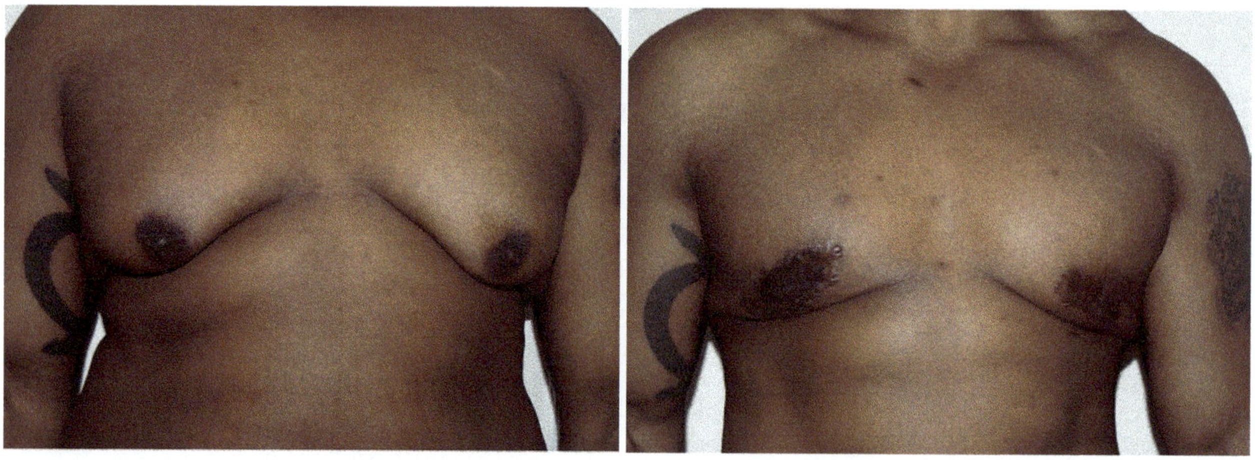

Fig. Unilateral keloid scar formation after gynecomastia and mastopexy surgery in a patient of African origin with skin type 6

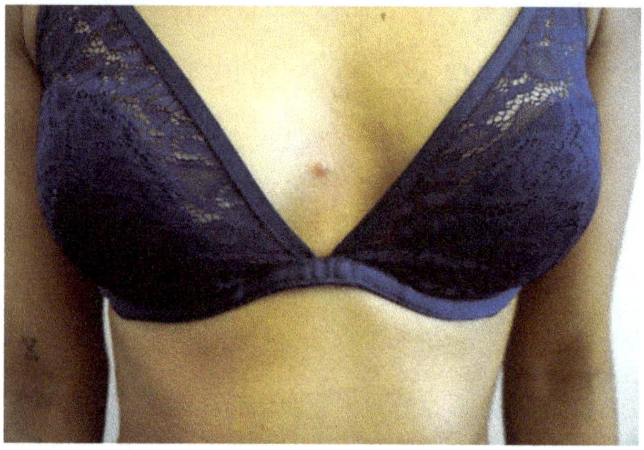

Fig. Nodular keloid scarring after a needle prickle of presternum skin

The patient needs to be fully informed and should have the time to weigh the risks versus the benefits of a procedure. Procedural planning and early preventative interventions can change the balance toward a more acceptable final outcome.

Modification of Lifestyle

A patient's lifestyle choices can have important effects on their postoperative recovery, including scarring. It is important to assess these types of risks and to advise the patient on the steps to be taken before and after surgery. Furthermore, as some patients may not fully follow proposed lifestyle modifications, it is wise for the surgeon to plan on compliance tests and to enter these into the patient's medical record prior to surgery.

It is well known that smoking tobacco products has a detrimental effect in the perioperative period by exposing tissue to the effects of nicotine, carbon monoxide, hydrogen cyanide, and nitric oxide. These all impair wound healing. There are numerous retrospective and prospective cohort studies of levels 2 and 3 evidence demonstrating the relationship between smoking and delayed postoperative healing.

That said, there are studies with level 1 evidence showing ameliorating effects on surgical outcomes when preoperative smoking is discontinued for 4 weeks or longer prior to surgery [9]. When embarking on a smoking cessation protocol, patient compliance should be checked with a carbon monoxide breath or urinary cotinine test just prior to surgery.

Heavy use of alcohol can cause vasodilatation and increase perioperative bleeding. Patients should be advised to refrain from drinking alcoholic beverages for 2 weeks before and after their surgery. A blood test for gamma-glutamyl transferase (GTT) can establish whether a patient is abstaining and compliant with the recommendation.

A balanced diet and supplements of vitamin D, zinc, and iron have a positive impact on postoperative healing.

Substance abuse can have complex effects that potentially include reducing a patient's compliance to preoperative protocols, and this can also decrease their immunity. These types of issues are serious enough; however, it should be noted that in some regulatory contexts, individuals suffering from addictions might not be considered capable of giving a valid consent to cosmetic surgery.

Physically fit, active, and psychologically stable individuals tolerate surgery better and recover faster [10].

In summary, it is important that the patient be informed that their surgical outcome will depend on lifestyle. This should be particularly emphasized for those who need to make changes prior to surgery.

Psychological Assessment and Expectations Management

Evaluating a patient's psychological state of mind can be challenging for cosmetic surgeons; however, it is an essential component of every presurgical consultation. It is important to evaluate a patient's motivations for surgery for several reasons. First, it can give an indication of whether they will be apt to follow the key pre- and postsurgical advice they have been given to optimize their surgical outcomes. Second, it can help identify those patients who may have unreasonable expectations and give an indication of the likelihood of them becoming combative or litigious (regardless of the outcome). Finally, it is a required step in determining whether a patient suffers from body dysmorphic disorder (BDD), which, depending on the regulatory context, could potentially legally disqualify them from surgery.

Psychological assessment and expectations management is a difficult process, especially since most surgeons are not trained in how to do this. There are some common sense steps that can be used without too much difficulty. The first is to look for indicators of psychological imbalance during the consultation process. For example, note whether the patient is overly concerned with minor cosmetic defects. If this is the case, then even the most nominal scarring will likely be unacceptable to the patient.

Show the patient before- and after-photos for a broad spectrum of surgical outcomes, and ask them for feedback on which ones correspond to their hopes and expectations. If the patient indicates a strong preference for an unrealistic outcome for their body type and age, the surgeon should factor this observation into the score.

The consultation process should be used to determine the history of psychological treatments, as well as the patient's history of past cosmetic procedures. Although a patient may hide their psychological care, a physical examination will turn up scars that may be easily associated with past cosmetic surgeries. This can be used to begin a conversation about the patient's satisfaction with past procedures, and what revisions they have undergone.

Finally, the surgeon should always ask the patient for permission to contact their general practitioner (GP) for a confirmation of their medical history. If the patient refuses, this might be a warning flag, although it may simply be due to negative social perceptions of aesthetic surgery. However, if the patient's medical condition or medical history might possibly contraindicate a surgical procedure, it is essential that the patient obtain a letter from their GP indicating that undergoing surgery would be safe.

Realize that no psychological evaluation will be 100% effective. Some patients with psychological issues such as BDD will have learned how to game doctors with credible answers. Nevertheless, the surgeon must make a good effort at trying to provide the patient with an honest assessment while also avoiding harming patients who are at risk. There are some practical tools that can be considered for this.

First, consider making a video recording of all consultations with every patient. This will be the primary record of what was discussed, including facts presented about surgical risks, and indications of the patient's expectations.

Make liberal use of before- and after-photos. It can be quite difficult to understand a patient's perspective, and it is equally difficult for a patient to understand the likely outcomes without concrete examples. Particularly important is the patient's appreciation of scarring patterns and their acceptance of their inevitability. The before- and after-photos present an excellent opportunity for gauging the patient's sentiments on scarring.

Asking the patient for permission to contact their GP is an important step of the consultation process. The GP can often provide relevant information about the patient's medical history that is relevant to the safety of a surgical procedure.

Finally, it is worthwhile to be abreast of psychological risk factors for various segments of the population and to fold such statistics into the patient's overall evaluation. For example, some patients might not be open about their true motives for cosmetic interventions, and in some contexts, their aims might be controversial [11]. Recognized factors associated with a poor psychosocial outcome of aesthetic surgery include [12] the following:

- Being of a young age and of male gender
- Having unrealistic expectations of the procedure
- Having had previous unsatisfactory cosmetic treatments
- Exhibiting minimal deformity
- Motivations based on relationship issues
- A history of depression, anxiety, or personality disorder

For cases where the surgeon has a serious doubt about a patient, it makes sense to defer surgery while collecting more data. The surgeon can insist on a letter from the GP stating their opinion that it would be safe for the patient to undergo surgery. In highly borderline cases, it might make sense to ask the patient to undergo a psychological assessment before proceeding with treatment.

Prophylactic Measures in Cosmetic Surgery to Reduce Excessive Scarring

Scarring is an inevitable result of all surgeries; however, as already discussed, patients will be more critical and less accepting of scars from cosmetic procedures than for those obtained after surgeries for illness or injury. Even after extensive preoperative counseling, patients typically do not fully appreciate the realities of scarring. This means that cosmetic surgeons should make every effort to minimize scarring by utilizing all available tools and methods to optimize healing. This section reviews a range of current options.

Choice of Surgical Techniques

Careful planning is the best approach to achieving success for any surgery, and this is especially true for elective cosmetic procedures. The following discussion provides a list of points that should be planned for prior to surgery.

Meticulous surgical field preparation and antibacterial prophylaxis are crucial in mitigating risk of infection. Infiltration with local anesthetic and adrenaline, combined with a careful hemostasis, will help reduce bleeding during and after the operation. Both infection and hemorrhage can be detrimental to wound healing and should be avoided at all cost.

The surgeon must take care not to damage vascular dermal plexus when undermining skin and take into account blood supply via a vascular pedicle when lifting flaps and cutting through tissues. Inadvertently damaging local circulatory pathways will lead to skin necrosis and devastating consequences.

Incisions should be made bearing in mind the natural skin tension vectors. Avoiding crossing these will diminish the likelihood of wound dehiscence, scar widening, or hypertrophy. Similarly, avoid areas with tight skin such as the presternal, upper shoulders, and over the extensor surfaces of joints [13].

Try to strategically hide scars by placing incisions as much as possible in the natural creases of the skin or where imperfections can be disguised by clothing.

Finally, a cosmetic surgeon must handle tissues gently, approximate edges of the wound carefully, and make use of fine instruments and suturing materials. While closing tissue incisions, a surgeon should bear in mind how the tensile strength of the wound will evolve during the healing process. The tension strength of the wound, related to cross-linking of collagen, will only be 3% of that of a normal skin after roughly 1 week, 30% after 3 weeks, and 80% after about 12 weeks [14]. This should be reflected in the choice of suturing techniques and materials. Non-absorbable sutures can be removed after 7–10 days, but appropriate additional scar holdup is required during the first 3 months with adhesive tapes, dressings, and garments.

Methods to Control Better Healing

Postsurgical techniques to influence and optimize scar formation are varied. Some methods are well established, while others are still experimental. A brief review of modalities currently in use is summarized here.

- Compression garments to reinforce tensile strength across a wound and to reduce stretching and friction
- Adhesive tapes and plasters
- Topical flavonoids
- Botulinum neurotoxin type A (BoNTA)
- Platelet-rich plasma (PRP)
- Microneedling + topical applications
- Imiquimod
- Bioengineering and recombinant DNA

The first step in postsurgical scar optimization is the use of compression therapy. Although the effects are poorly understood, compression keeps wounds reinforced and prevents both stretching and friction. A wide range of compression and support garments are available. Pressure levels should be sustained at 15–40 mmHg for at least 23 h/day over a period of 6 months. This presents, however, a problem of patient compliance due to restrictiveness of such a regime.

This can be managed with the use of various adhesive tapes and plasters to cover the already closed wounds. These keep the scar undisturbed and protected and can be more comfortably used over a longer period of time. A randomized controlled study of 70 patients using a paper tape on their wounds showed this to be an effective strategy [15].

More specialized dressings and skin substitutes can be utilized to promote epithelization by creating matrix for a cellular migration, providing a protective barrier, and sustaining a moist environment. Silicone gel and sheets have been shown to reduce unfavorable scarring in randomized controlled studies [16, 17], but a meta-analysis of 13 trials involving 559 patients demonstrated only weak evidence that silicone can reduce the incidence of abnormal scarring in high-risk individuals [18]. That said, silicone softens the scar and makes it more comfortable for patients, and because of this, it may be worthwhile. It is recommended to use silicone dressing for at least 12 h a day for 2 months from 2 weeks after the surgery.

Topical flavonoids such as Contractubex (Merz Pharma, Frankfurt, Germany) or Mederma skin care gel (Merz Pharmaceutical, Greensboro, CA, USA) are used to keep scars soft and supple from the second week after surgery for up to 6 months. Their efficacy has been found to be controversial, but the dietary bioflavonoid quercetin can also improve scarring by suppressing fibroblasts proliferation via inhibition of SMAD intercellular transduction protein [19]. This reduces the actions of the transforming growth factor β (TGF-β) and reduces fibroblasts activity.

In clinical practice, cosmetic surgeons can use botulinum neurotoxin type A (BoNTA) immediately after wound closure. Injections of 15U of the preparation have been shown to improve scarring following 6 weeks after a facelift [20].

Platelet-rich plasma (PRP) has gained some popularity for skin anti-aging, chronic wound management, and scar therapy. Treating a wound bed with PRP has shown substantial benefits for better wound healing, an increased survival of fat grafts, and the acceleration of cartilage and bone grafts uptake in a systematic review of 15 randomized controlled trials and 25 case-controlled studies [21]. Platelet-rich fibrin also proved to be useful in aesthetic and reconstructive applications.

Also note that the repeated microneedling at a controlled depth and topical application of retinol and marine collagen reversed both atrophic and hypertrophic scars to a more even appearance after a year of treatment [22].

Attempts have been made to use Imiquimod 5% cream to prevent keloid recurrence after surgical excision. This topical immune-response modulator stimulates a proinflammatory cytokine interferon, which increases collagen breakdown. Imiquimod also alters the effects of apoptosis-associated genes. The preparation was used daily for a fortnight after a surgery. Later it was applied three times a week under a dressing for 1 month. The efficacy for this prophylaxis is still questionable, as the result of this double-blinded, placebo-controlled pilot study showed no significant difference in keloid deposition rates in the two groups [23].

Interesting research in tissue bioengineering is attempting to bring new methods to improved wound healing, with an objective of even achieving scarless regeneration. Promising results have been obtained using therapies based on TGF-β. A preparation of a recombinant version of this cytokine marketed as Juvista by Renovo Laboratory (Manchester, UK) has shown a 70% improvement in wound healing and scar appearance in a phase 2 trial. Other therapies developed by the same company include formulations of mannose-6-phosphate (M6P; marketed as Juvidex) and another preparation based on estradiol (marketed as Zesteem) [24].

In another study, a preparation of recombinant human TGF-β3, called avotermin, was injected before the skin was cut and again 24 h after wounding in healthy participants. A dose of 50 ng/100 μl of the drug per linear centimeter achieved 10% scar improvement in three double-blinded, placebo-controlled studies. However, the investigators had commercial interests in TGF-β3, which may weaken their claim. Nevertheless, they demonstrated a strict adherence to established protocols and research standards and conducted a rigorous statistical analysis [25].

Whatever methods be used to prevent unfavorable scarring, they must be initiated early enough to influence the processes of tissue healing. Failure to do so might lead to florid scarring that might subsequently be more difficult to treat.

Treatment of Scars Following Aesthetic Surgery

Pronounced scarring following surgery is common. Up to 40% might display hypertrophic scar features, and 6–16% of these will evolve into a keloid scar (especially for patients of African descent). Scar atrophy can result from wound infection and inflammation, but it is less common.

If, after all other precautions, a scar begins to display features of pathological healing, or is simply too noticeable, treatment plans are still available and can do much to remediate the situation. Management of scars after aesthetic surgery does not differ from any other scar treatment. The therapeutic approach can be divided into surgical and non-surgical methods.

Surgical Treatments

Traditionally, keloid and hypertrophic scars are excised, and tissue is manipulated to allow for more favorable healing afterward. Excision with a linear, tension-free closure should be used. If the defect is a large one, or the wound is in a high skin-tension area, a split- or full-thickness skin grafting with Z-plasty or W-plasty skin closure flaps is recommended (◘ Fig. 45.3). That said, hypertrophic scars tend to spontaneously regress for up to 12 months. This suggests that surgical revisions should probably not be made until after a 1-year time window.

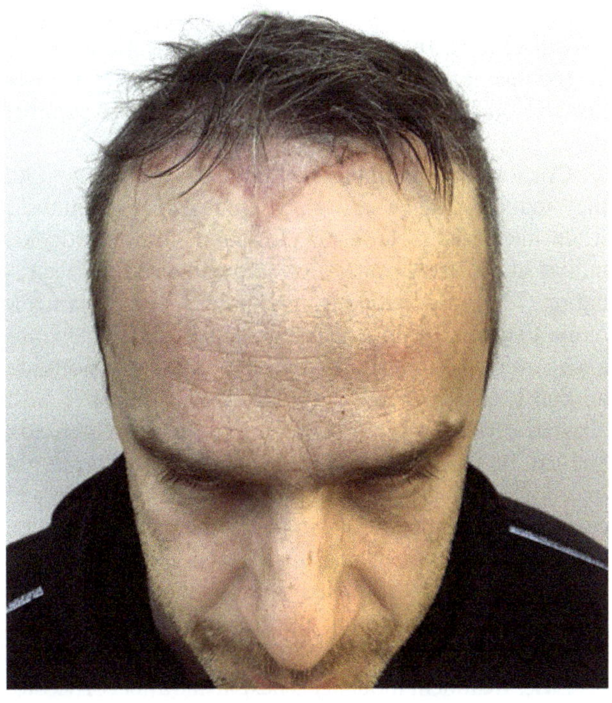

◘ **Fig.** Skin flap closure with W-plasty following a forehead lift with hair line advancement surgery

Hypertrophic scars rarely recur after excision, and as such, they require no adjuvant treatments following the removal. Keloid scars on the other hand can redevelop after excision. This will occur in more than half of all cases, and so will likely require additional therapeutic interventions. This should be undertaken immediately after their excision.

The most commonly used methods for controlling keloid scar recurrence include corticosteroid injections or radiotherapy. In recent years, a mixture of 5 fluorouracil (5FU) with triamcinolone has become popular. The cocktail is made of 3 ml of 5FU 50 mg/ml and 1 ml of the steroid containing 40 mg/ml triamcinolone. An amount of 1–2 ml of this mixture is used for postoperative tissue infiltration at the level of excision plane and below it. The treatment can be repeated after full epithelization of the wound. Postoperative pressure should be applied for 6 months afterward, and silicone gel should be used for 2 months.

Non-surgical Treatments

A broad range of treatments with no cutting of scars is available for cosmetic surgeons. Therapeutic choices vary from injectable preparations to interventions based on a variety of technologies. Whatever method is being employed, it should be done in a timely fashion with stepwise escalation to the next option if the current one is ineffective.

The first choice of non-surgical treatment for early keloid formation scars is intra-lesional corticosteroid injections. In most cases, steroid injections act as a second-line modality for hypertrophic scars if less-invasive options, such as silicone dressings and support tapes, fail.

Corticosteroids suppress inflammation in the wound; they reduce collagen and glycosaminoglycans synthesis, while increasing collagen degradation. Glucocorticoids inhibit fibroblasts proliferation and enhance their degradation. The most commonly used preparation is triamcinolone 40 mg/ml. A dose of 10 mg or 40 mg is injected into a scar, every 1–2 months. Usually two to three sessions are all that is required. Scars become flatter and softer with alleviation of symptoms, but a recurrence rate is common and can be as high as 50%. Side effects of corticosteroid injections are telangiectasia and dermal atrophy. Topical corticosteroid preparations in the form of creams can be massaged into post-blepharoplasty scars. Corticosteroid tapes are sometimes applied after aesthetic surgery for breast reduction. However, efficacy of topical corticosteroids for scar reduction has never been proven.

Laser treatment modality is next in line after corticosteroids. Pulsed-dye laser (PDL) with a wavelength of 585 nm is most commonly used for treating scars as a stand-alone intervention or in addition to other treatments. Pulse-shots at a fluency of 3.5–5.5 J/cm^2 are fired to cover the entire scar, making sure the shots do not overlap. Treatments are repeated four to six times every 3 weeks. Hyper- and hypopigmentation, blistering, and small bruises are possible after the treatment but tend to be transient.

It is sometimes possible to destroy scar tissue by subjecting it to subzero temperatures. For example, cryotherapy with liquid nitrogen is an option. Rarely used to improve scars caused by cosmetic surgery, it can be nevertheless be useful for pretreatment before repeating injections of corticosteroids in smaller scars. This is especially the case if laser is unavailable or has proven to be ineffective.

Recalcitrant scars can be subjected to radiotherapy. This method is mostly combined with the surgical excisions but is rarely used in aesthetic practice. The methods of radiotherapy choice include superficial X-rays, electron beam therapy, and low or high-dose-rate brachytherapy. They all can be utilized, but not for breast or tummy tuck scars due to their potential for carcinogenic side effects.

Atrophic tissue healing is another type of pathological scarring, leading to a volume loss and an indented surface formation. The treatment objective is to restore the tissue deficit and to reinforce thinning and hollowing of the scar surface. For the former, corrections are made with fillers and fat grafts. The latter can be achieved with stimulating therapies such as microneedling, Sculptra injections, free-floating PDO, or gold threads. An example study using a controlled depth microneedling approach proved to be effective for both atrophic and hypertrophic scars [22]. Early keloid scars can also respond to this type of intervention (◘ Fig. 45.4). This suggests that all pathological scars may have similar pathways for regression.

Another promising modality for treatment of scarring is botulinum neurotoxin type A (BoNTA). Keloid can be treated successfully with diluted BoNTA and the technique for that is described in ▶ Chap. 8.

Long-Term Management of Patients with Scars After Cosmetic Surgery

Even with a conscientious effort made by both the patient and the surgeon to control and optimize scarring, some patients will find it difficult to accept their outcomes. These patients may be especially psychologically vulnerable if their scars are located in areas easily seen. Examples include the eyelids after a blepharoplasty or in front of the ears after pretragal incision used during rhytidectomies.

The surgeon has some responsibility to help these types of patients come to terms with their scars. The

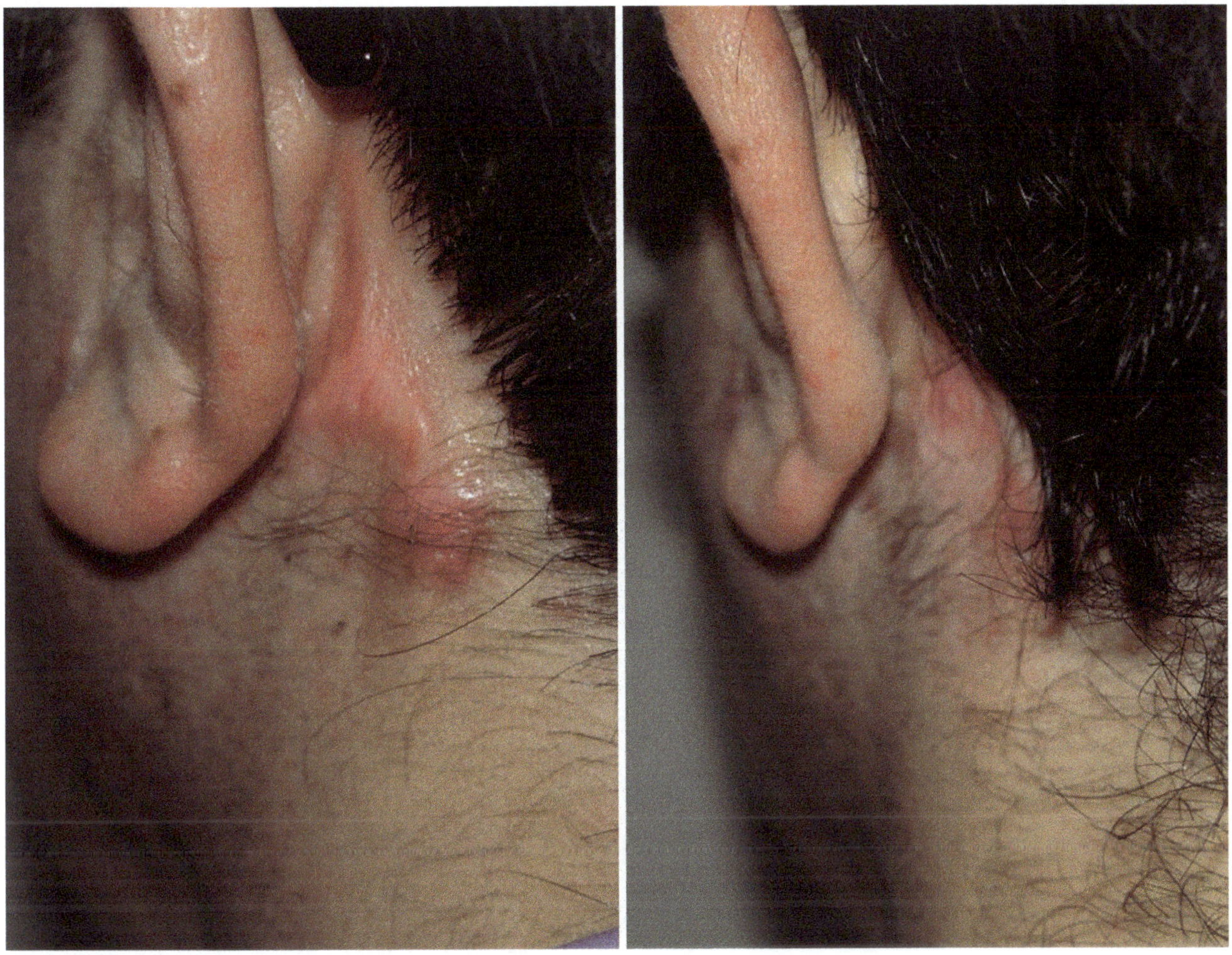

Fig. Keloid scar following rhytidectomy was improved by using microneedling and topical retinol

process will likely involve a combination of approaches, including counseling, cognitive behavioral therapy, camouflage makeup, and medical tattooing. A multidisciplinary approach to the psychological rehabilitation of the patient will likely be needed to succeed. The surgeon should be empathetic to the patient's perspective and be prepared to help with what can often be a lengthy and arduous process.

Conclusion

Scarring after cosmetic surgery is the same as that from accidents, disease, or other types of surgical procedures. The context, however, is completely different. Patients primarily choose aesthetic surgery for non-essential health reasons. Because of this, when poor scarring occurs, cosmetic surgeons are at much higher risk for patient dissatisfaction and potential legal action.

A wide variety of therapeutic and prophylactic methods are available for the management of posttraumatic and postsurgical cicatrix. Thus, the main point of this chapter is that surgeons should put into place pre-, intra-, and postsurgical processes to mitigate scarring risks.

Finally, regardless of the objective severity of cosmetic surgical scars, this is an important component of a patient's perception of the success of the procedure. Surgeons should take an active role in providing patients with information and compassionate support.

Take-Home Messages

- Always bear in mind that a scar following aesthetic surgery impacts a patient far more than its objective evaluation and it negatively contributes to the overall perception of otherwise successful treatment.
- Carefully evaluate the potential risk of scarring and take appropriate measures to reduce it prior to surgery.
- Manage patient expectations by providing sufficient explanation of the range of potential outcomes.
- Avoid offering elective cosmetic surgery to people at high risk of very poor scarring or to those with highly unreasonable expectations.
- Plan and execute an appropriate surgical technique.
- Employ prophylactic measures and treatments in a timely fashion.
- Take active measures to minimize the formation of keloid and hypertrophic or atrophic scarring should they occur.
- Keep careful records (written and video) of the consultation process, surgical techniques, and postsurgical treatments, making specific mention of the management of scarring.
- Provide emotional and medical support to a patient, who is troubled by a scar after her or his aesthetic surgery.

References

1. International Society of Aesthetic Plastic Surgery (ISAPS) Statistics 27 June 2017, Hanover, Germany. https://www.isaps.org/wpcontent/uploads/2017/10/GlobalStatistics.PressRelease.
2. Stewart KJ, Stewart DA, Coghlan B, Harrison DH, Jones BM, Waterhouse N. Complications of 278 consecutive abdominoplasties. J Plast Reconstr Aesthet Surg. 2006;59(11):1152–5.
3. Nava MB, Rancati A, Angrigiani C, Catanuto G, Rocco N. How to prevent complications in breast augmentation. Gland Surg. 2017;6(2):210.
4. Stone C. Scar revision costs, Unsightly Claims. Personal Inj Law J. 2011:15–9. https://www.medicalandlegal.co.uk/wp-content/uploads/2012/05/Scar-Revision-cost-in-Personal-Injury-Law-Journal.pdf.
5. Saldanha O, Salles A, Llaverias F, Saldanha C. Predictive factors for complications in plastic surgery procedures-suggested safety scores. Rev Bras Cir Plást. 2001;29(1):105–13.
6. Bayat A, Bock O, Mrowietz U, Ollier WE, Ferguson MW. Genetic susceptibility to keloid disease and hypertrophic scarring: transforming growth factor beta1 common polymorphisms and plasma levels. Plast Reconstr Surg. 2003;111(2):535–43.
7. Keeling BH, Taylor BR. Keloids and non-diabetic kidney disease: similarities and the APOL1–MYH9 haplotype as a possible genetic link. Med Hypotheses. 2013;81(5):908–10.
8. Brown JJ, Ollier WE, Thomson W, Bayat A. Positive association of HLA-DRB1*15 with keloid disease in Caucasians. Int J Immunogenet. 2008;35(4–5):303–7.
9. Rinker B. The evils of nicotine: an evidence-based guide to smoking and plastic surgery. Ann Plast Surg. 2013;70(5):599–605.
10. Levett DZ, Edwards M, Grocott M, Mythen M. Preparing the patient for surgery to improve outcomes. Best Pract Res Clin Anaesthesiol. 2016;30(2):145–57.
11. Macgregor FC. Selection of cosmetic surgery patients: social and psychological considerations. Surg Clin N Am. 1971;51(2):289–98.
12. Honigman RJ, Phillips KA, Castle DJ. A review of psychosocial outcomes for patients seeking cosmetic surgery. Plast Reconstr Surg. 2004;113(4):1229.
13. Son D, Harijan A. Overview of surgical scar prevention and management. J Korean Med Sci. 2014;29(6):751–7.
14. Buchanan PJ, Kung TA, Cederna PS. Evidence-based medicine: wound closure. Plast Reconstr Surg. 2016;138(3S):257S–70S.
15. Atkinson JA, McKenna KT, Barnett AG, McGrath DJ, Rudd M. A randomized, controlled trial to determine the efficacy of paper tape in preventing hypertrophic scar formation in surgical incisions that traverse Langer's skin tension lines. Plast Reconstr Surg. 2005;116(6):1648–56.
16. Gold MH, Foster TD, Adair MA, Burlison K, Lewis T. Prevention of hypertrophic scars and keloids by the prophylactic use of topical silicone gel sheets following a surgical procedure in an office setting. Dermatol Surg. 2001;27(7):641–4.
17. Chan KY, Lau CL, Adeeb SM, Somasundaram S, Nasir-Zahari M. A randomized, placebo-controlled, double-blind, prospective clinical trial of silicone gel in prevention of hypertrophic scar development in median sternotomy wound. Plast Reconstr Surg. 2005;116(4):1013–20.
18. O'Brien L, Pandit A. Silicon gel sheeting for preventing and treating hypertrophic and keloid scars. Cochrane Database Syst Rev. 2006;(1):CD003826.
19. Phan TT, Lim IJ, Sun L, Chan SY, Bay BH, Tan EK, Lee ST. Quercetin inhibits fibronectin production by keloid-derived fibroblasts. Implication for the treatment of excessive scars. J Dermatol Sci. 2003;33(3):192–4.
20. Chambers A. Effects of botulinum toxin a observed during early scar formation following rhytidectomy: controlled, double-blinded pilot study. Am J Cosmet Surg. 2018;36(2):78–84.
21. Sommeling CE, Heyneman A, Hoeksema H, Verbelen J, Stillaert FB, Monstrey S. The use of platelet-rich plasma in plastic surgery: a systematic review. J Plast Reconstr Aesthet Surg. 2013;66(3):301–11.
22. Chambers A. Unified approach to the treatment of hypertrophic and atrophic scars: a pilot study. Am J Cosmet Surg. 2016;33(4):176–83.
23. Berman B, Harrison-Balestra C, Perez OA, Viera M, Villa A, Zell D, Ramirez C. Treatment of keloid scars post-shave excision with imiquimod 5% cream: a prospective, double-blind, placebo-controlled pilot study. J Drugs Dermatol. 2009;8(5):455–8.
24. Rhett JM, Ghatnekar GS, Palatinus JA, O'Quinn M, Yost MJ, Gourdie RG. Novel therapies for scar reduction and regenerative healing of skin wounds. Trends Biotechnol. 2008;26(4):173–80.
25. Bush J, So K, Mason T, Occleston NL, O'Kane S, Ferguson MW. Therapies with emerging evidence of efficacy: avotermin for the improvement of scarring. Dermatol Res Pract. 2010;2010:690613.

18

Clinical Case: Earlobe Keloid

Luc Téot

Contents

Medical History

Medical History

A 23-year-old Asian-origin young male came after a long period of keloid of the left ear, secondary to a minor trauma during childhood. The patient was treated by three sequential surgical excisions followed by a recurrence, the last one being followed by YAG laser.

The patient abandoned the possibility to be adequately treated by any therapy during 7 years and was examined at the clinic (◘ Figs. 61.1 and 61.2).

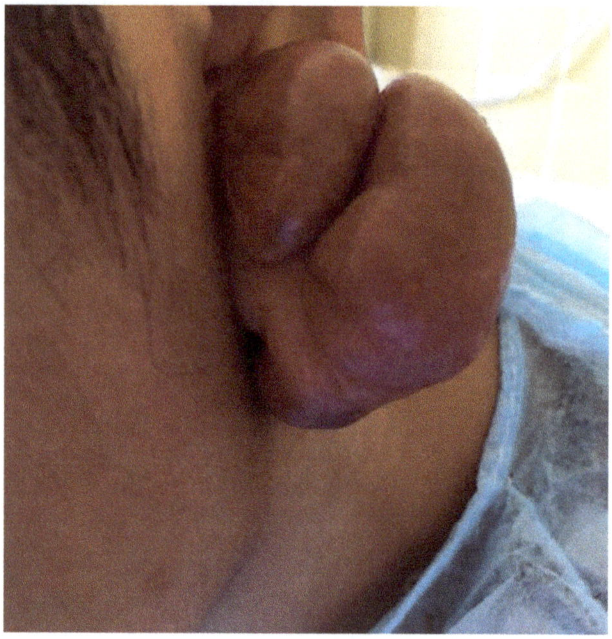

◘ **Fig.** Earlobe keloid at presentation (anterior view)

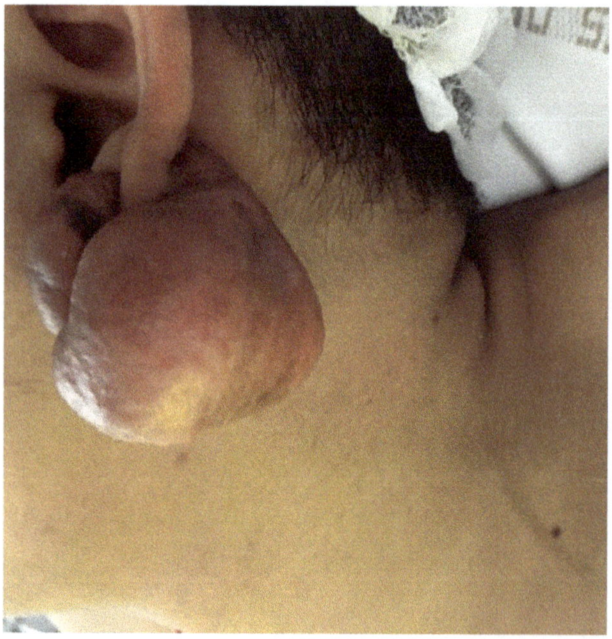

◘ **Fig.** Earlobe keloid at presentation (posterior view)

❓ Questions to Medical History

- Is Asian origin a predetermining factor for earlobe keloid?
- Is keloid growing permanently or does it stop with age?
- Is there any guideline for surgical management of keloid?

▪▪ Intervention 1

A series of 10 5-FU injections (5 mL) at a dosage of 50 mg/mL was administered at 3 weeks of interval.

The procedure was standardized as follows:

- EMLA cream application 2 hours before injection
- MEOPA (hilarant gas able to disconnect the patient from pain) administration during injection
- Hypnose adjuvant therapy during injection (hypnose works to deviate the attention of the patient and present a growing interest particularly on patients submitted repeatedly to painful stimulation) (◘ Figs. 61.3 and 61.4)

❓ Questions: Procedure 1

- Why 5-FU injections instead of corticosteroid injection?
- What is the rationale of the dose (50 mg/mL)?
- How painful is the procedure?

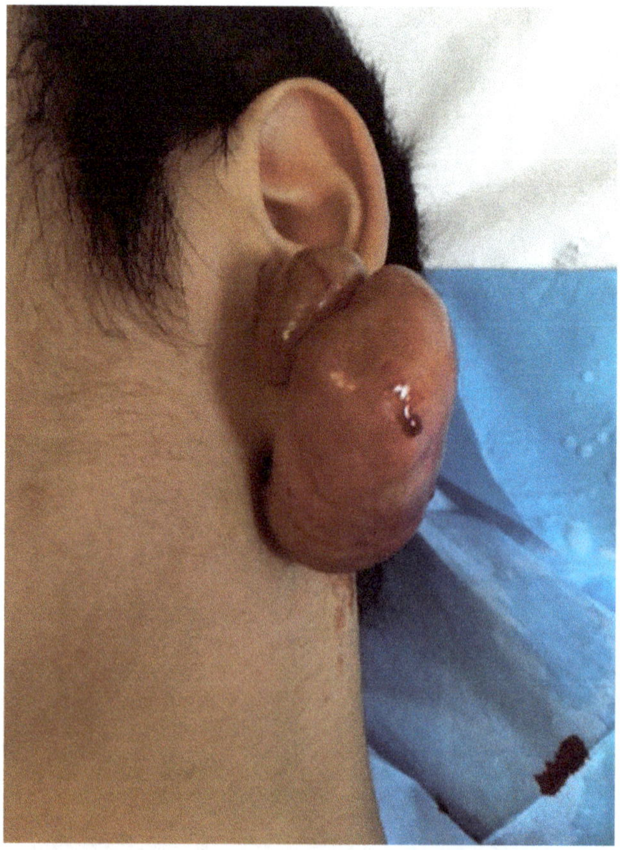

◘ **Fig.** Inflammatory aspect during 5-FU injections (anterior view)

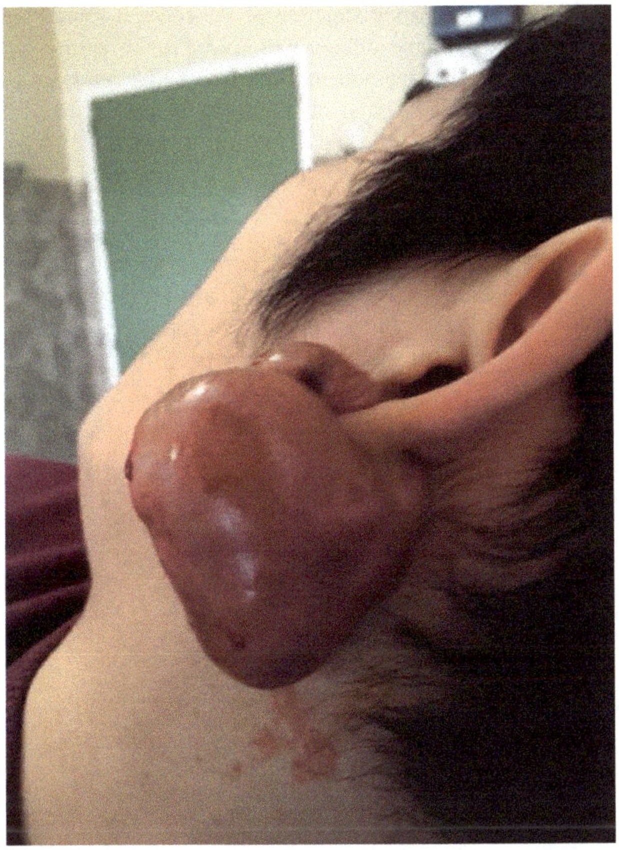

Fig. Inflammatory aspect during 5-FU injections (posterior view)

Intervention 2

A surgical excision was administered with reconstruction of the earlobe with a combined approach anteriorly and posteriorly to the earlobe. A compression was made at fashion to ensure the mechanical situation during the 12 months postoperative period. The results were good with no recurrence. The scar presented redness after 3 months postoperation and then this inflammation was resolutive with time (Figs. 61.5 and 61.6).

Late Postintervention Questions

- Why to choose not to apply any postoperative therapy?
- What about the loss of substance of the ear?
- Is there a need for complementary surgery?
- Is further surgery contraindicated?

Answers

The prevalence of earlobe keloid is higher in the Asian skin than in the Caucasian skin even if the global risk of keloid is higher in the black-skin population. Keloids are, contrary to hypertrophic scars, growing permanently, reaching enormous sizes when left apart without adapted treatment.

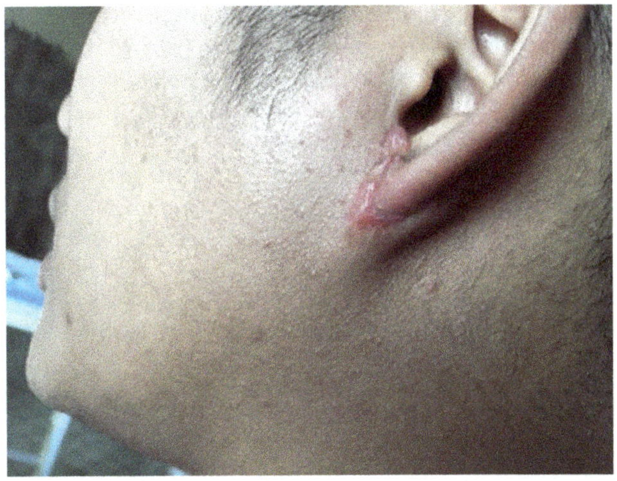

Fig. Aspect of the ear 3 months postopertion, and some inflammation is still present

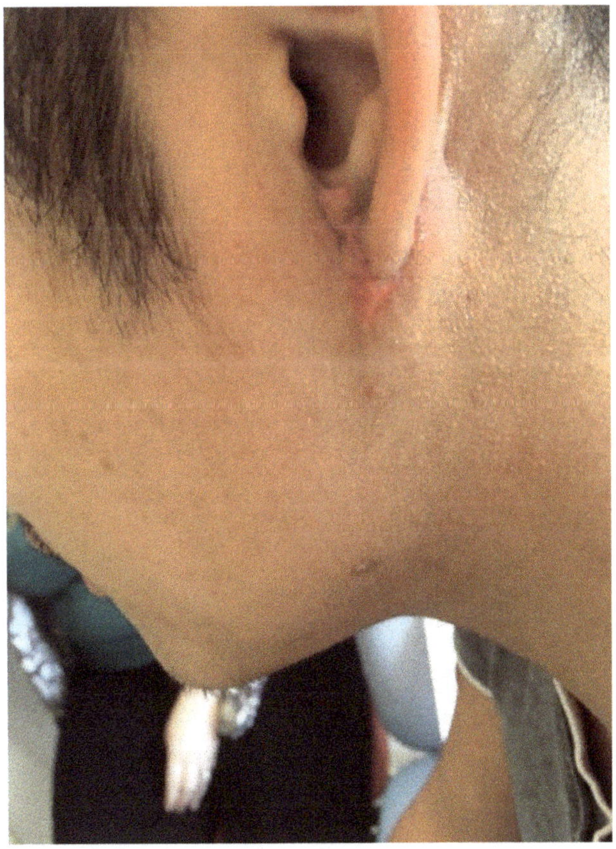

Fig. Aspect at 14 months postoperation: the scar is stable and no recurrence occurred

Guidelines of surgical scar management mention the need for a combination of techniques, and most of them are being proposed after surgery (radiotherapy, cryotherapy, laser). Cryotherapy has also been proposed as an alternative to surgery. In this case the preoperative management using antimitotic agents was proposed to limit the fibroblast postoperative proliferation 5-FU is used at a high dose (50 mg/mL) as suggested by several authors without systemic complications and the rhythm of injections (every 3 weeks) limits the risk of local skin necrosis.

This strategy limits the risk of recurrence after surgery and is proposed as a new option, in combination with preoperative injections and a close checkup of the local situation during 1 year.

The major inconvenience is pain induced by the injection, and pain management needs combined therapies (EMLA, MEOPA, Hypnose). During the surgical procedure the loss of substance of the earlobe had to be treated by reapproximation of the edges, a source of limited cosmetic difference compared to the contralateral side, but the patient refused to be reoperated, considering the high risk of worsening of the scar and of recurrence of the keloid.

Take Home Message

This clinical case reports the interest of a combined strategy using sequential intralesional chemotherapy before surgery in order to limit the rebund effect in highly proliferative ear keloids.

19

Scars in Pediatric Patients

Anne Le Touze

Contents

Introduction/Background

Healing Specificities in Children
Fetal Healing
Pediatric Peculiarities in Healing
How to Manage Wound Healing in Children

Pathological Scars
Clinical and Histological Aspects
Easing Factors
Prevention and Treatment

Defective or Disgracious Scars

Scars and Growth

Conclusion

References

Introduction/Background

A child is not a miniature adult. Although physiological healing process is not different in children, their growth potential gives them some specificities in terms of healing and scaring. Disturbance of healing process or inappropriate wound treatment will lead to pathologic scar. Pathologic scars can disrupt growth in children.

Healing Specificities in Children

Fetal Healing

Experimental and clinical studies point that fetal healing is scarless [1]. Fetal healing mechanisms are still poorly known, although many endogenous and exogenous factors seem to differ from those of adult healing mechanisms. The main difference probably lies at the level of the immune system and the inflammatory response. All these studies concern different animal species and any extrapolation towards human species should be cautious.

Macrophages are known to be the major agents of the inflammatory response and tissue regeneration process in adults. In early gestation, healing process is accomplished with poor influx of macrophages, while the influx of macrophages in the wound is more important at the end of gestation [2]. The embryo seems to be able to heal without macrophages, and therefore without undergoing inflammatory response. Nevertheless, the embryo is able to respond to inflammatory stimuli [3]. Explanation for this paradox could be the immaturity of the inflammatory system, but we need further exploration to understand this ambiguity.

Collagen is scarce in the healing wound due to the lack of response of the fibroblasts to transforming growth factor beta 1 (TGFβ1). TGFβ1 induces glycosaminoglycan synthesis all along gestation: glycosaminoglycan is much more important than collagen in the scar matrix in fetus [4].

Amniotic fluid provides the fetus with an environment rich in growth factors necessary for its development. High concentration of hyaluronic acid in the amniotic fluid has been supposed to be the extrinsic and intrinsic factor of non-inflammatory fetal healing [5]. Further experimental studies need to prove that the quality of fetal wound healing is due to intrinsic factors [6]. Even if scarless fetal healing mechanisms are uncertain, absence of inflammatory response seems to be the key point.

Nevertheless, at the end of gestation, inflammatory response appears and scar becomes visible. Further exploration of fetal healing and better knowledge should allow for promising clinical applications.

Pediatric Peculiarities in Healing

Very few data on this subject is available in the literature. Nevertheless, "healing behavior" is peculiar and varies all along childhood [7].

- 0–6 months

  Infants before the age of 6 months heal very fast and with very discreet scar. It happens as if the inflammatory response was immature, therefore attenuated. Perhaps some phenomena of prenatal period are perpetuated after birth.
- 2 years – teenage

  On the contrary, the inflammatory expression of the scar dominates this period, and the phenomena of remodeling seem amplified, major, and disabling. The few comorbidities of healthy organisms and the physiological mechanisms linked to growth are an undeniable asset for the good evolution of the child's wounds. Scarring is often very fast but can be explosive. Hypertrophic scaring could be considered as physiological at this age, as it is constant.
- 6 months – 2 years

  The evolutive pattern of scar is unpredictable at this age, sometimes still discreet, sometimes already very inflammatory.

How to Manage Wound Healing in Children

As the inflammatory response is constant and "explosive," the healing process must be carried out over a short period of time to prevent excessive production of collagen.

Except for children under palliative care, most of the wounds can undergo surgery: mechanical cleansing, suturing, grafting, flaps. Before, instead of or after surgery, we use dressings or negative pressure wound therapy (NPWT).

Management of pain is essential and difficult: pain and fear are often entangled; level 2 painkillers are not recommended before 12 years old. Therefore, level 3 painkillers are often necessary but to be administrated in health institutions. Inhalation of 50–50% N_2O–O_2 mixture and any adjuvant technique of analgesia may be useful (hypnoanalgesia, video distraction, virtual reality, etc.) [8, 9].

Surgical techniques have to be adapted according to age, psychomotor development, thickness of teguments, and potential of growth. Thinner sutures are used with young children. Rapid absorbable sutures that generate an inflammatory response are to be avoided on exposed areas. On the contrary, intradermal slow absorbable sutures are a good option to avoid marks. Cyanoacrylate

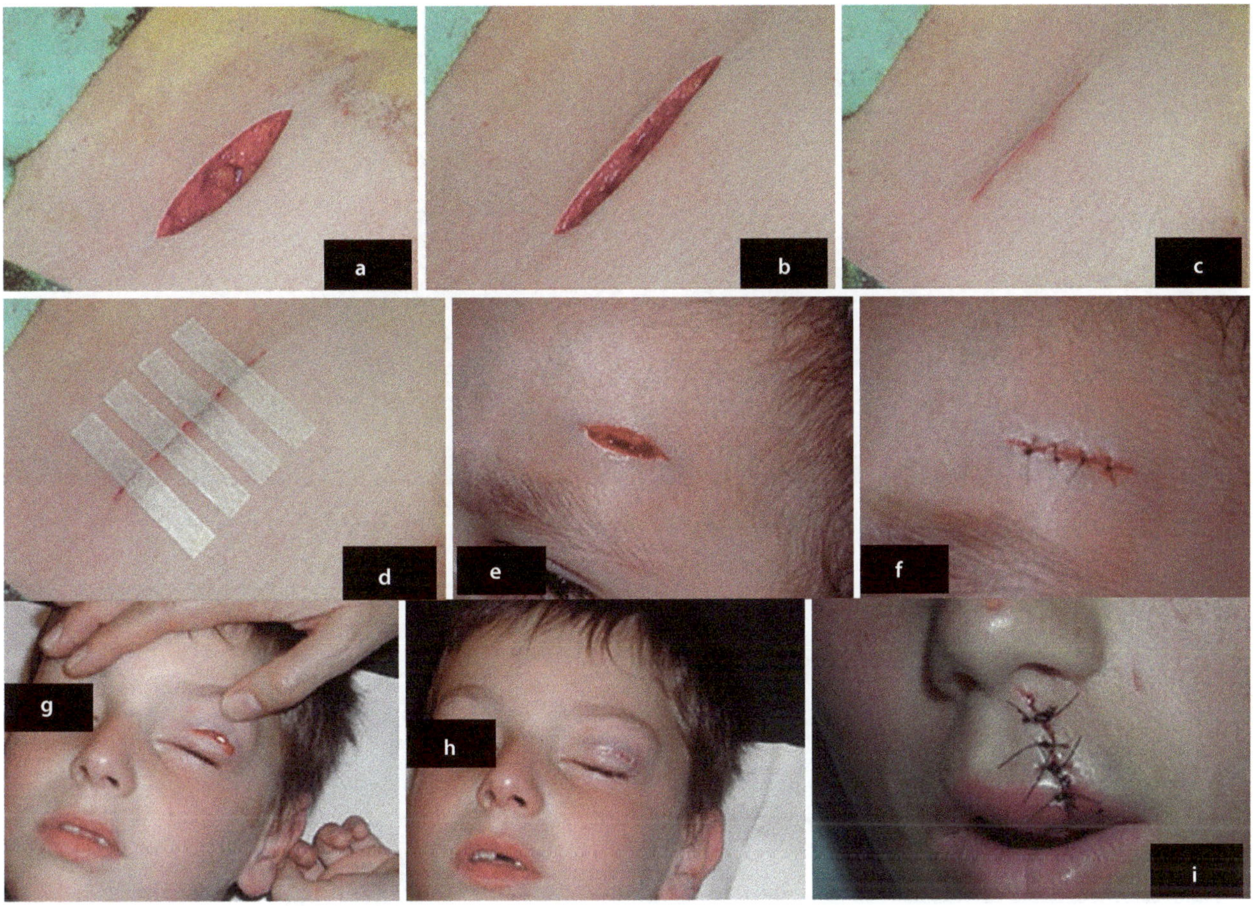

Fig. a–d: Good-quality intradermal suture; **e** and **f**: good-quality epidermal suture; **g** and **h**: cyanoacrylate tissue adhesive; **i**: poor-quality epidermal suture, too thick sutures and under wedging

tissue adhesive may be used but is appropriated for very superficial wounds (Fig. 46.1).

Dressings have to be painless at removal, easy to apply. It is better to realize dressing with hand rather than with forceps because it is quicker and less frightening. Topics should be elementary; healing is rarely a problem in pediatric practice as child's body continuously synthesizes tissue for growth. Therefore, NPWT is most often rapidly effective, preparing wound to be grafted. Flap indications are therefore less frequent in pediatric practice than in adult practice.

Pathological Scars

Scar is the result of the healing process. Ideal scar is thin, flat, white, supple, elastic, and painless, but it exists and is perfectly identifiable under microscope (Fig. 46.2).

Pathological scars are due to dysregulation of healing phenomena, especially due to the dysregulation that occurs during the modeling phase. This results in prolonged or definitive inflammation and are called hypertrophic or keloid scars [10].

Clinical and Histological Aspects

At the beginning of their evolution, it is not possible to distinguish hypertrophic scars from keloid scars: both remain very inflammatory beyond the normal period, red, hot, tense, and itchy. Only the evolution can distinguish them (Fig. 46.3).

- Hypertrophic scar: despite a marked and prolonged inflammation period, the inflammatory signs will eventually be amended, leading to scar enlargement and fibrosis resulting in a thick scar. Histologically, collagen is abundant, is immature (collagen III in excess), is organized in more flat bundles than in a normal dermis, and contains nodules. Secretion of transforming growth factor β (TGFβ) and platelet derived growth factor (PDGF) is abundant. Fibroblasts are numerous, responsible for the secretion of collagen in excess. Mast cells are numerous, secreting histamine which is probably responsible for pruritus.
- Keloid scar: evolution goes on forever, leading to extension of lesions beyond the initial limits of the scar, with persistence of inflammatory signs. Sometimes, telangiectasia appears at the surface of the scar. Histologically,

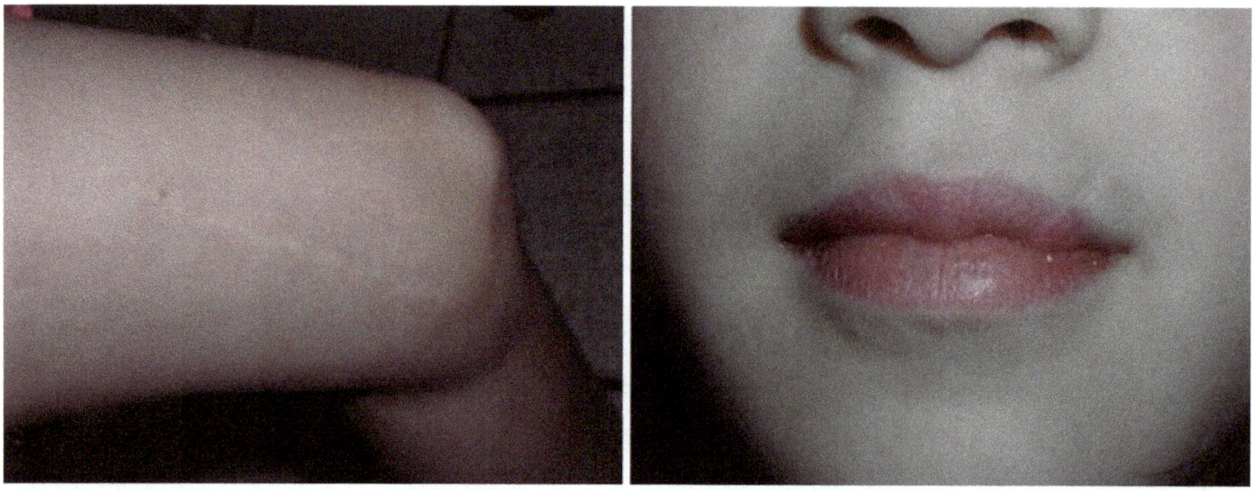

Fig. "Ideal" scars

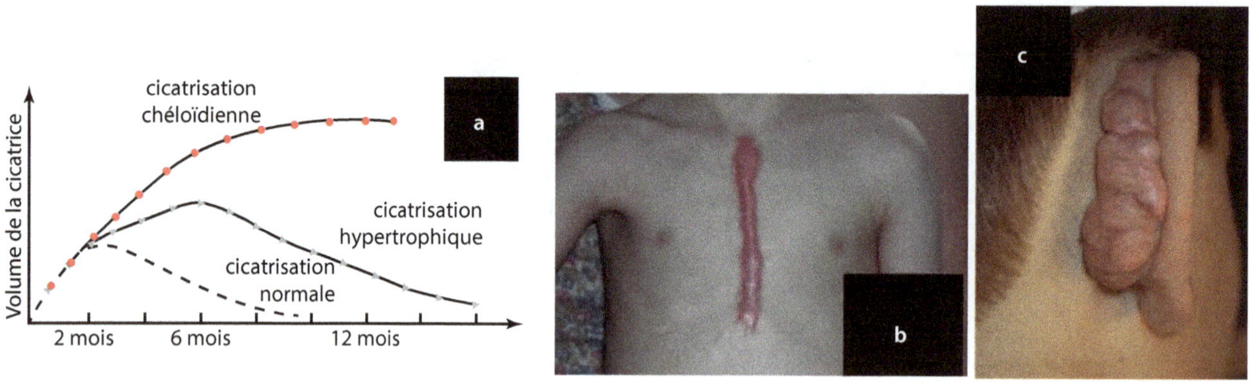

Fig. Pathological scars: **a**: evolution diagram; **b**: hypertrophic scar; and **c**: keloid scar

we found the same characteristics as for hypertrophic scar but with a complete disorganization of the collagen arrangement: there are no more beams but collagen fibers randomly connected and poorly oriented.

Easing Factors

Most often, pathological scars occur on a particular field. Although the causal link is not always obvious, there are several factors that contribute to the same scar.

- There is no male or female predominance. The sex ratio for pathological scars is equal to 1.
- There is no evidence of hereditary factor. However, some authors have questioned about the hereditary characters of keloid scars [11].
- Nevertheless, the ethnic origin seems to be decisive. A preponderance of keloid scars is observed in subjects with pigmented skin (Black, Asian, Métis, etc.). Some studies submit biological hypotheses related to the characteristics of pigmented skins, but there is no evidence at the moment.
- The age of the patient is a determining factor. Hypertrophic and keloid scars are exceptional in the elderly and are very common in young people and around puberty. It is therefore essential for pediatric surgeons to be familiar with this scar pathology.
- The location of the wound plays a clear role: the scapular region, the ear area, and the midline of the trunk (presternal and medio-abdominal) are particularly concerned by the development of pathological scars.
- The types of wounds, such as deep burn, soiled wounds, and presence of foreign bodies in the wound, will prolong the cleansing phase and therefore the inflammatory phenomena.
- Hormonal factors: the preponderance of pathological scars at the time of puberty, the impact of pregnancy on scars, and the regression of hypertrophic scars at the time of menopause seem to evoke the role of estrogen. Some studies have looked at the use of antiestrogens in the treatment of hypertrophic scars [12].

Although all these factors may have been suggested as favoring pathological scars, only the age, the ethnic factors, and the location of the wound are really the determining factors. Mechanism of occurrence of these pathological scars is not yet totally understood.

Prevention and Treatment [13]

Treatment is often disappointing. Many treatments have been proposed, but they are quickly abandoned as they are ineffective. The physio-pathological approach of mechanisms has helped rationalize treatments, particularly by acting on inflammation. Nevertheless, the results often remain below the expectations of the patient and the physician.

Prevention, especially in high-risk population such as pediatric patients, is often effective.

- Prevention of pathological scars
- To be really preventive, treatment must be applied as soon the wound is healed: a few days after primary closure or as soon as epimerization is achieved in secondary closure.
  - Reduce inflammation
    - Decrease healing time by activating mechanical cleansing.
    - Decrease healing time by using surgical means of cover (grafts, flaps).
    - Use non-absorbable or slow absorbable intradermal sutures for which inflammatory response is less intense.
    - Massage of recent scars reduce edema and mechanically dissociate molecular aggregates. Therefore, massages have a real mechanical action. Massages are most often made with an emollient cream because they are better tolerated. However, massages would be just as effective as without cream.
    - Pressure therapy will also reduce edema, inducing a relative tissue hypoxia, thereby minimizing local inflammation. Silicone sheets act in a same way on inflammation [14] (◘ Fig. 46.4).
  - Reduce tension on the scar
    - Use Langer's or Borges's lines in surgery.
    - Reduce tension on scar by using strips and splinting adjacent joints.
- Treatment of pathological scars

Some treatments are well established, even if their efficacy is disappointing. Other treatments are rather perspectives and subject to current studies. However, the evolution of these scars is sometimes so hopeless for the patient that minimally invasive techniques deserve to be tempted, even if their efficacy is very inconsistent.

Several techniques can be associated either simultaneously or successively.

When a scar becomes inflammatory, the earlier the treatment will be initiated, the more effective it will be.

Preventive techniques can be used as treatment techniques, but they will not be so effective.

- Massages
- Pressure therapy (◘ Fig. 46.5)
- Silicone sheets
- Steroids have been used for a long time to treat pathologic scars.

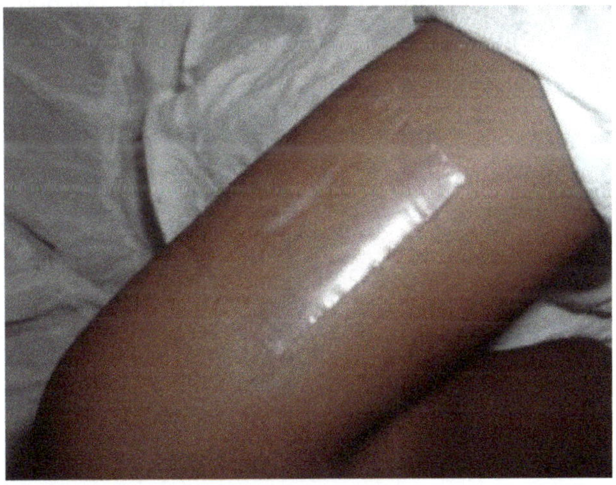

◘ **Fig.** Silicone sheet on hypertrophic scar

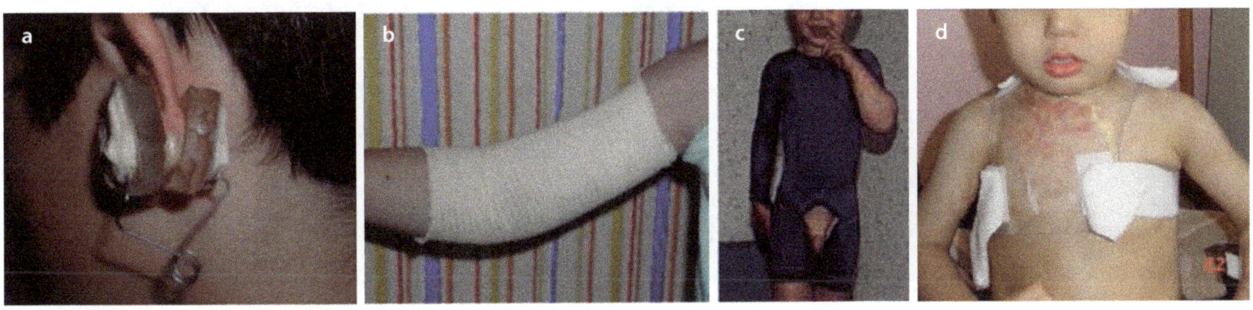

◘ **Fig.** Different devices for pressure therapy

They can be used as topic (cream or ointment) or in situ injections.

Local application may be dangerous in children, as the dose of absorbed steroids is difficult to evaluate. An overdose in steroids can lead to a partial or complete Cushing syndrome, which may occur due to abusive local application of corticoids.

For this reason, we prefer local injections of steroids in pediatric practice, using steroids of delayed action with minimal general effects. Injection is proceeded with dermo-jet or syringe and needle after local anesthesia (◘ Fig. 46.6). Nevertheless, it is often more comfortable to do so under general anesthesia in day surgery unit. Injections can be repeated until at least 2 months between two injections so as not to overload the scar with steroids. The only contraindication is the local infection. Most of the time, flattening of the scar and disappearance of functional signs (pain, pruritus) are observed.

However, it is necessary to be cautious because steroid overload results in epidermal thinning and appearance of telangiectasia.

- Cryotherapy [15] may be used with inconsistent results: it may be used by contact or with freezing needles (◘ Fig. 46.7).
- Surgery will induce more inflammatory reactions. Therefore, surgery on its own will not solve the problem: it must be a step in a therapeutic scheme, associating several techniques, and must be proceeded only at the end of the scar maturation, when the inflammatory phenomena have calmed down.

  Intralesional excision is the only way to prevent recurrence, but it does not mean that it consistently gives the expected result. The volume of the scar will decrease, which will improve comfort and release functional effects, and perhaps the residual scar will be more receptive to the complementary treatments that are necessary to avoid recurrence.

  An injection of delay-steroids can be performed in the dermis of the banks of the excision wound before closing by non-absorbable sutures. Pressure therapy will be prescribed systematically as soon as healing is achieved (10 days).
- Radiations (X-rays, radium, iridium) may be proposed, but they are not to be used in pediatric practice because of carcinogenic risk.
- Anti-neoplastic substances [16] have been the subject of research in recent years: Interferons, mitomycin C, bleomycin, 5-fluorouracil [17] are all molecules that are used as injections in situ, either alone or in combination with corticosteroids. These treatments have to be used very carefully and when there is no other therapeutic possibility in pediatric practice because of their interaction with growth.
- Laser therapy has been tried on pathological scars [18] and is easy to use in pediatric practice under contact local anesthesia.
- Finally, it may be wise, in some situations, to allow time for inflammatory phenomena to decrease spontaneously before initiating aggressive therapies. This implies to support the patient because the evolution often seems hopeless.

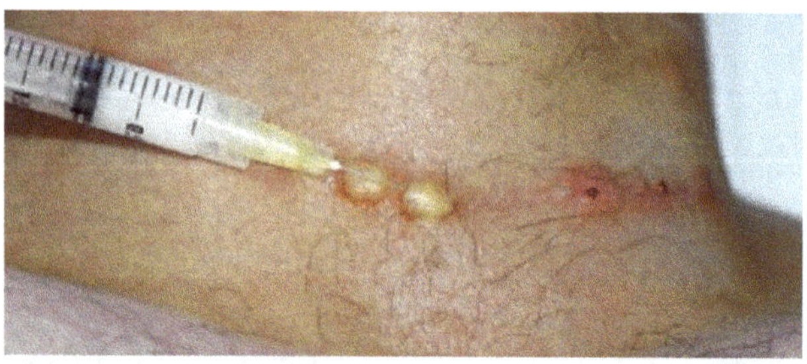

◘ **Fig.** Intralesional injection of steroids

Multiple treatments are proposed for these pathological scars due to their uncertain efficacy and the difficulty in achieving results that satisfy the patient (and the physician).

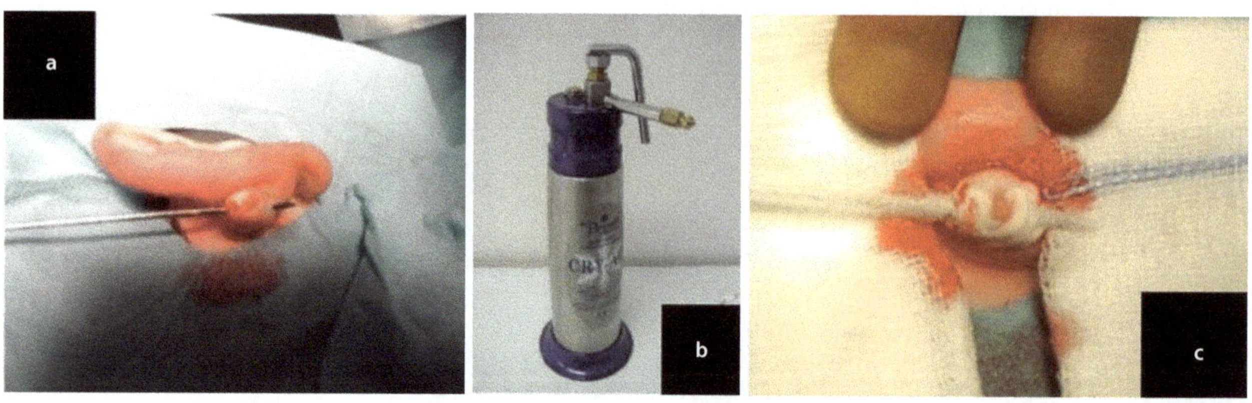

◘ **Fig. a–c**: Cryotherapy

Defective or Disgracious Scars

Some scars are defective or disgracious and do not disturb the healing process: hypotrophic or enlarged scars, adherent scars, dyschromic scars, tattooed scars, granuloma, technical defects, etc.

All scars that present defects but no pathology of the healing process can be corrected by surgery, irrespective of the technique used: surgical recovery, adipocytes transplantation (Coleman technique), dermabrasion with or without vaporization of autologous keratinocytes, etc. However, it will be necessary to wait at least until the end of the maturation phase to consider secondary surgery.

Deciding what is the best time to practice this surgery is sometimes difficult in pediatric practice. Apart from functional indications for which the question hardly arises, the indications are most often aesthetic. It is then necessary to ensure the child's actual motivations and that this is not a parental request.

If the child is voluntary, a "contract" must then be passed with the child or teenager emphasizing three key points:

- The disgracious scar will be replaced by a scar that hopefully will be of better quality. There is no magic rubber for scar.
- Postoperative scar management (e.g., strips, silicone, possible splint, and refraining from sportive activities) is constraining but necessary for a good result.
- If the patient is not able to undergo scar management, surgery is useless.

All these scar anomalies can be corrected, but it is of course essential to prevent and avoid them.

Scars and Growth

During the first 2 years after healing, the scar matures. Contraction of the scar is current and normal due to the action of myofibroblasts. After this period of time, the scar is quiet and more or less definitive.

In pediatric practice, the patient will grow with the scar. This may induce tractions because the scar is fibrous and does not grow as much as the patient. If this is not corrected, it may induce bending because of asymmetric growth.

Psychomotor development may be disturbed by scars. Physicians should be aware that psychological impact of scars evolves over time all along childhood and teenage. Therefore, pediatric patients with scars have to be followed all along their growth period to detect the need for scar surgery, whether it is for functional purpose or for aesthetic and psychological purpose.

Conclusion

Healing physiology is not different in children but the importance of inflammatory mechanisms makes the resulting scar different. Hypertrophic scar is physiological in pediatric practice and has to be prevented.

Take-Home Messages

- Obtain rapid closure of wound in children.
- Always prevent hypertrophic scaring in pediatric practice.
- Follow-up children with wide scars until end of growth.

References

1. Longaker MT, Adzick NS. The biology of fetal wound healing: a review. Plast Reconstr Surg. 1991;87:788–98.
2. Hopkinson-Woolley J, Hughes D, Gordon S, Martin P. Macrophage recruitment during limb development and wound healing in the embryonic and foetal mouse. J Cell Sci. 1994;107:1159–67.
3. Oztürk S, Deveci M, Sengezer M, Günhan Ő. Results of artificial inflammation in scarless foetal wound healing: an experimental study in foetal lambs. Br J Plast Surg. 2001;54:47–52.
4. Kishi K, Nakajima H, Tajima S. Differential responses of collagen and glycosamınoglycan syntheses and cell proliferation to exogenous transforming growth factor beta 1 in the developing mouse skin fibroblasts in culture. Br J Plast Surg. 1999;52(7):579–82.
5. Longaker MT, Adzick NS, Hall JL, Stair SE, Crombleholme TM, Du BW, Bradley SM, Harrisson MR, Stern R. Studies in fetal wound healing, VII. Fetal wound healing may be modulated by hyaluronic acid stimulating activity in amniotic acid. Br J Plast Surg. 1990;25:430–3.
6. Longaker MT, Whitby DJ, Ferguson MW, Lorenz HP, Harrisson MR, Adzick NS. Adult skin wounds in the fetal environment heal with scar formation. Ann Surg. 1994;219:65–72.
7. Le Touze A. Cicatrisation normale et pathologique. In: Captier G, editor. Chirurgie plastique de l'enfant et de l'adolescent. Montpellier: Sauramps Medical; 2015.
8. Jeffs D, Dorman D, Brown S, Files A, Graves T, Kirk E, Meredith-Neve S, Sanders J, White B, Swearingen CJ. Effect of virtual reality on adolescent pain during burn wound care. J Burn Care Res. 2014;35(5):395–408.
9. Burns-Nader S, Joe L, Pinion K. Computer tablet distraction reduces pain and anxiety in pediatric burn patients undergoing hydrotherapy: a randomized trial. Burns. 2017;43(6):1203–11.
10. Lee HJ, Jang YJ. Recent understandings of biology, prophylaxis and treatment strategies for hypertrophic scars and keloids. Int J Mol Sci. 2018;19(3):711.
11. Marneros AG, Norris JE, Olsen BR, Reichenberger E. Clinical genetics of familial keloids. Arch Dermatol. 2001;137(11):1429–34.
12. Gragnani A, Warde M, Furtado F, Ferreira LM. Topical tamoxifen therapy in hypertrophic scars or keloids in burns. Arch Dermatol Res. 2010;302(1):1–4.
13. Monstrey S, Middelkoop E, Vranckx JJ, Bassetto F, Ziegler UE, Meaume S, Téot L. Updated scar management practical guide-

lines: non-invasive and invasive measures. J Plast Reconstr Aesthet Surg. 2014;67(8):1017–25.
14. O'Brien L, Jones DJ. Silicone gel sheeting for preventing and treating hypertrophic and keloid scars. Cochrane Database Syst Rev. 2013;(9):CD003826.
15. O'Boyle CP, Shayan-Arani H, Hamada MW. Intralesional cryotherapy for hypertrophic scars and keloids: a review. Scars Burn Heal. 2017;3:2059513117702162.
16. Shridharani SM, Magarakis M, Manson PN, Singh NK, Basdag B, Rosson GD. The emerging role of antineoplastic agents in the treatment of keloids and hypertrophic scars: a review. Ann Plast Surg. 2010;64(3):355–61.
17. Ren Y, Zhou X, Wei Z, Lin W, Fan B, Feng S. Efficacy and safety of triamcinolone alone and combination with 5-fluorouracil for treating hypertrophic scars and keloids: a systemic review and meta-analysis. Int Wound J. 2017;14:480–7.
18. Jin R, Huang X, Li H, Yuan Y, Li B, Cheng C, Li Q. Laser therapy for prevention and treatment of pathologic excessive scars. Plast Reconstr Surg. 2013;132(6):1747–58.

20

Clinical Case Reports: Scar Prevention by Laser Treatment in Mastopexy with Implant

Vincent Hunsinger, Martin Lhuaire, Ibrahim Dagher, and Laurent Lantieri

Contents

Introduction

Case Report Number 1

Case Report Number 2

Discussion

References

Introduction

Breast ptosis is one of the most common conditions treated by plastic surgeons with more than 100,000 operations each year just in the USA. While its causes are not clearly defined, age, history of significant weight loss, higher body mass index (BMI), larger bra cup size, the number of pregnancies, and smoking history are known to be significant risk factors [1]. Treatment consists generally in mastopexy and/or breast augmentation with implant fitting. The mastopexy procedure is generally considered a reliable aesthetic procedure with less than 2% of unsatisfactory breast shape [2]. In addition to operative risks related to any surgery performed under anesthesia, some complications specific to breast plasty and breast implant may occur such as hematoma, infection, wound healing delay, wound dehiscence, necrosis of the areola, necrosis of the skin, disruption of the implant and silicon leakage, rare case of anaplastic large cell lymphoma, and poor quality of the scars, including hypertrophic scar or keloid [1]. The overall complication rate of mastopexy reaches 10% and the most represented complications are scar related, with 3% of hypertrophic or unaesthetic appearance [2]. The patients' perspective is also essential when evaluating scar cosmetic appearance as it might differ from the ones of the surgeon [3, 4]. In particular, their expectations at short term (inflammatory stage) and long term (1 year) are of equal importance as they usually wish to regain a normal appearance skin as soon as possible and desire sustainable results [3, 4]. To minimize the aesthetic impact of surgical scars, many different strategies have been identified, such as compressing devices, sun protection, silicone dressing, or laser treatment [5, 6]. According to the recent guidelines, prevention of abnormal scar formation should always be a first priority [5–7]. Preventive measures adapted to the patients' risks and needs (possibly including combined therapies) and early intervention are well recognized for their positive outcomes [5–7]. In particular, laser therapy seems to gain each year broader and broader application in this field [8]. Ten years ago, a new approach based on a preventive treatment of scars called Laser-Assisted Skin Healing (LASH) was developed by Pr Mordon (INSERM U703; University of Lille Nord, France), and clinically evaluated by the teams of Pr Magalon (Department of Plastic and Reconstructive Surgery, APHM, Marseille, France) and Dr. Capon (Plastic and Reconstructive Surgery Department of Pr Martinot and Pellerin, CHRU, Lille, France) [9]. Performed immediately after surgery, a laser shot induces a controlled elevation of skin temperature, which activates the overexpression of chaperone proteins (Heat Shock Protein 70) [9, 10]. These proteins then activate tissue regeneration by shortening the inflammatory stage of the wound healing process and hasten scar maturation [9]. This technique, performed during the earliest stage of the healing process for a maximum impact, gave promising results. In 2016, a new laser system was marketed on the basis of this LASH technique. The 1210-nm laser diode (UrgoTouch®, Laboratoires Urgo Medical, Chenove, France) was an automated, portable laser providing a controlled elevation of skin temperature, due to its scar control system technology. The wavelength of the system allows its use on patients with all skin phototypes, including Fitzpatrick scale phototypes V and VI. The performance and safety of this new device were assessed in a 1-year follow-up double-blinded randomized controlled trial (RCT), undertaken on patients undergoing breast reduction: The "SLASH" study [11]. This high-quality-level study was conducted in France and coordinated by Pr Casanova at the University Hospital of Marseille. A total of 40 women (with phototypes II to VI) undergoing bilateral breast reduction were enrolled by the five surgeons involved in the study and treated with the portable 1210-nm laser on one randomly assigned breast, while the controlateral one was used as the study control. The unique laser-treatment session was performed on the suture incisions, in the operating room, while the patient was still under the general anesthesia. According to the results of this clinical study, based on both subjective assessments (with the validated modified Observer Scar Assessment Scale (mOSAS) score) and objective measurements (with software analysis of three-dimensional [3D] pictures of the scars) the 1210-nm automated laser system provided significant improvements of the cosmetic aspect of the scars at short term (6 weeks), medium term (6 months), and long term (12 months) (◘ Fig. 59.1). These aesthetic improvements, notably in terms of volume, surface, and roughness, were strengthened with the blind expression of patients' preference for their laser-treated scars. Of note, in the subgroup of dark skin-type patients (phototypes V–VI), the results also favored the laser treatment, with 53% and 16% mean reductions of the scar volume and surface, compared to the control scars.

I have personally used this laser treatment (◘ Fig. 59.2) in many different indications in my current practice and I propose to report here two cases of breast hypotrophy and ptosis treated by mastopexy with implants associated with the laser treatment.

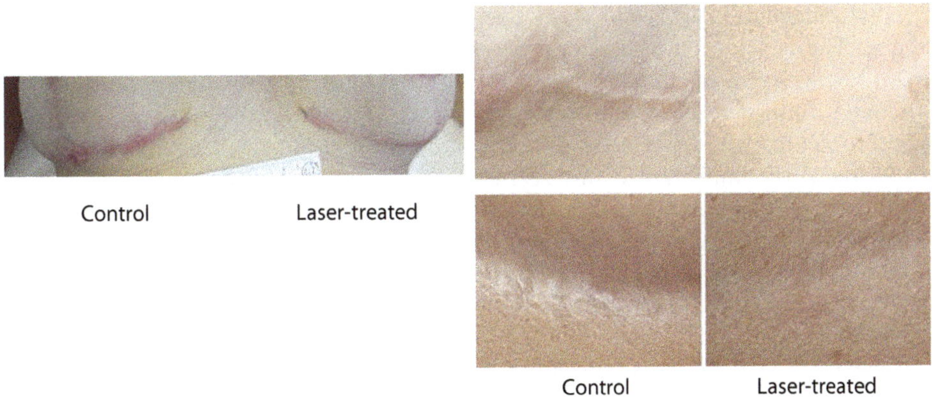

Fig. On the left, a two-dimensional (2D) photograph of the inframammary scars of a patient, 6 months after her breast-reduction procedure. The horizontal scar of one breast was randomly assigned to receive in the operating theatre, the day of the surgery, the laser treatment while the other scar of the controlateral breast was used as a control. On the right, 3D photographs of internal or external extremities of the scars treated or not with the laser in two different patients, 12 months after the procedure. (Reproduced from the double-blind RCT "SLASH" with the courtesy of Pr. Casanova, coordinator of the clinical trial)

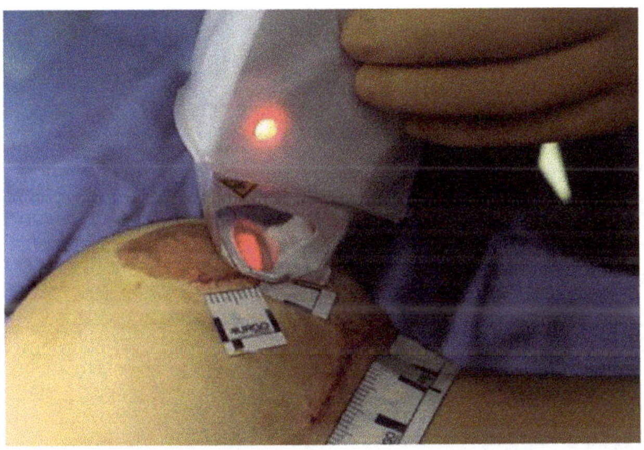

Fig. The 1210-nm laser diode laser system UrgoTouch® procedure. The laser treatment (only one pass over the incision) is performed in the operating theatre, when patients are still under general anesthesia. The target cutaneous zone is secured by the application of safety strips containing high-technology microchips. These microchips enable the laser shots and prevent any overdose. The sterile strips are positioned along the sutures just before the laser shot. The laser shot duration is determined and controlled by the laser software itself, based on the patient's skin temperature detected by the embedded pyrometer of the device. This technology ensures the automatic discontinuation of the shot when the target skin temperature (53 ± 3°C) is reached, ensuring both patient safety and reproducibility of the shots. Neither preliminary parameter settings nor adjustments are required for laser shots. A training to the laser is received before its first use

Case Report Number 1

Description

A 37-year-old woman with bilateral breast hypotrophy and ptosis was seen in consultation seeking for breast lift. Physical examination revealed 85C-sized breasts with grade 2 ptosis based on the Regnault classification (Nipple areola complex [NAC] 2 cm below the submammary fold) and asymmetry (with a left breast more voluminous and ptosic than the controlateral one). The patient (1.70 m, 58 kg, BMI 20) had recently lost 15 kg and reported a previous 95C breast size. She had three children and no prolonged breastfeeding period. The patient had no history of surgery, allergy, or medications, but was a current smoker.

A bilateral breast lift with retropectoral implants and laser treatment was proposed to the patient. The benefits and risks related to the procedure were explained, together with the necessity to quit smoking, before the patient gave her written consent.

Methods

The surgery was performed in November 2017, under general anesthesia and orotracheal intubation. The patient had received antibioprophylaxy and perioperative compression stockings and she underwent preoperative marking. A similar procedure was followed for both breast. Infiltration of local anesthetics (naropeine 7.5 mg/mL + xylocaine/adrenaline 1%) was done in the targeted zone. The incision on each breast was made under the future nipple-areola complex flap, with a glandular transection, until it reached the pectoralis muscle. The retropectoral area was dissected to develop the submuscular pocket at the implant size and a sizer was used for the mastopexy. The breast was lifted using inverted-T scar and a superior NAC pedicle technique. The round micro-textured breast implants prefilled with silicone gel were then placed in its pocket (LSM RM 345, Sebbin) and the satisfying shape and volume of the breast were checked. Surgical incisions were sutured according to local standard procedures, using common surgical sutures (Monocryl™ 3/0 and 4/0 and Vicryl™ rapide 4/0, Ethicon) compatible with the laser use, according to the laser manufacturer's instructions.

The safety strips of the laser were positioned along the sutured incisions. The laser shot duration was determined and controlled by the laser software itself, based on the patient's skin temperature detected by the embedded pyrometer of the device. The laser treatment procedure was rapid and went unremarkable. After the laser treatment, the sutured incisions were secured with 2-octyl cyanoacrylate adhesive (Dermabond®, Ethicon) and covered by a dry dressing, before adding the postoperative compressive bra.

Postoperative care recommendations included daily shower and dressing change after cleaning of the sutured incisions with an antiseptic solution. The patient was asked to wear postoperative compression bra for 4 weeks after the surgery and received a prescription for analgesics. Sport activity resumption was allowed 3 months after the surgery.

▪▪ Results

No complication was reported during the procedure and the early postoperative course. One month after the surgery and the laser treatment, the cosmetic aspects of the scars were already satisfying and the patient was pleased with this short-term outcome (◘ Fig. 59.3).

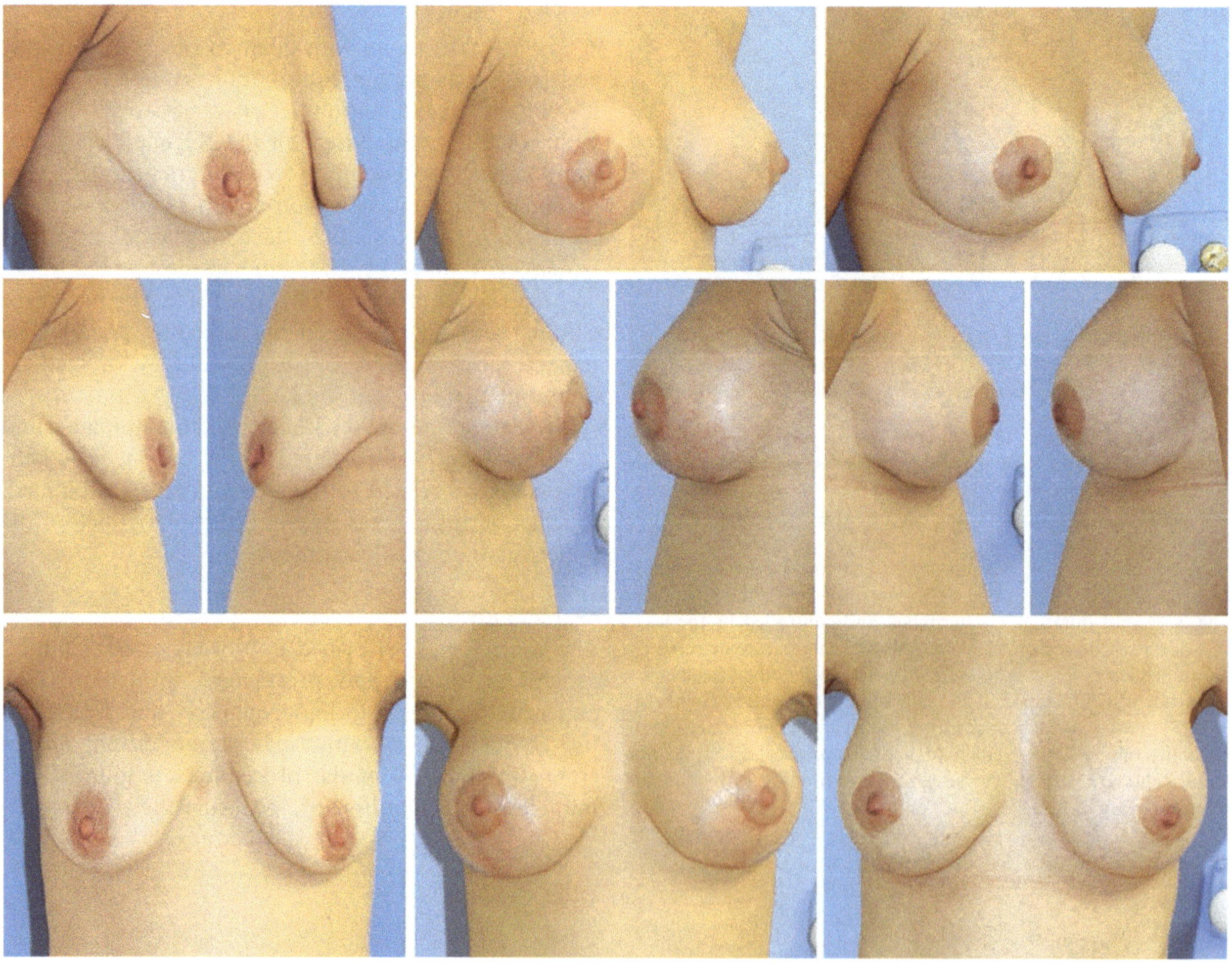

Pre-operative ptosis 1 month 18 months

◘ **Fig.** Eighteen months' follow-up of the patient: anterolateral, lateral, and anterior views of the preoperative ptosis and of the breasts 1 month and 18 months after the surgery and the laser treatment

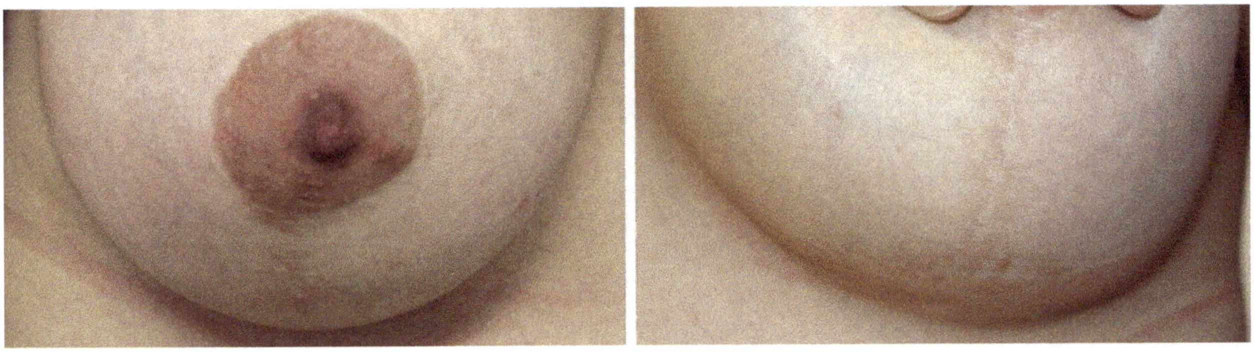

Fig. Enlarged photographs of periareolar and vertical scars of each breast, 18 months post-surgery

At the 18-month postoperative visit, the horizontal, vertical, and periareolar scars became very discreet and the patient expressed her complete satisfaction for her new breasts (Figs. 59.3 and 59.4).

Case Report Number 2

Description

The second case report relates to a 26-year-old woman (1.64 m, 60 kg, BMI 22) seen in consultation for breast lifting after weight loss. The patient presented a bilateral breast hypotrophy and grade 2 ptosis (NAC 1 cm below the submammary fold). The breasts were asymmetric (more voluminous and ptosic left breast). The patient currently had B-cup breasts and wanted a breast augmentation to reach plain C-cups. The review of the medical and surgical history of the patient revealed a sleeve-gastrectomy in March 2013, no allergy, no particular familial medical history, and no current medications, but she was a current smoker. A bilateral breast lift with retropectoral implants and laser treatment was proposed to the patient. She was informed that she had to quit smoking and the benefits and risks related to the procedure were explained to her. The surgery was scheduled in January 2018, once the written consent of the patient was obtained.

Methods

The surgery was performed under general anesthesia and laryngeal mask. The procedure was globally similar to the one reported in Case 1. The glandular transection reached the pectoral muscle plan. The submuscular area was dissected to develop the implant pocket. Inverted-T incision and superior NAC pedicle technique was used and the round micro-textured breast implants prefilled with silicone gel were positioned in their pocket (LSM RS 270, Sebbin, for the right breast, and LSC 72330, Sebbin, for the left breast). The shape and volume of the breasts were checked and judged satisfying. The surgical sutures and laser treatment were performed as previously described. After the laser treatment, the sutured incisions were secured with steri-strips and covered by a dry dressing, before adding the postoperative compressive bra. The global procedure (including surgery and laser treatment) lasted 2 hours. The drains were removed the day after the surgery. Postoperative care recommendations were similar to the ones given in Case 1.

Results

No complication was reported during the procedure and the postoperative course. Two months after the surgery, the interest of an early laser treatment on the inflammatory stage of the wound healing process was noticeable. At the 12-month postoperative visit, the scars were barely detectable. The cosmetic aspects of the scars were very satisfying and the patient was pleased with the results of the procedure, at both the short-term and long-term visits (Figs. 59.5 and 59.6).

Discussion

To my knowledge, this is the first time the use of the automated 1210-nm laser diode UrgoTouch® is reported in mastopexy associated with retropectoral implant. The short- and long-term cosmetic results reached after a unique session, realized in the operating theater the day of the surgery, were very satisfying from both the surgeon' and the patient's point of view, and consistent with the results reported in the "SLASH" RCT conducted in the breast-reduction indication.

I first tried this laser treatment in October 2016 in a revision of breast and abdominoplasty in a patient of dark phototype skin presenting at my consultation with very wide scars. The aesthetic outcomes of the scars at 10 months were very satisfactory and the patient said that she was happy with the result obtained. Subsequently, I have treated the scars of more than two hundreds of patients in different indications: secondarily to breast

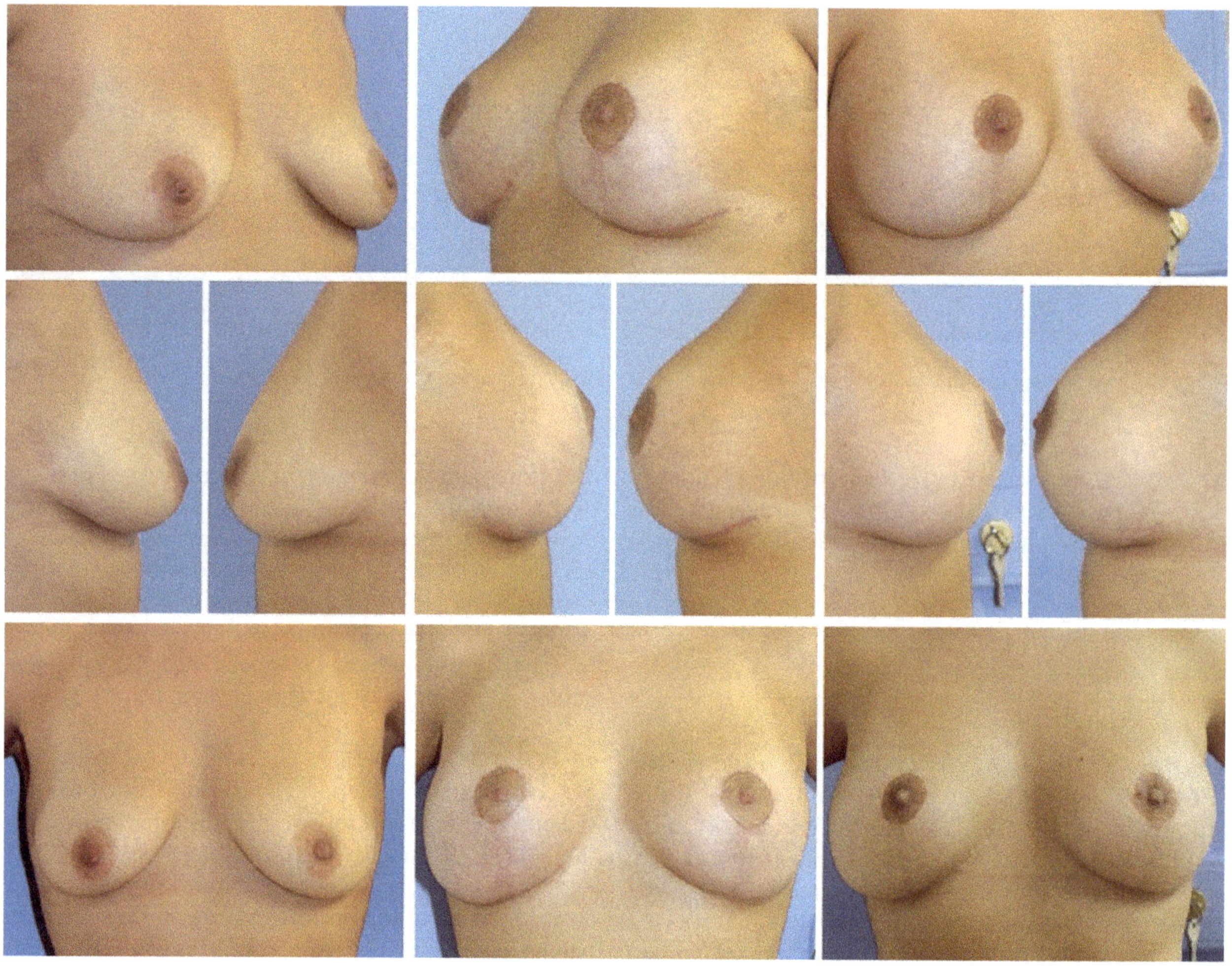

Pre-operative ptosis 2 months 12 months

Fig. Twelve months' follow-up of the patient: anterolateral, lateral, and anterior views of the preoperative ptosis and of the breasts 2 months and 12 months after the surgery and the laser treatment

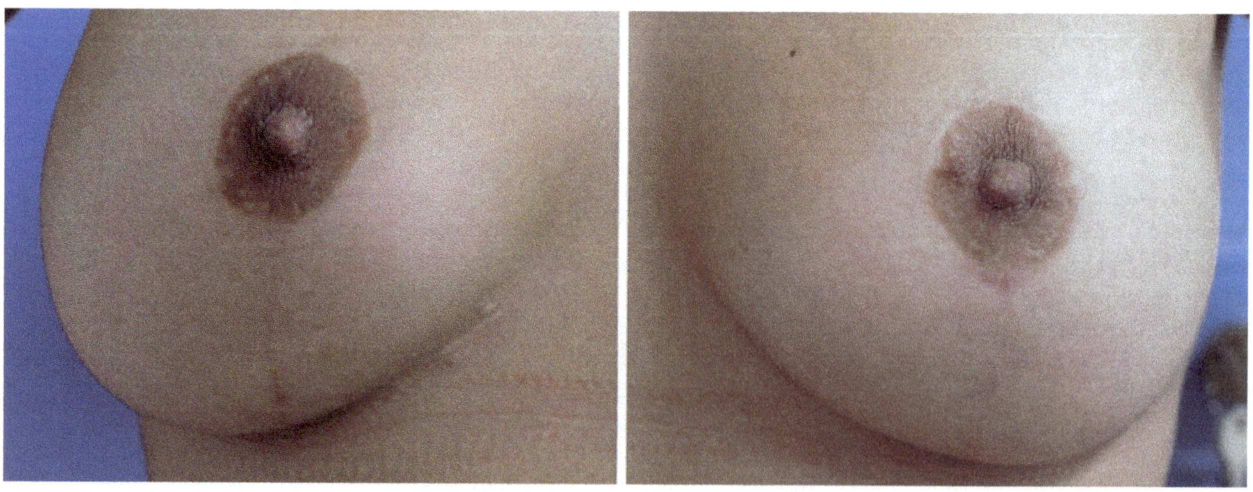

Fig. Enlarged photographs of periareolar and vertical scars, 12 months post-surgery

augmentation operations [12], breast plasty, ptosis cure, prosthesis repair, abdominoplasty, brachioplasty, body lift, or gynecomastia, without any particular complication. The laser procedure takes a minimum amount of time (a few minutes, depending on the length of the scars), and I agree with the surgeons of the "SLASH" study who have judged the portable laser very easy to use. Indeed, the absence of parameter setting or adjustment really simplifies this type of procedure.

I always explain the limits of the procedure to my patients during the consultation prior to the surgery and laser treatment, in order to clear unrealistic expectations. Consequently, till today, none of my laser-treated patients were dissatisfied and their testimonials, collected in postoperative consultation or on my medical office's website, are all very positive. While this laser treatment can potentially be offered to all my patients, at the beginning I mainly proposed this procedure to patients with skin at risk or anxious by the scar result of their future operation, but now, it often happens that patients arrive at consultation demanding for it. The contraindications of the use of the laser 1210-nm laser diode UrgoTouch® are available in the manufacturer's instruction for use.

Reflective Questions

- Are there predetermining factors and risk for abnormal scarring?
- What are the guidelines for prevention and treatment of surgical scars and laser treatment?
- What are the contraindications for laser treatment?
- What is the position of laser procedure in your scar prevention strategies?
- How long does a laser treatment take? What formation is required for laser use?

Take-Home Messages

- Different strategies have been identified to minimize the aesthetic impact of surgical scars and prevention of abnormal scar formation should always be a first priority.
- The performance and safety of the automated, portable, 1210-nm laser diode UrgoTouch® treatment reported in real-life practice are consistent with the ones established in the randomised controlled trial SLASH.
- An early and unique laser-treatment session with UrgoTouch® significantly improves the cosmetic aspect of the surgical scars.
- Patients treated with the laser procedure expressed their satisfaction both at short-term and long-term follow-up visits.

References

1. Rinker B, Veneracion M, Walsh CP. Breast ptosis: causes and cure. Ann Plast Surg. 2010;64(5):579–84.
2. Di Summa PG, Oranges CM, Watfa W, Sapino G, Keller N, Tay SK, Chew BK, Schaefer DJ, Raffoul W. Systematic review of outcomes and complications in nonimplant-based mastopexy surgery. J Plast Reconstr Aesthet Surg. 2019;72(2):243–72.
3. Celebiler O, Sönmez A, Erdim M, Yaman M, Numanoglu A. Patients' and surgeons' perspectives on the scar components after inferior pedicle breast reduction surgery. Plast Reconstr Surg. 2005;116(2):459–64.
4. Godwin Y, Barron EJ, Edmunds MC, Meyer M, Bardsley A, Logan AM, O'Neill TJ, Wood SH. A comparison of the patient and surgeon opinion on the long-term aesthetic outcome of reduction mammaplasty: have we improved over 15 years? J Plast Reconstr Aesthet Surg. 2014;67(7):932–8.
5. Gold MH, McGuire M, Mustoe TA, Pusic A, Sachdev M, Waibel J, Murcia C. International Advisory Panel on Scar Management. Updated international clinical recommendations on scar management: part 2—algorithms for scar prevention and treatment. Dermatol Surg. 2014;40(8):825–31.
6. Meaume S, Le Pillouer-Prost A, Richert B, Roseeuw D, Vadoud J. Management of scars: updated practical guidelines and use of silicones. Eur J Dermatol. 2014;24(4):435–43.
7. Monstrey S, Middelkoop E, Vranckx JJ, Bassetto F, Ziegler UE, Meaume S, Téot L. Updated scar management practical guidelines: non-invasive and invasive measures. J Plast Reconstr Aesthet Surg. 2014;67(8):1017–25.
8. Le Fourn B, Boagaert P. Secondary surgical and medical treatment of scars [Traitement secondaire chirurgical et médicales des cicatrices]. Ann Chir Plast Esthet. 2019; https://doi.org/10.1016/j.anplas.2019.07.013.
9. Capon AC, Gossé AR, Iarmarcovai GN, Cornil AH, Mordon SR. Scar prevention by laser-assisted scar healing (LASH): a pilot study using an 810-nm diode-laser system. Lasers Surg Med. 2008;40(7):443–5.
10. Souil E, Capon A, Mordon S, Dinh-Xuan AT, Polla BS, Bachelet M. Treatment with 815-nm diode laser induces long-lasting expression of 72-kDa heat shock protein in normal rat skin. Br J Dermatol. 2001;144(2):260–6.
11. Casanova D, Alliez A, Baptista C, Gonelli D, Lemdjadi Z, Bohbot S. A 1-year follow-up of post-operative scars after the use of a 1210-nm laser-assisted skin healing (LASH) technology: a randomized controlled trial. Aesthet Plast Surg. 2017;41(4):938–48.
12. Hunsinger V, et al. Minimally invasive inframammary breast augmentation (MINIBA). Accepted for publication in the 2019 December issue in Plastic and Reconstructive Surgery.

21

Genital Scars

Ursula Mirastschijski

Contents

Epidemiology and Etiology of Genital Wounds

Genital Skin Anatomy and Microstructure
Development of Genital Organs and Homology Between Sexes
Anatomy of Male and Female Genitalia
Microstructure of the Genital Skin

Pathophysiology of Genital Wound Healing, Lymphedema and Scarring
Skin Architecture and Biomechanics
Moist Environment and Bacterial Colonialization
Hormonal Influences

Acute Wound Repair of Genital Skin After Trauma

Chronic Inflammatory Diseases of the External Genitalia and Tissue Fibrosis
Lichen Sclerosus et Atrophicus/Balanitis Xerotica Obliterans
Behçet's Disease
Chronic Inflammation due to Foreign Body Reaction
Congenital and Acquired Genital Lymphedema and Tissue Fibrosis

Treatment of Genital Wounds and Scars
Treatment of Acute Wounds and Tissue Defects
Treatment of Genital Wounds and Scars After Burn Injury
Gender Reassignment Surgery
Treatment of Chronic Genital Skin Diseases
Lymphedema Treatment

Postoperative Management for Scar Prevention

Conclusion

References

Background

Excessive scarring of the genitalia is uncommon despite the fact that approximately 30% of men are circumcised worldwide with minor complication rates and no mention of scarring. After burn injury, severe scarring is commonly seen in the perineal or suprapubic area but rarely occurs to the outer genital organs. Skin anatomy, inflammatory response, and hormonal metabolism differ between the genitals and the extragenital skin and might therefore account for differences in wound healing and scarring. Owing to the high regenerative potential of genital skin, the management of genital wounds aims at the stabilization of the local tissue with infection control and demarcation of necrotic tissue. Reconstruction of tissue defects and scars comprises plastic surgical skin tissue transfer, including flap surgery and the restoration of the urinary and sexual function in an interdisciplinary context.

- **The objectives of this chapters are as follows**
  - To give an overview on the epidemiology and cause of genital scarring
  - To point out specific features of genital skin anatomy
  - To inform on the pathophysiology on skin wound healing, lymphology, and scarring of the outer genitals in women and men
  - To describe management of genital wounds and tissue defects
  - To give an overview on conservative and surgical treatment of genital wounds and scars

Epidemiology and Etiology of Genital Wounds

Since the ancient times, male circumcisions have been practiced by many communities mainly as a purity or religious ritual (◘ Fig. 47.1). Female genital mutilation (FGM)/cutting is still a common practice in many African countries, no matter the religious background of the people. Little is known on the incidence and severity of scarring in the genital area despite the fact that 30% of all men on the earth are circumcised [37].

Aside from circumcisions and ritual cuttings, other types of injuries, infections, tumors, skin diseases, and malformations can lead to abnormal wound healing and scarring of the genital skin. Due to the multitude of causes for genital trauma with subsequent scarring, a general incidence for genital scars is difficult to provide. As a consequence, I will first describe different origins for genital tissue defects with special focus on cutaneous wound healing and scarring of the outer genitalia, that is, the vulva, the scrotum, and the penis. For wound repair of the urinary system or the vagina and uterus, I would like to refer to the corresponding urological or gynecological literature and textbooks.

- **Causes for genital scarring and fibrosis**
  - Trauma, for example, burns, injuries to the pelvic area, autoerotic injuries, genital self-mutilation
  - Sequelae of any type of infections, for example, Hidradenitis suppurativa/acne inversa, Fournier gangrene, viral infections, and sexually transmitted diseases

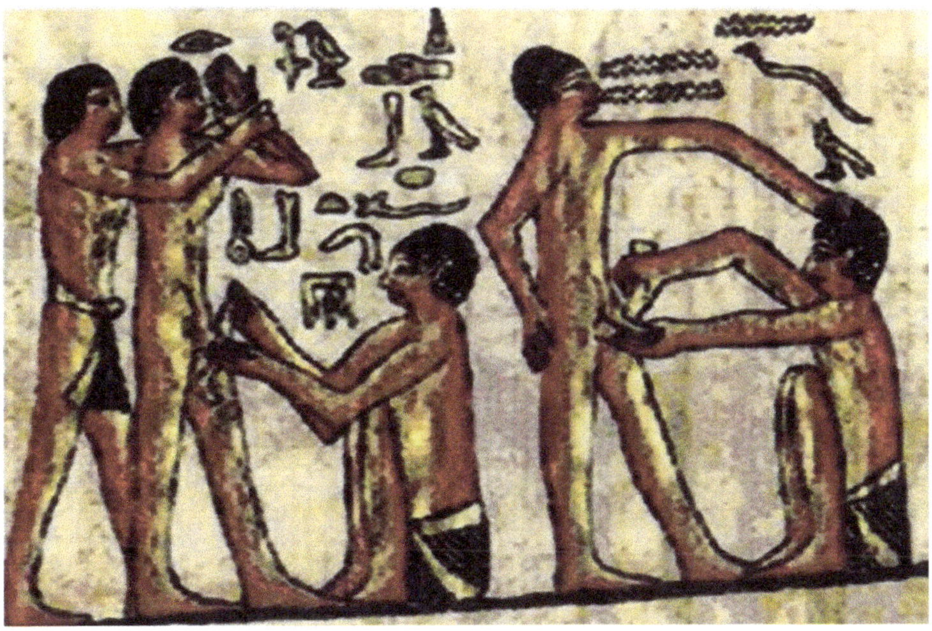

◘ **Fig.** Ritual act of *cir cumcision*: relief in the tomb of *Ankhmahor* at *Saqqara (sixth dynasty, 2345 BC.*

- Dermatological diseases, for example, various inflammatory autoimmune diseases (e.g., Behçet's syndrome or Crohn's disease with ulcerations, pyoderma gangraenosum), bullous skin diseases, lichen sclerosus et atrophicus (LSC), lichen planus
- Religiously/culturally motivated, for example, circumcisions, FGM/-cutting, or self-inflicted procedures, for example, piercings, tattoos, foreign body insertion
- Iatrogenic/surgical interventions, for example, aesthetic surgery, cosmetic procedures, including foreign body application; circumcision for phimosis; treatment of malformations; genital reassignment surgery
- Tumors followed by oncological surgery with/without radiation therapy
- Lymphatic disorders: congenital (Milroy's or Meigs' disease) or acquired (e.g., after tumor surgery, lymph node excision, irradiation; infectious: filariasis)

The literature search for causes of genital wounds that result in scarring yields some information on burns or combat injuries with concomitant affection of the genital organs. The incidence of burn injury to the genitalia is rare with around 1.5% [15] but associated with a higher mortality rate with 17% in comparison to non-genital burns (4.7%) [12]. In contrast to perineal and inguinal scar contractures that are a common sequela after burns to the lower abdomen and groin area, excessive scarring is rarely attributed to the outer genital organs (◘ Fig. 47.2).

The shift from high velocity to more explosive weapons during the end of the twentieth century and the use of improvised explosive devices resulted in more genital injuries in military conflicts than noticed before [1]. Genitourinary trauma accounted for only 5.3% of all combat-related injuries being mostly associated with severe polytraumatic incidents (62.1%). There are no reports on scarring after this type of injury.

Infections are quite common in the genital area. With several body orifices being anatomically located in close relation, a multitude of commensal microbia is constantly present. In case of small lesions, lacerations, or immune incompetence of the host, germs can penetrate into deeper tissue layers and cause severe infections, for example, abscesses or gangrenes with high mortality rates. Predisposed patients develop chronic infections of the sweat glands and hair follicles in the groin and genital area, also called hidradenitis suppurativa or acne inversa. Without appropriate treatment, they develop fistulas with recurrent infections and subsequent scarring to the perineal crease. The annual prevalence of hidradenitis suppurativa is around 1% with an estimate of 70 million patients worldwide [14].

Fournier gangrene is a life-threatening necrotizing fasciitis of the genitalia with an incidence of 1.6/100,000 patients that affects mostly men (10:1) [18]. The only sufficient cure is the radical surgical debridement of the entire infected and necrotic tissue with accompanying antibiotic treatment. Massive tissue losses can be the consequence with plastic surgical reconstruction after successful elimination of the infection. Because the tissue defects have a tendency to spread over the groin area as well, scar contractures are found as remnants of this type of genital infection (◘ Fig. 47.3).

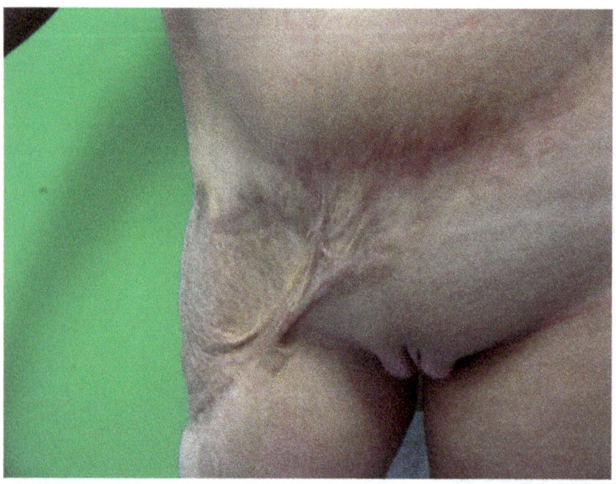

◘ **Fig.** Inguinal scar contracture with impairment of the abduction of the right leg but without involvement of the big labia after severe burn injury

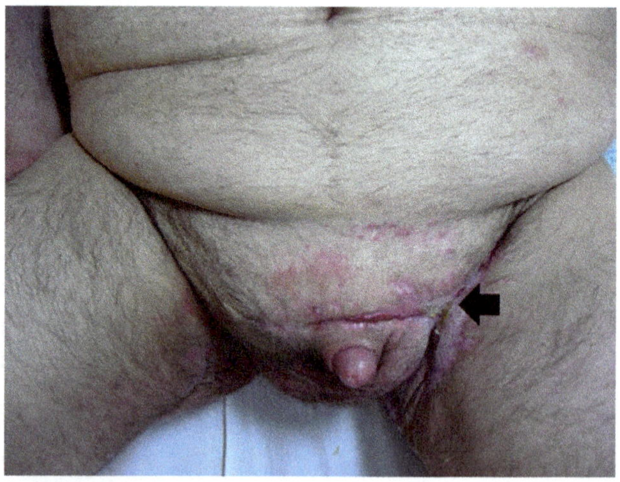

◘ **Fig.** Inguinal hypertrophic scarring with scar contractures after hidradenitis suppurativa and recurrent inguinal infections that culminated into a Fournier gangrene with vast tissue excision and postoperative scarring. The resulting scar contractures impaired the abduction of the left leg. Please note the instable scar with recurrent ulceration between the prepubic area and the left inguinal crease adjacent to the contracture (arrow). Aside from severe scarring, a buried penis grade III is present. No scarring of the penile skin or glans but of the pubic skin and groin is present

The incidence of autoerotic or self-inflicted genital injuries has not been determined but is extremely low and patients present sporadically. Genital lesions can derive from blunt, strangulating, or penetrating trauma and go as far as to incomplete or total amputations. Self-inflicted genital injuries can derive from neurotic, psychotic, and various other types of mental disorders or associated diseases and are seen in gender dysphoric conditions.

It appears that the genital skin tends more to chronic ulcers or fistulas seen in various dermatological diseases or infections than to healing with excessive scar formation. Despite reports on scarring after Behçet's syndrome, it seems that the genital skin heals with atrophic rather than hypertrophic scarring. Of note, excessive swelling of the outer genitalia is another feature that occurs typically after trauma or surgery and that differs to skin wound repair of other body areas. Genital lymphedema can be idiopathic and associated with congenital malformations but is also present after cancer therapy and infections, for example, filariasis. Chronic genital lymphedema can ultimately lead to severe fibrotic conditions and elephantiasis.

The genitalia differ in several regards from other body sites. Urogenital and anal orifices and the surrounding skin are colonized by resident microbia in a moist environment, there is abundant highly elastic skin around the external genital organs that is loosely fixed to the pelvic bone, and the cutaneous microstructure, inflammatory reaction, and hormonal responsiveness are different compared to other tissues. In the following sections, all these features and their influence on genital wound repair and scarring will be elucidated in detail.

Genital Skin Anatomy and Microstructure

For a better understanding why genitalia behave differently to skin from other body sites, the macro- and microstructure of the genital skin and organs, including lymphatics, are important and will be described in the following paragraphs. The knowledge of the anatomy is the prerequisite for the appropriate conservative and surgical treatment.

Development of Genital Organs and Homology Between Sexes

Female and male outer genitals derive from the same embryological origins with different development depending on the sex of the infant. The development of the external genitalia is presented in detail in ◘ Fig. 47.4, which depicts the common origin of respective anatomical entity at the embryonic stage and further differentiation into male and female genitalia during the fetal period. ◘ Table 47.1 summarizes the homologous anatomical and microscopic structures.

Anatomy of Male and Female Genitalia

The main anatomical differences between genital and skin of other body areas are the lack of fat tissue to the scrotum, penis and labia minora, the absence of hair to the penile and small labia skin, and the reduced or missing cornified epidermal layer of the epithelium of the prepuce and the small labia. With regard to biomechanics, the genital skin is highly elastic and flexible because it lacks a firm attachment to underlying structures, for example, bones or cartilage. A subcutaneous smooth muscle layer, also called Dartos muscle or Tunica dartos that is found in the scrotum and big labia, is reminiscent of the subcutaneous carnosus muscle in fur bearing animals and enables a gliding between the skin and the underlying connective tissue. Of note, the anatomic relict of the carnosus muscle in humans is the Scarpa fascia that is found in most other parts of the body underneath the subcutaneous fat layer. The genitalia are devoid of fat and the Scarpa fascia. Instead, the Dartos fascia is found here. An illustration of the genital anatomy for both sexes is shown in ◘ Figs. 47.5 and 47.6.

▪ **Summary: Differences Between Genital and Nongenital Skin**

Genital skin differs from other regions:

- No subcutaneous fat tissue, no Scarpa fascia; instead tunica dartos with smooth muscle cells (scrotum and big labia) or dartos fascia with loose attachment of the skin (penis)
- No tight attachment of the skin to underlying bone or cartilage
- Little or no keratinizing epithelia—mucous surfaces of small labia, glans, and prepuce
- Reduced hair growth—skin of scrotum and big labia
- Moist environment due to mucous surfaces and a multitude of mucous secreting glands
- Constant microbial contamination—cutaneous, genitourinary, and intestinal flora

Microstructure of the Genital Skin

The skin is the largest organ of the human body that protects us against biological (e.g., microbial), chemical (e.g., acids, bases), physical (e.g., irradiation, pressure), thermal (heat, cold), and other threats, including exsic-

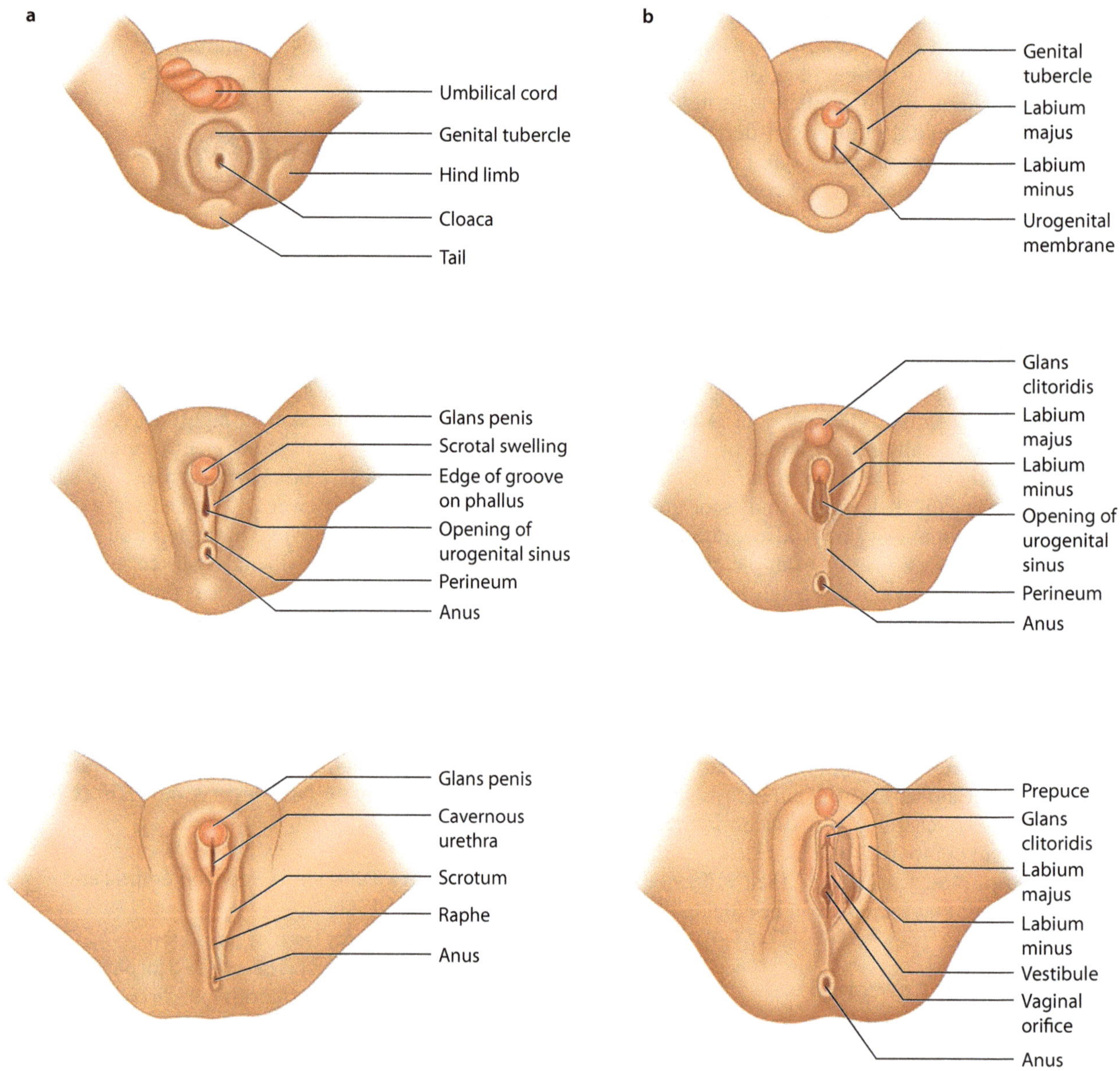

Fig. Development of the external genitalia in **a** men and **b** women

cation. We sense our environment by touching things and we are simultaneously protected by pain receptors in the skin. We regulate our body temperature via the cutaneous vasculature, and we communicate with other people via mimics or smell—all provided by our intact skin. To ensure its protective function, the skin possesses an intricate architecture that can vary depending on the body site, for example, eyelid, back, palms, oral cavity, or genitals. The general micro-structure of the skin comprises three different entities, that is, the epidermis, the dermis (cutis) consisting of the upper/papillary and the lower/reticular dermis, and the subcutaneous fat layer. Epidermis and dermis are separated from each other by a basement membrane that is also the limit for vasculature. The epidermis is free of vessels and nourished by means of oxygen diffusion. The subcutaneous fat is separated from the deeper fat by a superficial fascia, called Scarpa fascia. In the genitalia, this superficial fascia is called Colles (women) or Dartos fascia (men). This anatomical structure is of importance because it serves as a fixation point between fat layers whereas it provides elasticity and sliding properties to the genital skin.

The cutaneous surface of moist environments is characterized by the absence of the cornified layer and

Table Homology of male and female genitalia

Male	Female	Microscopic structure of the skin
Glans penis	Glans clitoridis	Multilayered, nonkeratinizing epidermis, dermal tissue with abundant innervation
Penile foreskin	Clitoral prepuce	Outer face of foreskin: epidermis with cornified layer; Inner face: nonkeratinizing epidermis; mucous epithelium; no subcutaneous fat tissue
Frenulum penis	Frenula clitoridis (pair)	Nonkeratinizing, mucous epithelium, no fat tissue
Penile shaft skin	Small labia	Penis: epidermis with cornified layer Labia: outer surface with thin cornified layer; inner surface: no cornified layer Both sexes: no hair; no subcutaneous fat tissue; many elastic fibers; Penis: highly flexible attachment to underlying tissue via Dartos fascia (fascia penis superficialis)
Scrotal skin	Big labia	Hair bearing epidermis (labia: only outer surface), epidermal cornified layer Labia: subcutaneous fat layer and smooth muscle cells Scrotum: no fat, but contractile tunica dartos with smooth muscle cells and myofibroblasts

hair follicles. Instead, different types of glands, for example, apocrine and eccrine, secrete fluids that moisturize the surface and protect the mucous epithelium (Figs. 47.7, 47.8, and 47.9).

Pathophysiology of Genital Wound Healing, Lymphedema and Scarring

Cutaneous scarring with tissue fibrosis is the result of a postnatal wound healing process. The longer the duration and the excessive the inflammatory response in the healing course, the more likely is the development of aberrant scarring and severe tissue fibrosis. However, scar formation varies depending on the body site, the skin architecture and anchorage to underlying structures.

Little is known about the pathophysiological processes of genital cutaneous wound repair except for the general clinical statement that genital wounds heal fast, with enormous swelling and almost invisible scarring. In the following, I will describe features that are different between the genitalia and the skin of other areas of the body and that influence acute wound healing or chronic scarring (Fig. 47.10). It is beyond the scope of this chapter to include urethral, vaginal, or anal epithelial repair; tissues that derive from different developmental origins and with differential healing behavior (e.g., ulcerations, adhesion or fistula formation) compared to genital skin.

Skin Architecture and Biomechanics

The genital skin has to master many challenges, for example, fast volume changes during sexual activity, sex steroid sensitivity with permanent hormonal changes, the presence of several body openings with constant commensal microbial presence, and infectious threats deriving from sexual contacts. In that context, it is breathtaking to understand the extraordinary adaption of the genital skin to its multiple tasks. To encounter aforementioned challenges, it is excellently equipped anatomically and physiologically to address specific features of the genital microenvironment.

Notably the male genital skin has to manage fast volume changes that occur during sexual activity and for thermal regulation of the testes. These physiological tasks are addressed by several means: (i) abundance of skin tissue on both the penile shaft and the scrotal sac, (ii) the Dartos fascia on the penile shaft and the Tunica Dartos with the Dartos muscle in the scrotum, and (iii) a high amount of elastic fibers in the dermis. In all three items, the genitalia differ from skin of other body areas that is firmly attached to the underlying structures by a rather immobile fat layer. High skin elasticity and abundance of tissue are the prerequisite for tension-free acute wound healing with unapparent scars—optimal repair conditions present in the genitalia. A drawback is the tendency of the outer genitals to enormous swelling and edema after surgery or trauma. The good side is that due to its elasticity and intricate lymphatics, the swelling of the genital tissue resolves as fast as it occurs in healthy subjects.

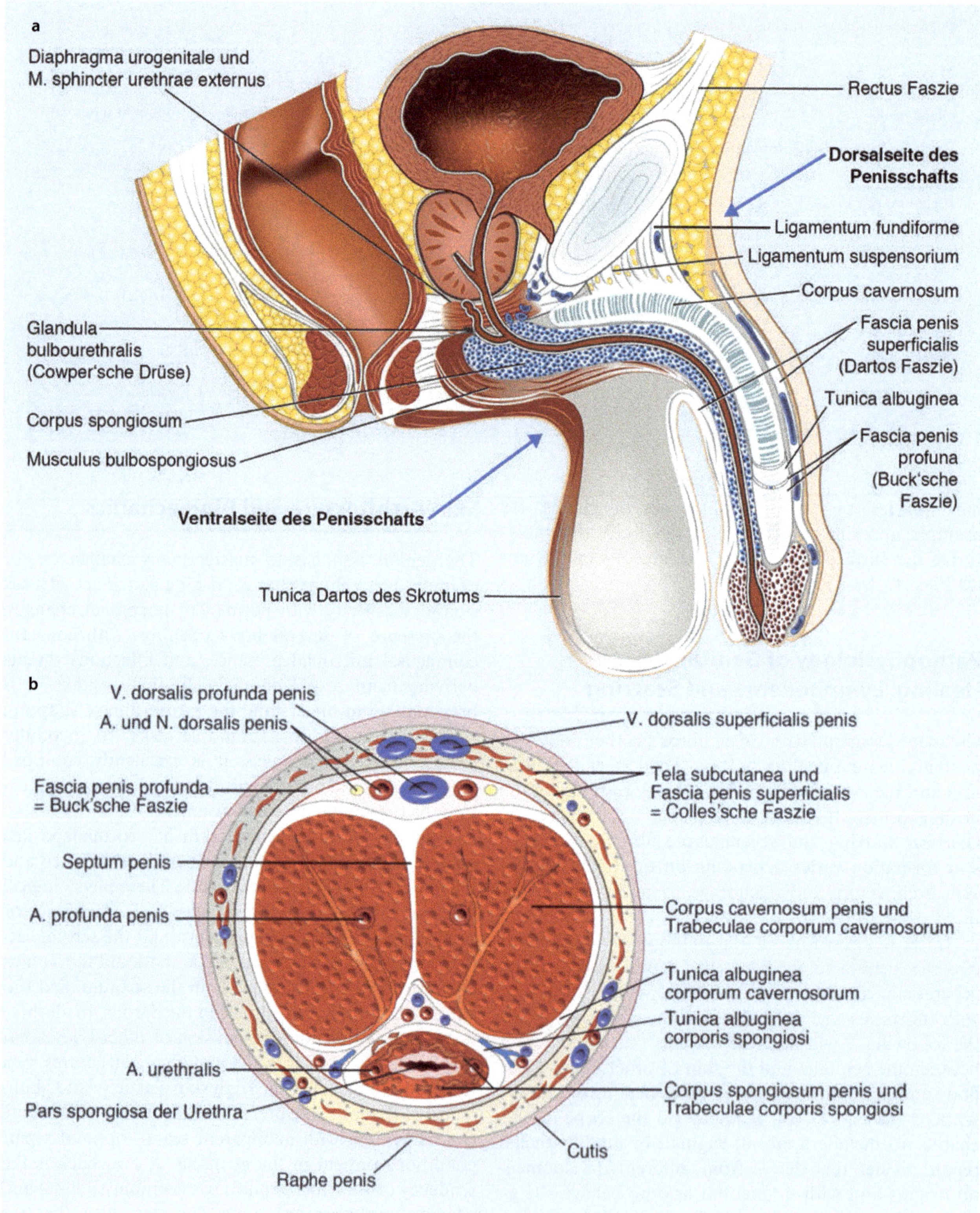

Fig. Anatomy of the male external genitalia. Of note, no fat tissue is present in the penis or scrotal tissue underneath the skin. (Source: Mirastschijski & Remmel, Intimchirurgie, Springer Verlag, 2019)

Moist Environment and Bacterial Colonialization

Urethral, vaginal, and anal orifices are transition zones between mucous membranes and keratinizing skin. As depicted previously, parts of the genitalia are covered by little or nonkeratinizing squamous epithelia. The secreted fluids of multiple glands prevent the exsiccation of mucous membranes and provide a moist microenvironment. It is an established fact that moist wound healing contributes to faster wound closure and reduced scarring.

The proximity of the genital skin to different orifices is Janus sided. Aside from the beneficial moist milieu, bacterial load and stringent body fluids such as urine bear constant threats to the fragile mucosal skin lacking the protective epidermal cornified layer. And again, the genital mucosal skin is well prepared to address both biological and chemical challenges. In contrast to other parts of the body, keratinocytes and fibroblasts of the

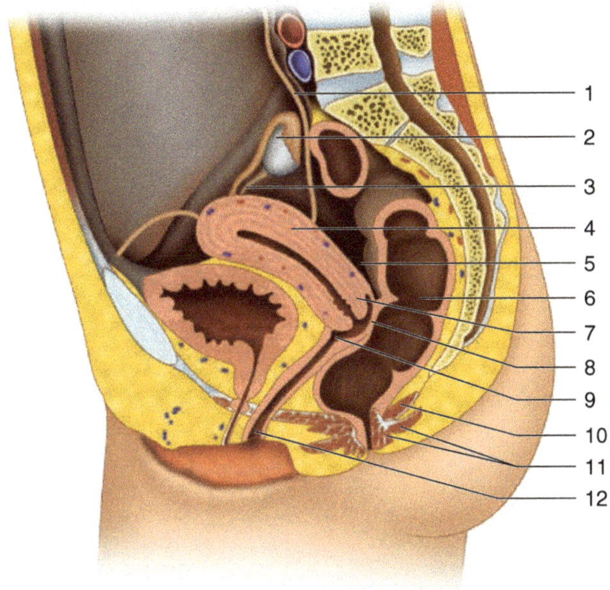

◘ **Fig.** Anatomy of the female external genitalia

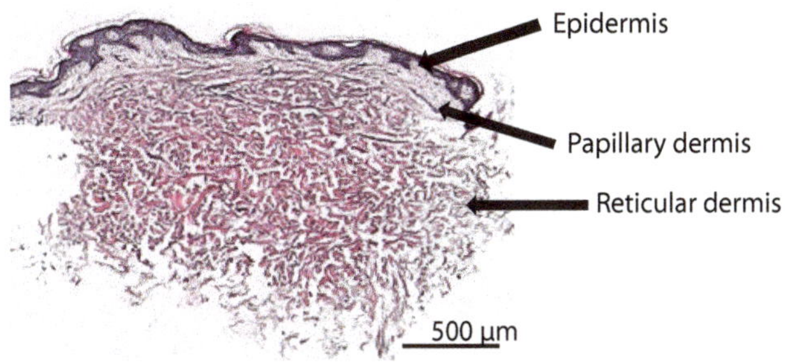

◘ **Fig.** Histological section from the abdominal skin stained with hematoxylin-eosin. (By courtesy of Dr. D. Jiang and Dr. Y. Rinkevich, Helmholtz Center Munich. © All rights reserved)

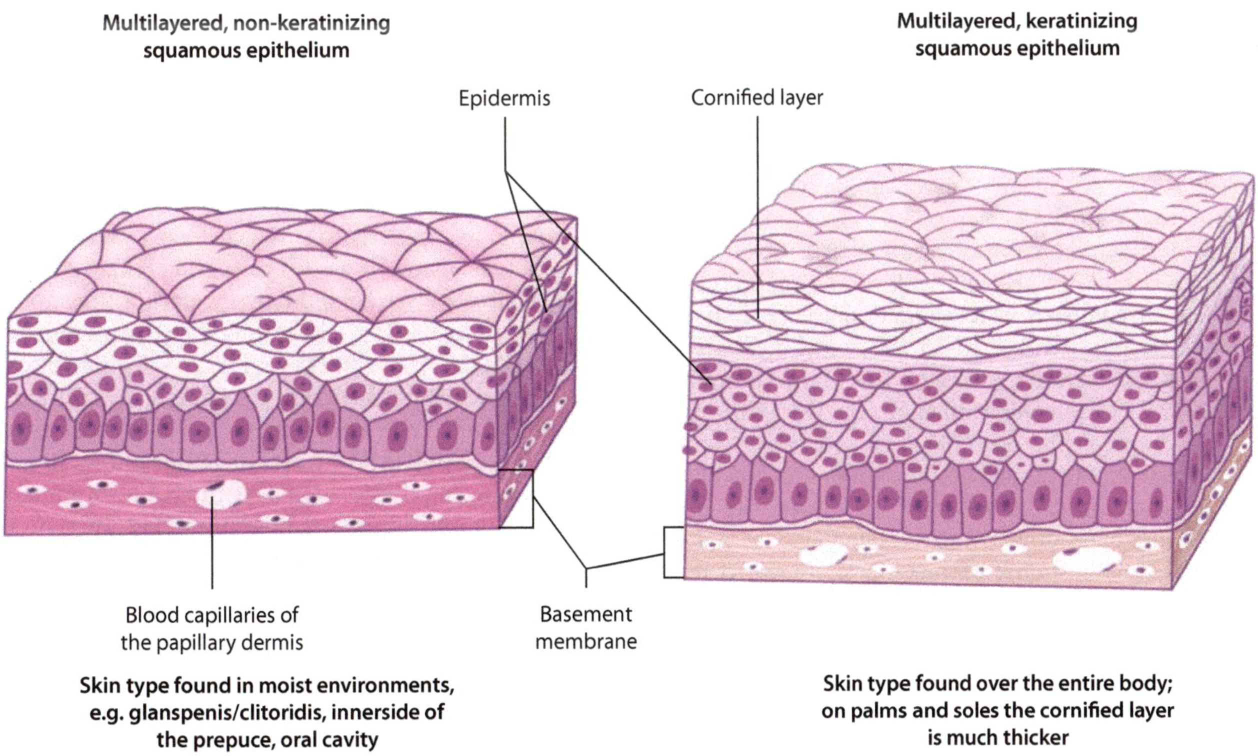

◘ **Fig.** Microstructure of nonkeratinizing and keratinizing skin

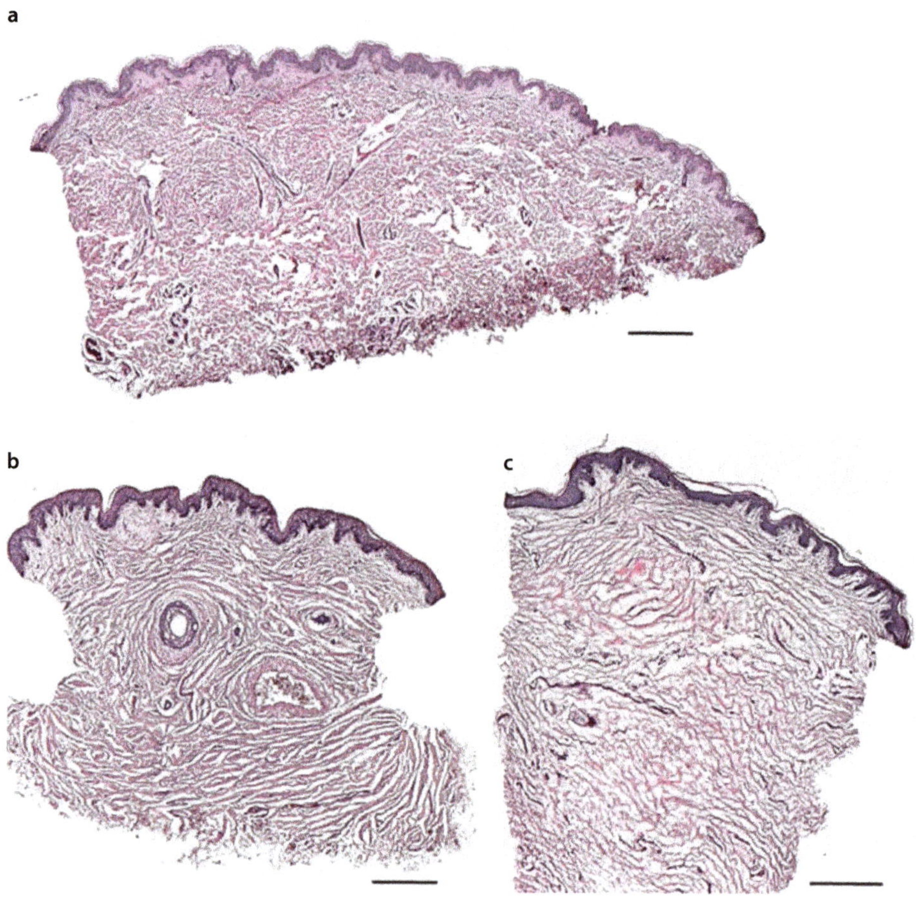

Fig. Microstructure of the skin from different body areas: **a** arm, **b** penis, and **c** small labia. Note the dense dermal structure with multiple vessels in **a** and lose collagen bundles in **b** and **c** with high similarity of penile and labial skin. Scale bar in all sections 500 µm. (Elastica-van-Gieson stainings; by courtesy of Dr. D. Jiang and Dr. Y. Rinkevich, Helmholtz Center Munich)

genital skin are equipped with a fast immune response to bacterial presence. By secreting antimicrobial peptides (AMPs) and defensins and with glandular mucous fluids, bacteria are held at a distance. The immune response is fast and so is the resolution with quick conversion of M1 to M2 macrophages and reduced expression of proinflammatory cytokines [38]. Upon injury, skin cells increase the interleukin (IL)-1α production 15-fold in comparison to vaginal epithelial cells with only threefold increase. IL-1β and tumor necrosis factor (TNF)-α were only secreted by cutaneous epithelia in contrast to mucous epithelial cells [9]. With regard to profibrotic mediators, TGF-β is significantly elevated in normal skin keratinocytes but not in mucosal epithelia and without induction of fibrotic processes in the underlying connective tissue. In summary, the reduced inflammatory response of mucosal epithelia to injury is sufficient to ensure wound closure without inducing serious scarring.

Hormonal Influences

Increased Aromatase Activity and Intracrine Estrogen Production

Hormone responsivity of tissues has profound impact on wound healing. Estrogens accelerate wound closure whereas testosterone delays healing [10]. Skin is a major source of extraglandular sex steroid hormones that are produced from circulating dehydroepiandrosterone (DHEA, [24, 28]) (◘ Fig. 47.11). The intracellular enzyme aromatase converts DHEA downstream into the weaker estrogen Estrone or via testosterone into the more potent 17β-estradiol. Both estrogens act via the estrogen receptors (ERs) α and β, and stimulate keratinocyte and fibroblast migration [11]. In genital fibroblasts, aromatase expression is androgen dependent. Interestingly, estrogens stimulate fibroblast contractility without increasing alpha-smooth muscle actin expression or myofibroblast differentiation [31]. Upon

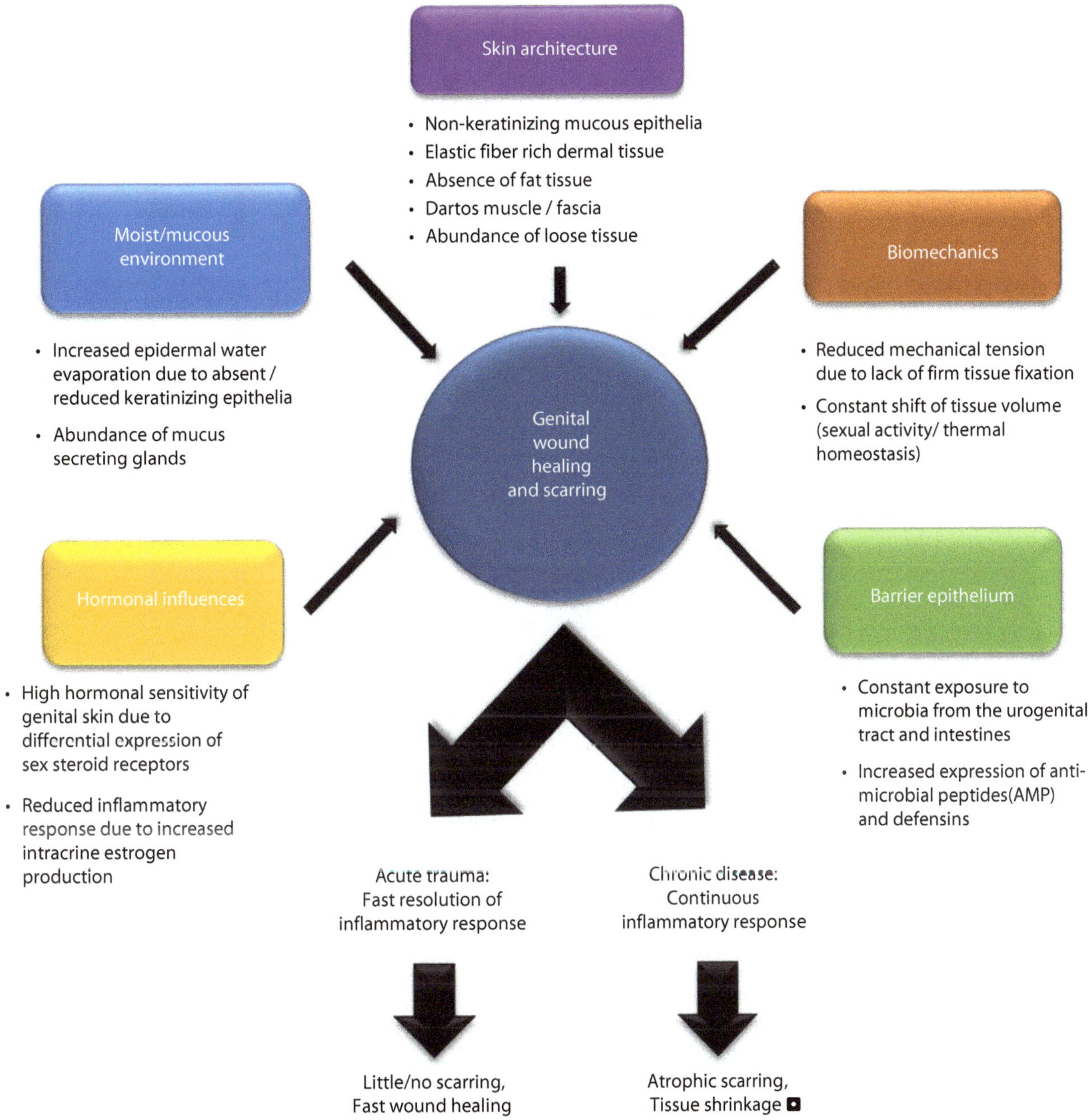

Fig. Factors that influence genital wound repair and differ from skin from other body regions

mechanical wounding, aromatase activity increases 400-fold in keratinocytes with increased intracellular bioavailability of estrogens. Testosterone reduces aromatase activity, albeit this effect is not present in case of low oxygen levels in tissues. Estrogens reduce the cellular inflammatory response via downregulation of the proinflammatory cytokine macrophage migration inhibitory factor (MIF) [6], by reduced TLR-4 mediated MAPK activation, by the reduction of macrophage infiltration into wounds and by dampening the proinflammatory signaling of IL-6 and TNF-α [5]. Of note, estrogens are also important antioxidants that reduce cellular oxidative stress and apoptosis and increase keratinocyte migration and collagen synthesis by dermal fibroblasts [38]. In menopausal women, cutaneous estrogen insufficiency manifests by atrophic skin changes and a diminished defense against reactive oxygen species.

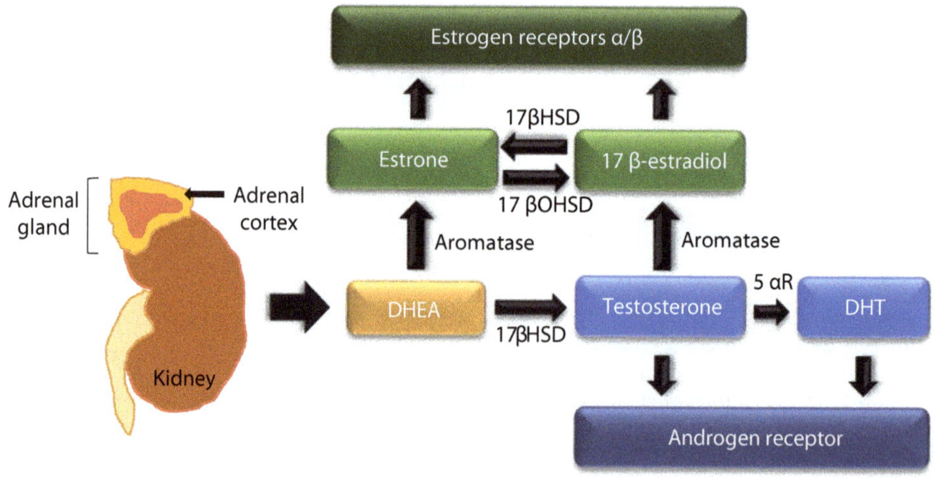

Fig. Simplified description of intracrine sex steroid hormone production by skin cells. Dehydroepiandros-terone (DHEA) is released by the adrenal cortex and further processed directly into estrogens by aromatase or into testosterone by 17-β-hydroxysteroid dehydrogenase (17-β-HSD). Estrone is reversibly oxidized into 17β-estradiol by 17β-OHSD. Testosterone can be either directly converted into the estrogen 17β-estradiol by aromatase or irreversibly converted into dihydrotestosterone by 5-α-reductase (5αR) [39]

Androgen and Estrogen Receptor Expression in Genital Skin

Estrogens act via estrogen receptors and testosterone via androgen receptors (ARs) that are expressed by many cell types. For instance, AR expression differs between genital and nongenital skin with upregulation in genital fibroblasts. In general, it appears that sex steroid hormone expression is higher in stromal cells than in epithelial cells, implying higher responsiveness of fibroblasts to hormonal influences. Aside from receptor expression, the binding capacity and metabolism of sex steroid hormones differs between different skin regions. Testosterone binding capacity of the AR is higher in genital compared to nongenital skin cells [39] from both sexes—independently of age—and testosterone degradation is up to 30 times faster in genital skin compared with nongenital skin [30].

Sex hormone receptor expression in genital skin differs between prenatal and adult genital skin due to the terminal differentiation of the external genitalia that is dependent on hormonal influences. In fetal skin, ARs are very similarly expressed in both sexes with the absence of ARs on the preputial skin, penile shaft/labia minora, and scrotal skin/labia majora. ARs are expressed in the tissue of the glans and inner prepuce of both sexes and in the stromal tissue of the labia.

ER was present in fetal female genital skin except for labia minora and majora [16] and prominent ER staining was found in the entire developing fetal penis including skin, glans, inner prepuce, and stromal cells [4]. Interestingly, ARs and ERs were colocalized in penile tissues.

Less detailed information is available with regard to adult genital skin. In women, ARs are found in keratinocytes and fibroblasts of the labia majora and minora and in the adjacent extragenital skin. ER immunopositivity was found in the labia minora and nongenital skin. There are no differences in sex hormone receptor expression between pre- and postmenopausal women. Progesterone receptors are not present in genital skin. In men, ARs were located to basal keratinocytes and stromal fibroblasts of the penile foreskin. No AR expression was found in nongenital cutaneous keratinocytes or fibroblasts but in fibroblasts of hair follicle papillae or in cells of pilosebaceous ducts and glands, skin structures that are influenced by androgens in their function and structure. The highest intensity of AR staining was noted in genital skin. ERs were similarly expressed in postnatal penile skin with localization to basal epithelia and stromal cells adjacent to the urethra and the urethra itself with age-dependent reduction [27]. Aromatase is not colocalized with estrogen receptors, and levels of aromatase, ERα, and ERβ decrease with age [27].

In summary, ARs and ERs are highly expressed in genital skin in contrast to skin of other body areas with fast binding and degradation of testosterone or conversion into estrogen by increased aromatase activity. A summary of hormonal differences between genital skin and nongenital skin is given in ◘ Table 47.2.

Acute Wound Repair of Genital Skin After Trauma

Depending on the type and severity of the injury, two main clinical symptoms characterize traumatized genitalia, namely enormous bleeding and swelling. When the hematoma resolves and the swelling disappears, wounds heal with almost no visible scarring even after major trauma. An example for invisible genital scarring is the fact that one-third of the male world population is circumcised [37] without any report of hypertrophic

Table Hormonal differences between genital skin and nongenital skin

	Genital skin	Nongenital skin
Androgen receptor	Higher expression in labia majora and minora Upregulated in fibroblasts and basal keratinocytes Colocalization with ER	Only present in hair follicles and pilo-sebaceous duct keratinocytes Low expression in extra-genital skin
Estrogen receptors	Highly expressed in penis and labia minora Restricted to basal keratinocytes and stromal fibroblasts Expression decreases with age	Lower expression compared to vulva or vagina Expressed by keratinocytes and fibroblasts Absence in skin appendages or blood vessels
Testosterone	Higher AR-binding capacity of testosterone 30 times faster degradation Reduced effect on aromatase activity in low-oxygen conditions	Higher rate of conversion into DHT Higher 5-α-reductase activity with irreversible formation of DHT
Estrogens	No conversion of 17β-estradiol into the weaker estrone Stimulate fibroblast contractility without alpha-smooth-muscle actin (ASMA) expression	Threefold increased metabolism of 17β-estradiol into estrone
Aromatase	Higher activity in fibroblasts with conversion of testosterone into 17β-estradiol Dose-dependent reduced activity by testosterone Aromatase expression androgen dependent	Expression in skin fibroblasts, keratinocytes of the outer root sheath and in terminal hair follicles and in cells of sebaceous glands and ducts

AR androgen receptor, *ER* estrogen receptor, *DHT* dihydrotestosterone

scarring to the preputial skin. Despite major trauma after female genital mutilation/cutting, the genital skin heals uneventfully if the girl survives postinterventional bleeding and infection. Cutaneous genital infections are disastrous and can rapidly lead to septic conditions with high lethality. Fournier gangrene is one example of necrotizing fasciitis of the genital skin with a mortality rate of 80% without surgery [18]. Obviously, the loose architecture of genital skin provides optimal means for rapid subcutaneous bacterial spreading leading ultimately to multiple organ failure and death.

The aforementioned characteristics of the outer genitalia with regard to architecture, fixation, microenvironment, hormonal influences, and reduced inflammatory response orchestrate the fast resolution of the acute wound healing process with reduced scar formation. Albeit the apparently scar-free wound healing properties of genital skin, there is one exception. The ventral part of the prepuce ends in the so-called frenulum that is fixed to stromal tissue of the ventral side of the glans bridging to the penile shaft. In case of excessive tissue removal during circumcision, the frenulum can shrink and pull the glans in direction of the penile shaft that is painful, gives discomfort during erection, and can cause reduced sensation of the glans penis (Fig. 47.12).

Chronic Inflammatory Diseases of the External Genitalia and Tissue Fibrosis

Several skin diseases with autoimmune background can affect the outer genitalia with chronic inflammation leading to tissue shrinkage and atrophy. Chronic lymphedema after tumor surgery and/or irradiation, with infectious background or due to congenital malformation of lymphatic organs, leads to tissue fibrosis and stiffening and to verruca-like epidermal changes in the long run. In the following, the most common chronic diseases and changes to the genital skin will be described in detail.

Lichen Sclerosus et Atrophicus/ Balanitis Xerotica Obliterans

Lichen sclerosus et atrophicus (LSC), also called balanitis xerotica obliterans in men, is the most common chronic dermatitis localized to the mucous membranes and skin of the genitalia. LSC is found in females and males with a ratio of up to 10:1 and has a double peak in females with occurrence in prepubertal and postmenopausal age. In men, LSC is the most common

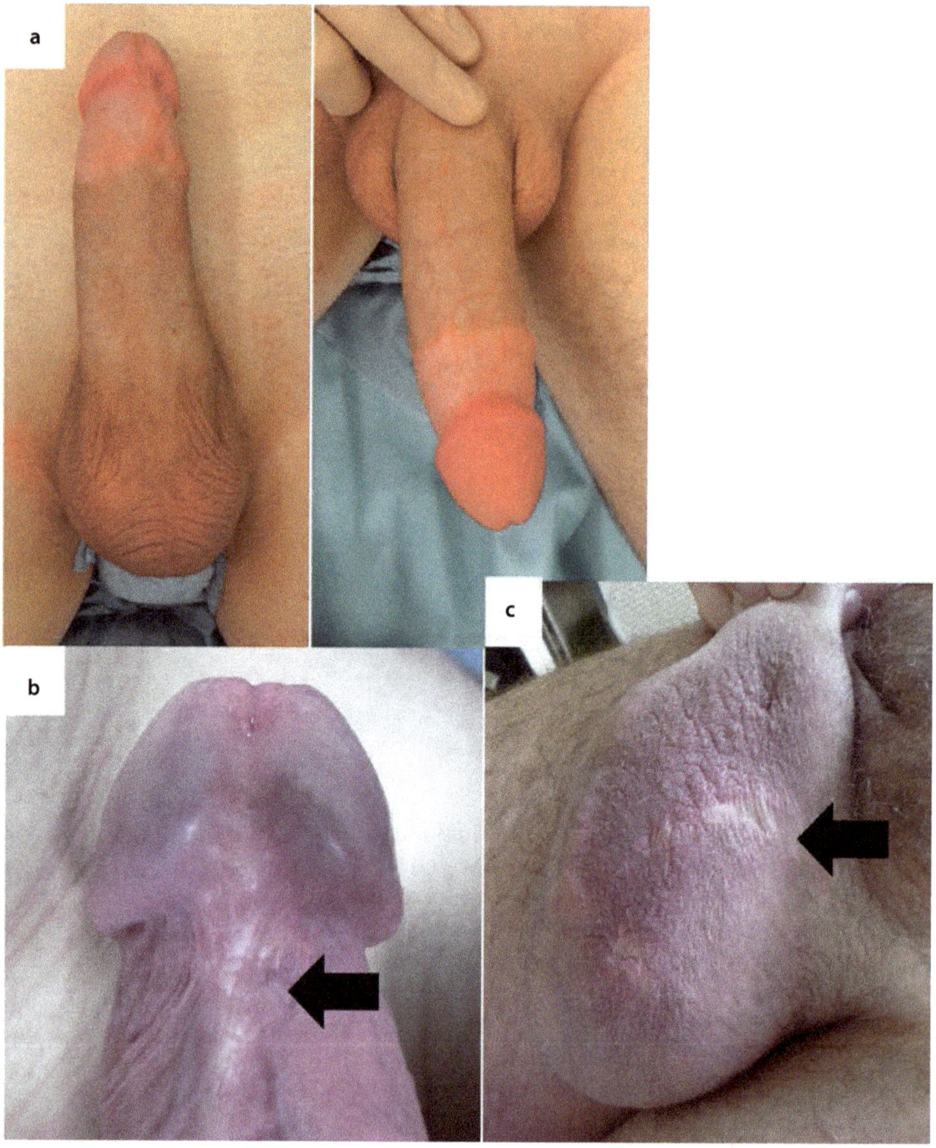

◘ Fig. Examples for scar formation to the male genitalia. **a** Invisible scar after circumcision. Note differential pigmentation of the outer penile skin and the remaining inner part of the prepuce. **b** Scar after excessive circumcision with shortening and scarring of the frenulum (arrow). **c** Scrotal scar (arrow) after multiple excisions of silicone granuloma and subcutaneous fibrotic tissue

cause of acquired phimosis [3] and affects the glans and the prepuce (◘ Fig. 47.13). Typical symptoms are a thickening of the foreskin that impairs retraction. Whitish plaques can extend over the entire glans with affection of the urethral meatus followed by stenosis and voiding problems. In females, the anogenital area is frequently affected forming an 8-shaped efflorescence around the vulva and the anal orifice with opaque plaques and papules. In chronic disease, these atrophic lesions can lead to a complete destruction of the vulva with resorption of the small labia, narrowing of the vaginal introitus and burying of the clitoris. The patients' quality of life is severely reduced due to chronic pruritus, pain, and obstipation resulting from painful defecation in women and painful erection and hygienic problems in men. Of note, LSC is associated with squamous cell carcinoma formation in 5% of women [17] and up to 30% of men [3]. Other LSC-associated diseases comprise autoimmune thyroiditis, vitiligo, or pernicious anemia. The etiology of LSC is not fully understood. An autoimmune origin with T- and B-cell-driven response to a yet unknown antigen is discussed because dense T-lymphocytic infiltrates with concomitant vasculitis and extensive tissue destruction are found in LSC-tissue sections. The glycoprotein extracellular matrix protein 1 (ECM 1) has been targeted as putative autoantigen because the symptoms of the autosomal recessive disorder lipoid proteinosis resemble acquired LSC with thickening and scarring of skin and mucosa [2]. Another related dermatosis, the Lichen planus, presents with similar symptoms and etiology that makes the initial differentiation between lichen sclerosus and lichen planus difficult [35].

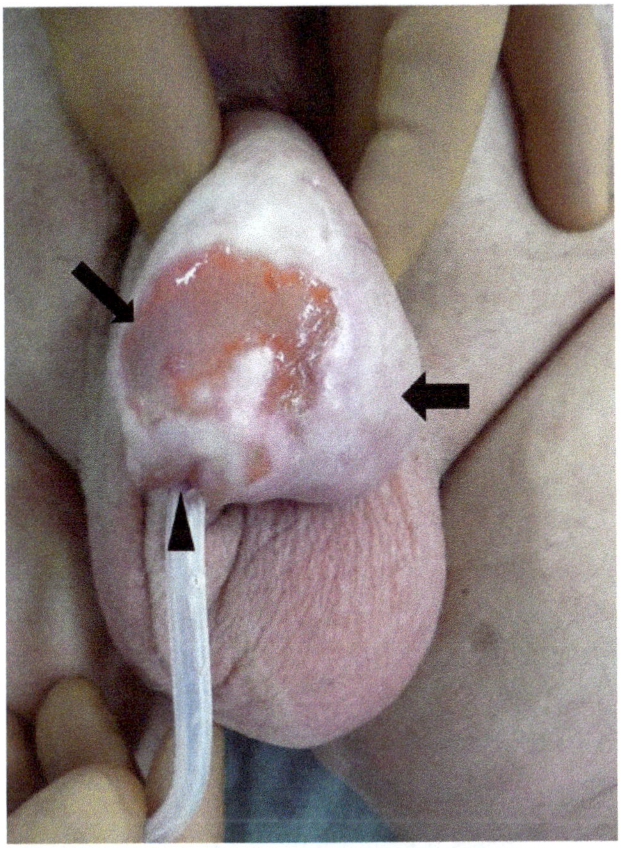

■ **Fig.** Patient with Lichen sclerosus et atrophicus to the penile glans and after several circumcisions and reconstruction of a buried penis. Note central ulceration (thin arrow) surrounded by opaque and shiny skin changes of the glans including meatal stenosis (arrowhead) and granuloma formation (thick arrow)

Behçet's Disease

Aphthous stomatitis (oral ulcers) and genital ulcers are common features of Behçet's disease. The etiology of the autoimmune vasculitis is unknown. The most common site for genital ulcer formation is the scrotum in men and the big labia in women. Interestingly, scrotal and big labia ulcers heal with normal, nonhypertrophic scarring whereas skin lesions on the small labia heal without scars similar to oral ulcers [22].

Chronic Inflammation due to Foreign Body Reaction

The size of the penis is of central importance for many men who build their self-confidence on the penile length. In that context it is not surprising that a plethora of different substances were used for penile enlargement over centuries. Vaseline, paraffin, liquid mercury, silicone (■ Figs. 47.12c and 47.14), or cod liver oil were injected in to the scrotum or under the penile skin for girth enhancement with catastrophic complications such as granuloma formation, infections, swelling, and local tissue necrosis [33]. Alternatively polymethylmethacrylate (PMMA) microspheres or autologous fat are used as fillers or silicone implants for permanent enlargement [19, 20]. The placement of permanent, alloplastic foreign body material in an environment populated by a variety of commensal microbes is risky due to the inherent danger of infection. In case of granuloma, tissue necrosis, or implant infection, the foreign material must be removed with subsequent tissue loss. Foreign body materials can initiate a chronic inflammatory process with cutaneous thickening and subcutaneous tissue fibrosis leading ultimately to a shrinkage of the entire penile shaft. Details of the surgical treatment after foreign body injection are shown in ■ Fig. 47.14.

Congenital and Acquired Genital Lymphedema and Tissue Fibrosis

Lymphedema is defined as low- (<1 g/100 ml) or high- (>1 g/100 ml) protein fluid retention in the interstitial space [8]. Congenital malformation of lymphatic vessels can cause chronic lymphedema. Acquired lymphedema occurs after surgery (■ Fig. 47.15) for various reasons (cancer, gangrene, foreign bodies, etc.), irradiation, or filariasis. The swelling is due to an imbalance of the production and absorption, including drainage of the lymph that can be caused by an obstruction, disruption, or insufficiency of the lymph vessels. Chronic lymphedema affects the surrounding tissue with fibrosis and the skin with rhagades and recurrent infections, blister formation, wart-like epidermal excrescences, and scarring.

Treatment of Genital Wounds and Scars

The manifold the causes for wounding and scarring to the genitalia are, the diverging are the treatments as well. The choice of the appropriate surgical technique is orientated on the depth, magnitude, and location of the defect and the quality of the surrounding tissue. Needless to say that the delicate genital anatomy of both sexes and the variety of tissue defects or scars that can extend over to adjacent body areas require highly skilled surgeons with expertise in reconstruction of the genitalia. Aside from defect closure, restoration of the voiding and sexual function are central to each reconstructive procedure and require often an interdisciplinary setting.

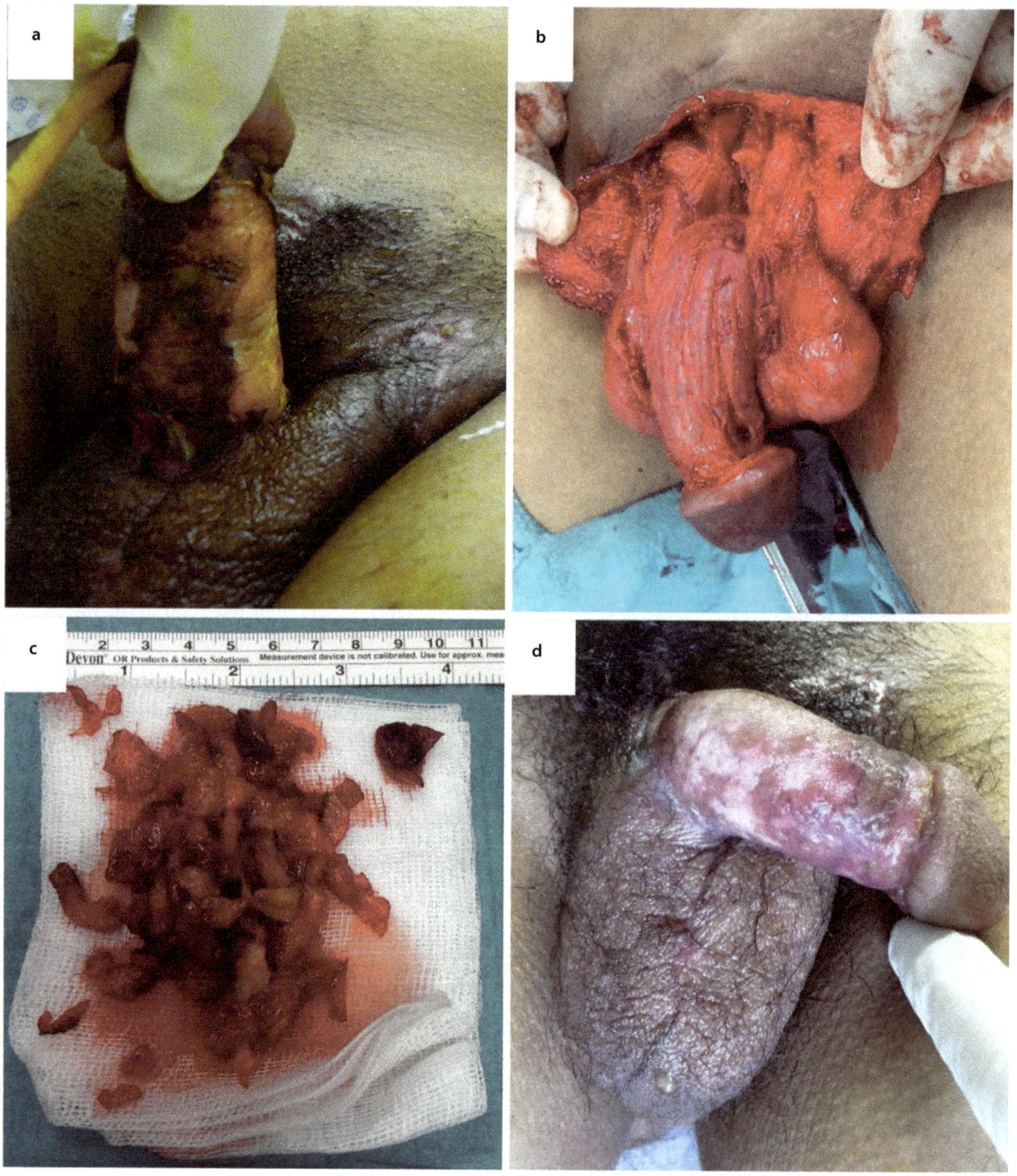

Fig. Penile skin necrosis after silicone oil injection. **a** Tis-sue necrosis over the entire penile shaft preoperatively. **b, c** Intraoperative situs **b** after meticulous excision of all foreign body material and granuloma **c**. **d** Postoperative result after full-thickness skin grafting with epidermal thickening and hypopigmentation 6 weeks after grafting

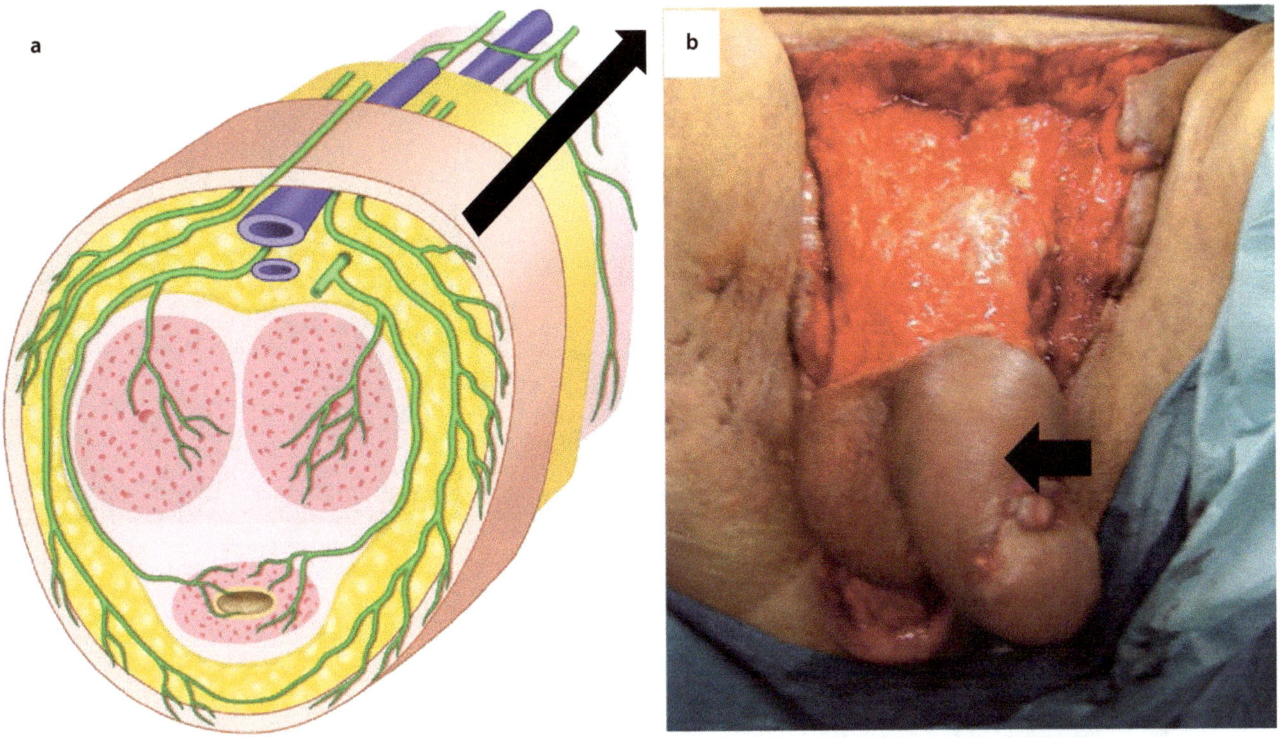

◘ Fig. Penile lymphedema **a** Penile lymphatic vessels and lymph drainage on the dorsal side of the penile shaft (arrow). **b** Fournier gangrene on the base of a chronic acne inversa with massive tissue resection of the prepubic and groin area after necrotizing infection with a multiresistant *Staphylococcus aureus* and different enterobacteriaceae. Note massive swelling of the penile shaft (arrow) with burying of the glans due to loss of dorsal lymphatic vessels and drainage pathways after debridement

Treatment of Acute Wounds and Tissue Defects

Small acute wounds and tissue defects are commonly closed primarily due to the abundance, elasticity, and loose fixation of the genital skin and tissue. For instance, primary closure of scrotal defects after up to 50% tissue loss is feasible, otherwise local or distant flaps (e.g., bilateral gracilis flaps; ◘ Fig. 47.16) or skin grafts are used to reconstruct the scrotal sac [18]. Superficial skin loss to the penile glans recovers by conservative treatment, and deeper tissue defects need skin grafting, for example, with oral mucosa or thin split-thickness skin [34]. Penile shaft defects can be elegantly closed using preputial flaps in case the patient is not circumcised. Otherwise, split-thickness or full-thickness skin grafts are the current state-of-the-art for penile shaft reconstruction. Drawback of free skin grafts is the lack of cutaneous elasticity and sensation. In case of abundant scrotal tissue, local neurovascular flaps (e.g., midline raphe scroti artery, MiRA-flap) can restore—at least in part—tissue texture and sensation [26].

The reconstruction of the female genitalia is similar as in men with primary closure of small lesions and flap surgery in case of larger tissue losses. An elegant procedure for reconstruction of the big labia is the anterior obturator artery perforator flap (aOAP) that is harvested from the groin area [29]. Interestingly, the flap tissue heals with minimal scarring once it is transferred to the vulva in contrast to its harvest site in the groin that is prone to hypertrophic scarring (personal communication with Prof. Dr. Uwe von Fritschen, Desert Flower Center, Helios Klinikum Emil von Behring, Berlin).

Treatment of Genital Wounds and Scars After Burn Injury

The golden standard for treatment of partial-thickness (deep second degree) and full-thickness (third degree) burns is debridement of the necrotic tissue with skin grafting. Due to its high regenerative potential, a more conservative approach is the current clinical practice for genital skin until full demarcation of the necrotic tissue. As mentioned earlier, the genitals are capable of

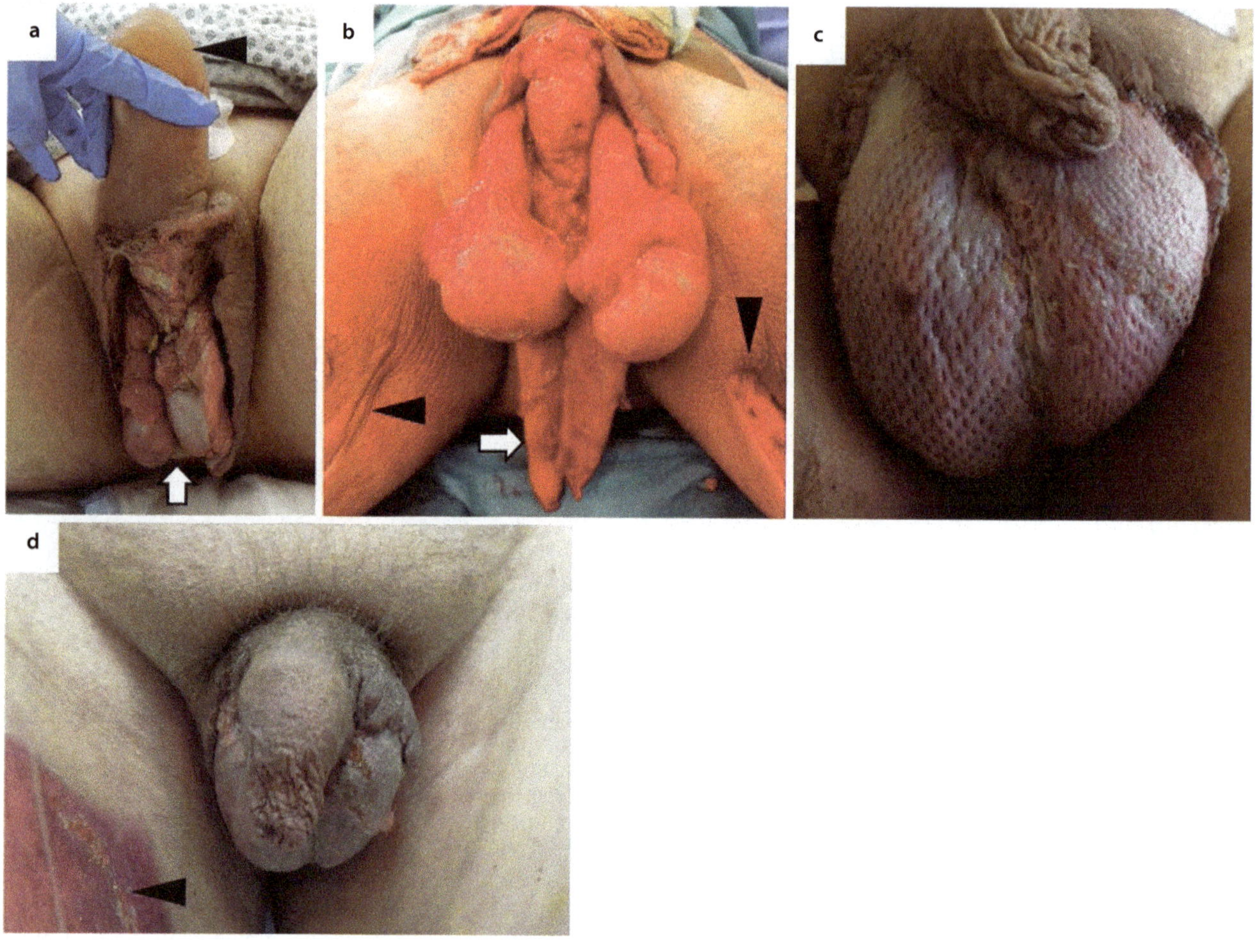

■ **Fig.** Plastic–reconstructive surgery of the scrotum with bilateral gracilis muscle flaps covered by a split-thickness skin graft. **a** Preoperative site with almost complete loss of the scrotal tissue. Both testes are exposed (white arrow) with lymphedematous swelling of the penis (arrowhead). **b** Intraoperative situs after debridement. Both gracilis muscles (white arrow) are mobilized and rotated into the defect by tunneling underneath the perineal crease. Harvest areas are depicted with arrowheads. **c** Postoperative site after 1 week with almost complete skin graft take. **d** Situation after 3 weeks with little scarring and a skin texture resembling the natural scrotal appearance. Note split-thickness harvest site to the right thigh (arrowhead)

compensating for rather large tissue losses with only minor scar formation [15]. In contrast, severe scarring and scar contractures are common to the groin and perineal area that can impair the movement of the lower extremities (■ Figs. 47.2 and 47.3). After scar excision, local skin flaps, for example, Z-plasties, are usually used for wound closure and tension release. In case of insufficient local tissue, distant, pedicled, or free flaps with microvascular anastomosis are standard procedures and belong to the repertoire of a plastic–reconstructive surgeon (■ Fig. 47.17). For further detailed information, the recently published textbooks for genital [25] or burn [13] reconstructive surgery are recommended.

Gender Reassignment Surgery

Genital gender reassignment surgery comprises the formation of a female vulva, including big and small labia, a clitoris with a clitoral hood and a vagina in male-to-female transsexuals and the formation of a penoid with functional elongation of the urethra and a scrotum in female-to-male transsexuals. Highly specialized surgeons perform these extraordinary procedures in an interdisciplinary context with astonishing results. Notably scarring is minimal despite extensive surgical intervention to the genitalia with relocation of ontogenetically homologous entities. My profound fascination for absent or minimal genital scarring derives from patients after gender reassignment surgery (■ Fig. 47.18).

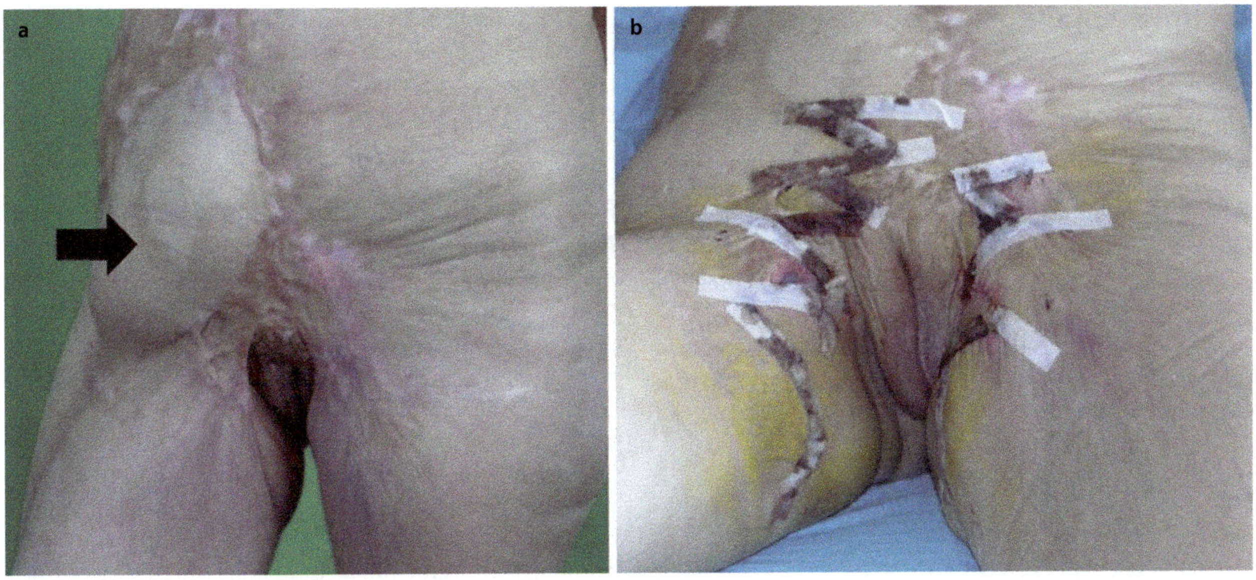

Fig. Scar contractures to the inguinal and perineal region after burn injury. **a** Preoperative situs with scar contractures span-ning over both groins that impair the range of motion of both legs. Of note, the genital area, including the big labia, is devoid of scarring. Previous reconstructive surgery included local tissue transfer for scar release to the right groin (arrow). **b** Postoperative situs after multiple Z-plasties

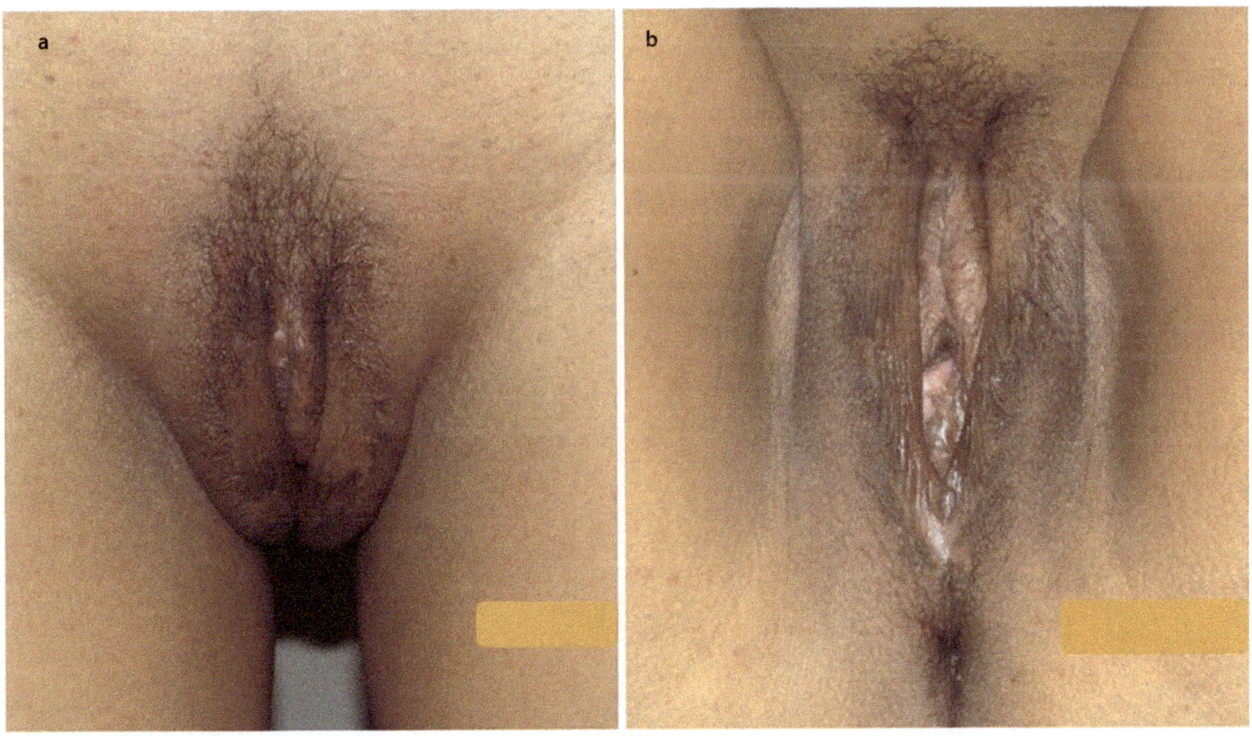

Fig. Male-to-female transsexual patient after genital reassignment surgery. Note construction of all vulvar structures with big and small labia, a clitoris covered completely by the clitoral prepuce and the vaginal entrance. **a**. ventral aspect, **b**. caudal aspect (By courtesy of Dr. Jürgen Schaff, PSC Munich)

Treatment of Chronic Genital Skin Diseases

Chronic genital ulcers can originate from autoimmune diseases, infections, pressure sores, etc. Describing details on the systemic rheumatologic treatment of autoimmune disorders is beyond the scope of this chapter. More information on diagnosis and therapy of dermatologic autoimmune disorders is provided in excellent reviews [7, 32].

LSC in women responds well to topical corticosteroid ointments whereas phimoses in men require surgical intervention. Circumcision with complete removal of the penile foreskin is the gold standard that leads to relapse-free recovery from LSC [3, 7].

Lymphedema Treatment

Depending on the underlying cause of noninfectious genital lymphedema, the treatment is primarily conservative with a complex decongestive physiotherapy (CDP), according to Földi [8]. To ensure permanent lymphatic drainage, compression therapy is recommended not only in patients with lymphedema but also in patients after genital reconstruction. Surgical intervention in secondary genital lymphedema is controversially discussed and should be limited to selected patients in the hands of experienced surgeons and physiotherapists [23, 36].

The treatment of filariasis is antimicrobial; in case of genital elephantiasis, surgical removal of penile and scrotal tissue is indicated for debulking although clinical studies on the postsurgical outcome are scarce [21].

Postoperative Management for Scar Prevention

Postoperative excessive scarring of the genitalia is rare and limited to free partial-thickness skin grafts to the penile shaft. In contrast, hypertrophic scarring and scar contractures are common to the perineal and inguinal area with postoperative compression therapy and mobilizing physiotherapy being imperative. With regard to the genitals, lymphedema formation is more common and an issue for intensive postoperative care. Standard or tailor-made individual compression garments are available and recommended for 3–6 months. Compression panties for women are available in different sizes. With regard to male compression therapy, the issue is more problematic due to difficulties in handling penile compression stockings and the fixation to the penile base. Our group has developed such a penile compression stocking in cooperation with highly qualified orthopedic technicians who produce individually tailored pressure garments for men after skin grafts or flap surgery with postoperative lymphedematous swelling. After a short training period, all men were capable of handling the stocking by themselves (◘ Fig. 47.19).

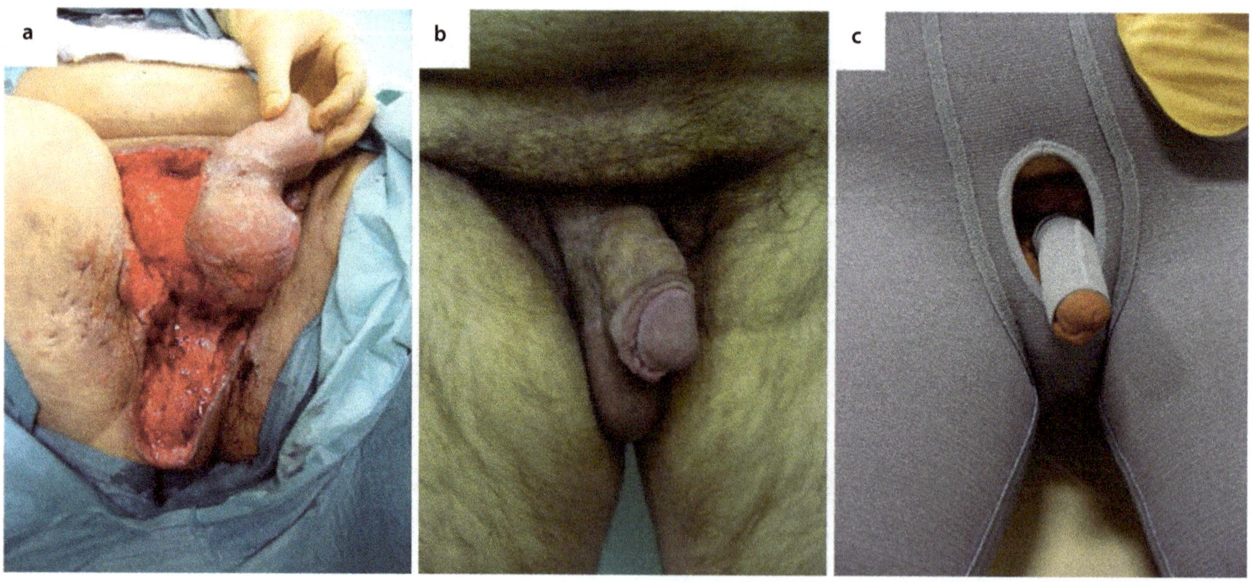

◘ **Fig.** Postoperative treatment after reconstruction of a genital and perineal defect after Fournier gangrene. **a** Preoperative site after multiple debridements. **b** Postoperative situation 4 weeks after defect closure with split-thickness skin grafts. **c** Adjuvant treatment with tailor-made pressure garments to prevent excessive scarring. Note separate compression panty for the perineal area and a tailor-made stocking for the penile shaft

We recommend the prescription of at least two pairs of garments to ensure daily changes and washing for better hygiene.

Conclusion

Hypertrophic scarring to the genitalia is uncommon, possibly due to the high regenerative potential of genital skin, the abundance and elasticity of the local tissue, and the rapid and reduced immune response to traumatic events. Chronic inflammatory diseases such as lichen sclerosus et atrophicus or chronic lymphedema lead to tissue fibrosis with epidermal thickening and to a shrinkage and atrophy with complete destruction of the genitalia in the long run. In contrast to the genital skin, hypertrophic scarring and scar contractures are frequently seen in body areas adjacent to the genitalia, for example, the groin or the perineal crease. The reconstructive procedures for scar release or tissue defect coverage should aim not only at defect closure but also at the functional restoration of micturition and sexuality and should exclusively be performed by experienced specialists preferably in an interdisciplinary setting.

Take-Home Messages

- Genital skin wounds heal fast and with almost invisible scarring.
- The anatomical microstructure of genital skin differs in its architecture and elasticity to skin from other body sites.
- Extensive tissue loss can be compensated—in part—due to the abundance of genital skin.
- The inflammatory response of genital skin is adapted to the permanent microbial colonialization with fast-onset and quick resolution.
- Androgen and estrogen receptors are highly expressed in genital skin. Genital wound repair benefits from hormonal responsiveness and increased presence of sex steroid hormones due to intracrine production by skin cells.
- Chronic inflammatory conditions caused by autoimmune disorders, infections, or foreign material can lead to severe tissue fibrosis followed by shrinkage and destruction of the outer genitalia.
- Chronic lymphedema manifests in enormous swelling of the outer genitalia with long-term tissue fibrosis and wart-like epidermal changes.
- Reconstruction of tissue defects or scar contractures should include the functional restoration of micturition and sexuality.
- Reconstructive interventions to the outer genitalia are complex and delicate and should exclusively be performed by experienced surgeons specialized in genital surgery.

References

1. Balzano FL, Hudak SJ. Military genitourinary injuries: past, present, and future. Transl Androl Urol. 2018;7:646–52.
2. Chan I, Liu L, Hamada T, Sethuraman G, McGrath JA. The molecular basis of lipoid proteinosis: mutations in extracellular matrix protein 1. Exp Dermatol. 2007;16:881–90.
3. Clouston D, Hall A, Lawrentschuk N. Penile lichen sclerosus (balanitis xerotica obliterans). BJU Int. 2011;108 Suppl 2:14–9.
4. Crescioli C, Maggi M, Vannelli GB, Ferruzzi P, Granchi S, Mancina R, Muratori M, Forti G, Serio M, Luconi M. Expression of functional estrogen receptors in human fetal male external genitalia. J Clin Endocrinol Metab. 2003;88:1815–24.
5. Crompton R, Williams H, Ansell D, Campbell L, Holden K, Cruickshank S, Hardman MJ. Oestrogen promotes healing in a bacterial LPS model of delayed cutaneous wound repair. Lab Investig. 2016;96:439–49.
6. Emmerson E, Campbell L, Ashcroft GS, Hardman MJ. Unique and synergistic roles for 17beta-estradiol and macrophage migration inhibitory factor during cutaneous wound closure are cell type specific. Endocrinology. 2009;150:2749–57.
7. Fistarol SK, Itin PH. Diagnosis and treatment of lichen sclerosus: an update. Am J Clin Dermatol. 2013;14:27–47.
8. Földi M, Földi E. Földi's textbook of lymphology. San Francisco: Elsevier; 2012.
9. Gallant-Behm CL, Du P, Lin SM, Marucha PT, Dipietro LA, Mustoe TA. Epithelial regulation of mesenchymal tissue behavior. J Invest Dermatol. 2011;131:892–9.
10. Gilliver SC, Ashcroft GS. Sex steroids and cutaneous wound healing: the contrasting influences of estrogens and androgens. Climacteric. 2007;10:276–88.
11. Gilliver SC, Ashworth JJ, Ashcroft GS. The hormonal regulation of cutaneous wound healing. Clin Dermatol. 2007;25:56–62.
12. Harpole BG, Wibbenmeyer LA, Erickson BA. Genital burns in the national burn repository: incidence, etiology, and impact on morbidity and mortality. Urology. 2014;83:298–302.
13. Herndon DN, editor. Total burn care. Philadelphia: Saunders Elsevier; 2018.
14. Isbir D, Cedidi C. Acne inversa inguinalis. In: Mirastschijski U, Remmel E, editors. Intimchirurgie. Berlin: Springer; 2019. p. 243–51.
15. Ismail Aly ME, Huang T. Management of burn injuries of the perineum. In: Herndon D, editor. Total burn care. London: Elsevier; 2018. p. 609–17.
16. Kalloo NB, Gearhart JP, Barrack ER. Sexually dimorphic expression of estrogen receptors, but not of androgen receptors in human fetal external genitalia. J Clin Endocrinol Metab. 1993;77:692–8.
17. Kirtschig G. Lichen sclerosus-presentation, diagnosis and management. Dtsch Arztebl Int. 2016;113:337–43.
18. Lehnhardt M, Wallner C, Daigeler A. Reconstruction of the male genitals after Fournier gangrene. In: Mirastschijski U, Remmel E, editors. Intimchirurgie. Berlin: Springer; 2019. p. 253–63.
19. Lemperle G, Casavantes L. Penisvergrößerung durch Injektion von PMMA-Mikrosphären. In: Mirastschijski U, Remmel E, editors. Intimchirurgie. Berlin: Springer; 2019. p. 79–89.
20. Lemperle G, Elist JJ, Jethon C. Penisvergrößerung mit dem Penuma-Silikon-Implantat. In: Mirastschijski U, Remmel E, editors. Intimchirurgie. Berlin: Springer; 2019. p. 69–78.
21. Lim KH, Speare R, Thomas G, Graves P. Surgical treatment of genital manifestations of lymphatic filariasis: a systematic review. World J Surg. 2015;39:2885–99.
22. Mat MC, Goksugur N, Engin B, Yurdakul S, Yazici H. The frequency of scarring after genital ulcers in Behcet's syndrome: a prospective study. Int J Dermatol. 2006;45:554–6.

23. Mcdougal WS. Lymphedema of the external genitalia. J Urol. 2003;170:711–6.
24. Mills SJ, Ashworth JJ, Gilliver SC, Hardman MJ, Ashcroft GS. The sex steroid precursor DHEA accelerates cutaneous wound healing via the estrogen receptors. J Invest Dermatol. 2005;125:1053–62.
25. Mirastschijski U, Remmel E. Intimchirurgie. Berlin: Springer; 2019.
26. Mirastschijski U, Schwenke C, Schmiedl A. Plastic-surgical reconstruction of the male genitals. In: Mirastschijski U, Remmel E, editors. Intimchirurgie. Berlin: Springer; 2019. p. 189–206.
27. Mowa CN, Jesmin S, Miyauchi T. The penis: a new target and source of estrogen in male reproduction. Histol Histopathol. 2006;21:53–67.
28. Nelson LR, Bulun SE. Estrogen production and action. J Am Acad Dermatol. 2001;45:S116–24.
29. O'dey DM, Bozkurt A, Pallua N. The anterior Obturator Artery Perforator (aOAP) flap: surgical anatomy and application of a method for vulvar reconstruction. Gynecol Oncol. 2010;119:526–30.
30. Pinsky L, Finkelberg R, Straisfeld C, Zilahi B, Kaufman M, Hall G. Testosterone metabolism by serially subcultured fibroblasts from genital and nongenital skin of individual human donors. Biochem Biophys Res Commun. 1972;46:364–9.
31. Pomari E, Dalla Valle L, Pertile P, Colombo L, Thornton MJ. Intracrine sex steroid synthesis and signaling in human epidermal keratinocytes and dermal fibroblasts. FASEB J. 2015;29:508–24.
32. Saccucci M, Di Carlo G, Bossu M, Giovarruscio F, Salucci A, Polimeni A. Autoimmune diseases and their manifestations on oral cavity: diagnosis and clinical management. J Immunol Res. 2018;2018:6061825.
33. Schill S, Panfilov DE, Mirastschijski U. Intimchirurgie beim Mann. In: Mirastschijski U, Remmel E, editors. Intimchirurgie. Berlin: Springer; 2019. p. 49–68.
34. Schwenke C, Melchior S. Peniskarzinom aus uro-onkologischer Sicht. In: Mirastschijski U, Remmel E, editors. Intimchirurgie. Berlin: Springer; 2019. p. 207–15.
35. Terlou A, Santegoets LA, Van Der Meijden WI, Heijmans-Antonissen C, Swagemakers SM, Van Der Spek PJ, Ewing PC, Van Beurden M, Helmerhorst TJ, Blok LJ. An autoimmune phenotype in vulvar lichen sclerosus and lichen planus: a Th1 response and high levels of microRNA-155. J Invest Dermatol. 2012;132:658–66.
36. Torio-Padron N, Stark GB, Foldi E, Simunovic F. Treatment of male genital lymphedema: an integrated concept. J Plast Reconstr Aesthet Surg. 2015;68:262–8.
37. Who. Male circumcision. Global trends and determinants of prevalence, safety and acceptability. In: Data ILC-i-P, editor. UNAIDS/07.29E/JC1320E. Geneva: WHO Press; 2007.
38. Wilkinson HN, Hardman MJ. The role of estrogen in cutaneous ageing and repair. Maturitas. 2017;103:60–4.
39. Zouboulis CC, Chen WC, Thornton MJ, Qin K, Rosenfield R. Sexual hormones in human skin. Horm Metab Res. 2007;39:85–95.

22

Psychological Impact of Living with Scars Following Burn Injury

Nancy E. E. Van Loey

Contents

Background

Psychological Problems After a Burn Injury

Psychological and Social Impact of Living with Scars
Body-Esteem and Self-Esteem Concerns
Social Self-Consciousness of Appearance

Factors Impacting Adjustment
Burn Severity and Scarring
Facial Involvement
Concealed Scars
Gender
Importance of Appearance

Interference of Psychological Problems with the Perception of the Scar

Management

Conclusion

References

Background

There is no getting around it: a severe burn injury is a major life event that can dramatically disrupt a person's life. The traumatic nature of the event, the long hospitalization and co-occurring high pain intensity, and the suddenly changed appearance can have a profound impact on those affected. Along with medical advances, more people with severe burns survive their injury and live with scars in a society where a high premium is placed on physical appearance and attractiveness. Scars resulting from burns can have a conspicuous look and may capture attention from the environment. When scars are hypertrophic, they are typically firm, raised, red, and have a rough surface. Hypertrophic scars can be difficult to conceal when they are located at visible body parts. Also, scars in less visible areas can pose a burden on someone's life in specific situations such as the swimming pool, or when the weather is warm and more revealing clothing is indicated at that time.

Living with scars may become even more complicated in the current society. Professionals and academics are concerned about the changing notions of normality related to appearance and the increasing demands of beauty. A recent paper [1] mentioned that an increasing amount of people in the UK consult the plastic surgeon or use cosmetic products to look as good as possible. Pictures on social media are manipulated to present persons in the best possible way. Body image and the perception of bodies are changing and result in increasing engagement in beauty practices that are justified by the new concept of normality. Unsurprisingly, living in a world that values beauty can be challenging for those with a visible difference. It can be particularly challenging for the individual himself or herself when there is a high personal standard placed on beauty. Also, society may be less acceptant toward those with a visible difference. Therefore, even minor scarring may increase the call for plastic surgery and cosmetic interventions. Underlying psychological problems may therefore be a point of attention.

This chapter has the general purpose to provide information about the psychological impact of a burn injury and psychological difficulties that may be encountered when living with scars. Because survival rates have increased, more people live with the physical and psychological consequences of burns. Consequently, appropriate psychosocial support and interventions that help burn survivors deal with scars, from a personal view and the view from the outside world, become increasingly important. Also, an understanding care environment including all professionals, that is, medical doctors, nurses, and physiotherapist, can improve outcomes. Learning objectives of this chapter include to know the prevalence rates of diverse psychiatric disorders that can develop in the aftermath of burn injury, to be aware of signals that may require an in-depth examination of underlying problems, to be aware that psychological problems can affect the perceptions of scar outcomes, to have some knowledge of risk factors, and, finally, to have knowledge regarding psychological treatment options to support people living with scars.

Psychological Problems After a Burn Injury

A burn event happens suddenly and can be life threatening. This may elicit a broad range of psychological reactions. Although it is documented that a substantial group of patients has pre-burn existing psychological problems sometimes being the cause of the injury, for example, self-harm during psychosis or suicide attempts, one may also develop severe and long-term psychological problems in response to the trauma or the adjustment process to a changed appearance. In the acute phase of burn injuries, there is a large focus on physical recovery. Along with wound healing and with the stabilization of the physical condition comes the realization that scars may be permanent and that appearance has changed. Facing this change may elicit feelings of grief and diminished body and self-esteem.

Severe psychological disorders may be encountered such as posttraumatic stress disorder (PTSD), depression, and anxiety. These disorders can become chronic when persons do not receive appropriate treatment. PTSD is included in the *Diagnostic and Statistical Manual of Mental Disorders, 5th Edition* (DSM-V) as a stress disorder and can develop in response to a traumatic event. PTSD comprises four symptom clusters: *intrusions* (intrusive thoughts and memories), *avoidance* of trauma-related stimuli, alterations in *arousal* and reactivity, and *negative alterations in cognitions and mood*. Initial higher levels of acute stress symptoms may be expected and can be regarded as normal reactions to a distressing event. For a substantial proportion of the patients, the high initial stress levels largely decrease within the weeks or months following the trauma. Severe symptoms of acute traumatic stress are reported in approximately 25% of patients admitted to a burn center. In a subgroup, however, they persist and become chronic. Prevalence rates of full PTSD after 1 year postburn are around 10% and another 15% may display severe symptoms that do not meet all criteria, that is, partial PTSD.

Depression is a disorder typically characterized by a negative mood and diminished interest or pleasure during a period of 14 days or longer. One to 4 years after the burn event, about 10% fulfilled criteria of major depression with a postburn onset. Generalized anxiety disorder (GAD) entails the presence of excessive anxiety and worry, is experienced as challenging to control, and is accompanied by physical or cognitive symptoms. GAD was also found to occur in about 10% of burn survivors after 1 year. This implicates that over time, the majority of people involved in a burn injury appear to adjust well and they will recover from initial high stress and depressive symptoms but a substantial subgroup will have long-term problems [2]. Clinical attention and screening is needed for PTSD, depression, and anxiety.

Psychological and Social Impact of Living with Scars

After a burn injury, when wounds are healing and scars start to develop, one has to adjust to this new situation in which appearance has changed. There are two perspectives that have a mutual influence: the individual perspective and the social perspective. The first refers to how people look at themselves and the latter perspective entails the social perspective.

Body-Esteem and Self-Esteem Concerns

People sustaining a burn injury can be faced with noticeable visible differences resulting from large wounds that lead to scarring. Besides an altered appearance caused by these scars, functional limitations can occur if they are located across joints. Both the visible and functional characteristics can diminish satisfaction with appearance and can cause negative self-perceptions and difficulties with social interactions that place people at risk to develop depression and (social) anxiety disorders. These psychological problems may be debilitating to daily functioning in key areas of living such as occupational functioning.

Important psychological concepts such as self-esteem and body-esteem can be damaged when a person is forced to live with visible differences [3, 4]. Self-esteem is a generic cognitive representation of the self. It is a multidimensional concept comprising the view of the person on the different abilities and characteristics. It influences how external information is processed, for example remarks or looks from other people. Body-esteem refers to the evaluation of one's own body and can be viewed as a part of self-esteem [5]. After acquired disfigurement, there is a change in body-esteem that a person needs to adjust to.

It is reasonable to expect that persons with more severe scarring have greater difficulty integrating the scars in daily life than a person with minor scarring. But objective characteristics such as severity of the burn injury in terms of body area affected, the number of surgeries needed, or the number of affected body parts are only modestly related to psychological well-being, indicating that psychological factors may be more important. One such factor, importance of appearance, showed to moderate the relationship between severity characteristics and body-esteem. This indicates that for those who attach little value to their appearance, scars have a lower impact on their body-esteem. For people who highly value appearance, scars negatively affect their body-esteem [6]. These aspects will be addressed in more detail below.

Social Self-Consciousness of Appearance

Scars can elicit negative reactions from the environment. This is well described after burns. Feelings of stigmatization is one of the documented social problems of living with scars. This feeling may result from reactions from other people such as prejudices, discrimination, being ignored, intrusive behaviors such as staring, intrusive questions and remarks, or even bullying [7]. People who have to deal with these reactions may develop a feeling of self-conscious and may perceive stigmatization which may affect self-esteem in a negative way. This in turn can induce avoidant behavior or sometimes (symptoms of) social anxiety. However, the impact of these reactions may differ across individuals. Some persons are more prone to feel stigmatized because of a stronger attentional bias toward stimuli that elicit fear. Psychological therapies can help dealing with these reactions and build self-esteem to increase quality of life.

Factors Impacting Adjustment

Burn Severity and Scarring

In general, the objective severity of scarring showed to be a poor predictor of psychological adjustment. Both small and large defects can elicit body image concerns and diminish satisfaction with appearance. Therefore, it has been argued that a person's subjective perception is a better starting point to assess how persons adjust [4]. However, the body of knowledge that shows (in)direct associations between injury severity and psychological problems is growing. One in-hospital study documented that there were no differences across groups with minor and severe burns, but dissatisfaction with appearance increased over time in the group with more severe burns [6]. Another study found that persons with severe burns showed to ruminate more often—rumination is considered a cognitive strategy in which perseverative negative thinking and impaired disengagement from negative stimuli is present—which in turn predicted the level of depressive symptoms [8]. However, permanent scarring can act as a reminder to the burn event and has the potency to maintain psychological problems. Particularly when persons developed posttraumatic stress symptoms in response to the burn event, changes in appearances can trigger re-experiencing the traumatic event, which is an important symptom of posttraumatic stress disorder [9]. This indicates that more severe burns, possibly associated with more functional problems, can partly drive psychological adjustment. This does not exclude the fact that less extensive scarring can also elicit appearance-related concerns. Paying attention to the role of the scars in personal life is therefore warranted.

Facial Involvement

The face is a key figure in identity and it plays a key role in personal communication and expression of emotions. Sustaining a severe facial burn can be a devastating experience as it affects issues that are central to identity and social interactions. It is commonly expected that persons with facial disfigurement have more problems compared to persons with scars located at body parts that can be covered with clothes. Although there is evidence that living with facial burns may be more distressing than non-facial burns, the evidence is not that straightforward. One of the explanations put forward as to why people with facial burns may adjust relatively well is that they get used to negative reactions and are therefore better able to anticipate these unwanted reactions. Still, it is well established that persons with facial injury are presented with certain social challenges. Unwanted social reactions include staring, intrusive questions and remarks, and prejudices. A study comparing persons with facial burns to persons with the face not involved found higher problems in several domains of functioning such as: emotions, that is, they perceived more anger and sadness, and they had more social problems due to appearance issues [10]. Examples are available illustrating that facial differences is given meaning by others, for example, a woman who is pitied because she is seen as a victim of abuse [11]. Due to these responses, the risk to develop social anxiety and avoidance, low mood, and difficulties with relationship may increase and remains a concern across the lifespan. This is illustrated by a quote from a 60-year-old man who was injured during childhood: *"There is a part of me that hasn't quite made the hurdle to 100% adjustment. I'm comfortable at home and work, and among my circle of friends. Going out among strangers brings good and bad days"* [12], p. 368.

Concealed Scars

Scars that can be covered with clothes trigger dilemmas such as when to show the scars or how to present yourself in certain social situations, how to deal with stares in the swimming pool and at the beach. This can lead to avoidance of these situations because of the reactions of others. Hidden scars can also affect intimacy and sexuality, topics still surrounded with taboo. Scars can impact the ability to enjoy intimacy because one may not feel attractive and avoid being touched.

Gender

It is suggested that women are more frequently concerned about their appearance and therefore find it harder to cope with visible differences. Little research provides direct support for this assumption but, in general, there is evidence that women (with facial burns) or with more severe burns have higher depression scores and are less satisfied with appearance [13]. These findings do not exclude the fact that also (young) men can be troubled by (facial) disfigurement and can question their physical attractiveness. There is, however, evidence supporting that women were more concerned about the change in appearance. Men predominantly reported an increased awareness of their whole body and not specifically their appearance. This may indicate there is, in general, a higher risk for women to develop appearance concerns compared to men because appearance is more valued by women.

Importance of Appearance

How persons view themselves is closely related to how they feel. The role of scars in psychological problems after burns is therefore not straightforward. A person's appraisal of his or her appearance constitutes an important factor of self-esteem. There is evidence for the importance that persons attach to appearance in the adjustment process after burns. Importance of appearance showed to predict distress of living with burn disfigurement [6].

Interference of Psychological Problems with the Perception of the Scar

There is ample evidence that scar evaluation by health care providers does not match that of the patient and is a poor predictor of satisfaction with the treatment by patients. This may be frustrating for both the patient and the health care provider. Understanding why these differences occur may diminish disappointment for both. Psychological problems such as depression can alter the way scars are perceived. As shown in a study [14], many patients with burns were well able to score scar characteristics within the same range as the professional. Persons scoring lower on self-esteem, however, rated their scars more troublesome, compared to the professional's view. This particularly concerned hypertrophy, possibly due to the fact that this characteristic is most conspicuous. This indicates that the psychological state influences how scars are viewed. Particularly the discrepancy between the patient's and professional's view may be a starting point to evaluate psychological factors.

Bradbury [11] underlines the importance of recognizing psychosocial issues in surgical decision-making. Having a realistic view on surgical outcomes in terms of what can be expected and psychosocial factors that may interfere with expectations and decisions is important. She proposed a three-staged approach in which individuals working with patients with visible differences all have some knowledge on influencing psychosocial factors, which forms the first stage of attention. If indicated, patients can be referred to, for example, a clinical nurse specialist trained in counseling skills. In the event therapy is needed, referral to a psychologist should be considered. It is emphasized that understanding psychological needs surrounding surgery is imperative to ensure that personal needs are met.

Management

Over the last decades, a number of interventions has been described that have the objective to help people dealing with challenges that result from living with a visible difference. Social skills training was among the first intervention programs aimed at expanding the arsenal of responses to a variety of reactions of people. Other therapies include cognitive behavioral therapy (CBT) in which dysfunctional cognitions, appraisals, beliefs, and assumptions are identified and changed in order to learn more useful ways of dealing with the visible difference [11]. CBT showed to have the strongest evidence of effectiveness and can support patients to come to terms with the visible difference, it can help in decision-making, and showed to be effective in overcoming social anxiety [3]. An online program called YPFaceIt, which includes elements of CBT and social skills training, has shown improvement in persons with a visible difference [15], although more research in larger groups is needed.

Besides psychological therapies, peer support groups have shown to be beneficial to well-being of burn survivors. Talking to a person who experienced a similar event and is faced with the same challenges increases empowerment. This was illustrated in the next quote: "*When you meet someone who really knows what you're going through, you can discuss things in a different way*" [16]. It is assumed that peer support groups can facilitate social sharing, which is a specific type of social support in which illness-related emotions are shared.

Conclusion

In sum, a burn injury can have devastating consequences in terms of psychosocial well-being. To predict who will adjust well after a burn injury comprises a complexity of factors that should be taken into account. It is an interplay of resilience and vulnerability factors; it involves a dynamic process over time. Some indications, however, may be points of attention for professionals in burn care. How persons cope with the consequences strongly depends on the significance they place on the value of their physical appearance. Objective factors such as gender, burn extent, and the extent to which the scars are visible all showed to have some relation but are poor direct predictors of dealing with the impact of scars. However, there are relationships that are worth considering. If there is a considerable deviation between the professional's and the patient's view on outcome, it is worth starting a dialogue with the aim to identify the causes. There is also a higher risk for women to struggle with visible differences as they, more frequently than men, value appearance and beauty; appearance may make up a larger part of their self-esteem and self-worth when compared to men. In men, functional problems may cause more problems.

The challenge for the health care provider is to be aware of signals that point to underlying psychological difficulties and judge to what extent another (surgical) intervention adds to the well-being of the patient. A staged approach of professionals with knowledge of psychosocial problems associated with visible differences should become more custom as it is now. It is only when the patient receives understanding, and whether it is clear for all parties what is going on in the patient, that compliance, decision-making, and outcome can be improved. Interventions focusing at psychological components may be indicated and can make a difference in the final outcome.

Take-Home Messages

- Pay attention to the role of the scars in personal life.
- A changed appearance can have psychological and social consequences.
- Pay attention to signals that indicate underlying psychosocial problems.
- Be aware of underlying psychosocial issues in surgical decision-making.
- Consider a stepwise approach to recognize psychosocial issues.

References

1. Widdows H, MacCallum F. The demands of beauty: editors' introduction. Health Care Analysis. 2018;26:207–219. Epub 2018/07/11.
2. Ter Smitten MH, de Graaf R, Van Loey NE. Prevalence and co-morbidity of psychiatric disorders 1–4 years after burn. Burns. 2011;37(5):753–61. Epub 2011/02/22.
3. Rumsey N. Psychosocial adjustment to skin conditions resulting in visible difference (disfigurement): what do we know? Why don't we know more? How shall we move forward? Int J Women's Dermatol. 2018;4(1):2–7. Epub 2018/06/07.
4. Rumsey N, Harcourt D. Body image and disfigurement: issues and interventions. Body Image. 2004;1(1):83–97.
5. Lawrence JW, Fauerbach JA, Thombs BD. A test of the moderating role of importance of appearance in the relationship between perceived scar severity and body-esteem among adult burn survivors. Body Image. 2006;3(2):101–11.
6. Thombs BD, Notes LD, Lawrence JW, Magyar-Russell G, Bresnick MG, Fauerbach JA. From survival to socialization: a longitudinal study of body image in survivors of severe burn injury. J Psychosom Res. 2008;64(2):205–12.
7. Shepherd L, Tattersall H, Buchanan H. Looking in the mirror for the first time after facial burns: a retrospective mixed methods study. Burns. 2014;40(8):1624–34. Epub 2014/04/20.
8. Van Loey NE, Oggel A, Goemanne AS, Braem L, Vanbrabant L, Geenen R. Cognitive emotion regulation strategies and neuroticism in relation to depressive symptoms following burn injury: a longitudinal study with a 2-year follow-up. J Behav Med. 2014;37(5):839–48. Epub 2013/10/16.
9. Macleod R, Shepherd L, Thompson AR. Posttraumatic stress symptomatology and appearance distress following burn injury: an interpretative phenomenological analysis. Health Psychol. 2016;35(11):1197–204. Epub 2016/10/18.
10. Ryan CM, Lee A, Stoddard FJ Jr, Li NC, Schneider JC, Shapiro GD, et al. The effect of facial burns on long-term outcomes in young adults: a 5-year study. J Burn Care Res. 2018;39(4): 497–506. Epub 2018/06/15.
11. Bradbury E. Meeting the psychological needs of patients with facial disfigurement. Br J Oral Maxillofac Surg. 2012;50(3): 193–6. Epub 2011/03/29.
12. Jones BA, Buchanan H, Harcourt D. The experiences of older adults living with an appearance altering burn injury: an exploratory qualitative study. J Health Psychol. 2017;22(3):364–74. Epub 2015/09/02.
13. Al Ghriwati N, Sutter M, Pierce BS, Perrin PB, Wiechman SA, Schneider JC. Two-year gender differences in satisfaction with appearance after burn injury and prediction of five-year depression: a latent growth curve approach. Arch Phys Med Rehabil. 2017;98(11):2274–9. Epub 2017/05/10.
14. Hoogewerf CJ, van Baar ME, Middelkoop E, van Loey NE. Patient reported facial scar assessment: directions for the professional. Burns. 2014;40(2):347–53. Epub 2013/10/22.
15. Williamson H, Griffiths C, Harcourt D. Developing young person's face IT: online psychosocial support for adolescents struggling with conditions or injuries affecting their appearance. Health Psychol Open. 2015;2(2):2055102915619092. Epub 2017/01/11.
16. Oster C, Kildal M, Ekselius L. Return to work after burn injury: burn-injured individuals' perception of barriers and facilitators. J Burn Care Res. 2010;31(4):540–50. Epub 2010/07/10.

23

Makeup Therapy for Scars

Joëlle Nonni

Contents

Definition

Characteristics

The Benefits of Medical Makeup
Psychological Impact
Social Impact

Medical Makeup
Step-by-Step Process
Using Color Correction Is the Best Solution to This Issue
Complementary Colors
The Value of Colors
Compact Foundation Creams
Fluid Foundation Correctors

Medical Makeup Classes

References

> Medical makeup is a solution to hide scars and burns on the face as well as body, to both men and women. The objective is to reduce the psychological impact and to improve the patient's self-image.
>
> Various studies have highlighted the positive effect of medical makeup on the patient's quality of life. With medical makeup, patient's self-confidence gradually comes back.

Definition

The priorities for medical makeup are different from those for cosmetic makeup, which is primarily concerned with fashion and trends. With medical makeup, first and foremost, camouflage solutions must be found that do not risk aggravating skin lesions, the objective being to reduce the psychological impact and to improve the patient's self-image. The aim is therefore not to create the "most beautiful makeup" but to find corrective products that are compatible with medical prescriptions, skin sensitivity, the expectations of the patient, and their ability to put on the makeup. Medical makeup is offered to both men and women and helps hide lesions on the face as well as the body.

Characteristics

- Makeup referred to as "medical" is formulated to guarantee complete safety even for damaged skin [1].
- Products are hypoallergenic and non-comedogenic and must contain a high sun-protection factor.
- The quality of textures is important to make it easier to apply the makeup and also to achieve a natural result.
- It is essential that the makeup be long lasting and resistant to water and sweat so that it lasts all day long. That being the case, the description of the product on the packaging should be checked to make sure they have all these qualities.
- The anhydrous forms, and stick and compact types are resistant because their outer oily phase is less miscible with water. For the other formulas, the addition of polymer increases the adhesion of the product to the skin and thus limits its migration into the water.
- By using makeup products that are resistant to water and perspiration, the makeup hold may be greater than 10 hours.
- However, one last important point should be emphasized: the makeup must be easy to remove so as not to cause a secondary irritation.

The Benefits of Medical Makeup

Various studies have highlighted the positive effects of medical makeup on the patient's quality of life, particularly in the case of treatment for scars.

Psychological Impact

By learning how to conceal their skin imperfections, patients:
- Find it easier to look at themselves in the mirror
- Regain a more realistic body image
- Enjoy taking care of themselves again
- Grow in self-confidence

The patient's self-esteem is boosted and they find it easier to look to the future.

Social Impact

After having concealed highly visible lesions, patients:
- Are less likely to notice the sometimes "intrusive" looks from other people
- Find other people look at them more approvingly again
- Maintain or return to social activities
- Are able to continue working if they wish to do so

Their relationship with others is improved, thus avoiding or putting an end to their sense of isolation.

Medical Makeup

Step-by-Step Process

Evaluation of Needs

The first step is to evaluate the needs and expectations of patients.

What products does the doctor recommend: emollient, sun protection, etc.?
- What does the patient want to conceal?
- Does the patient want a highly corrective or a lighter type of makeup?
- Does the patient usually apply makeup?
- Always remember to adapt the advice according to sex, age, habits, and preferences.
- And to give advice that the patient can easily replicate.

Makeup Base

Applying an emollient cream is essential for correcting a skin imperfection. Skin must be moisturized and supple to be able to spread the foundation easily. If the skin is not moisturized, the pigments contained in the makeup will stick to raised areas of the skin, the correction will not be even, and the makeup will not last for the entire day. If sun protection is required, apply this after the emollient cream, using it as the makeup base [2].

Color Correction

Thick makeup often gives the impression of a mask effect and sometimes gives burn patients' faces a frozen look. The makeup must therefore be lighter so that the patient does not feel their personality has been stripped away after having it applied [3].

Using Color Correction Is the Best Solution to This Issue

By experimenting with color, we can reduce the intensity of imperfections, which means less foundation needs to be applied therefore obtaining a more natural result.

Complementary Colors

The principle is to superimpose two complementary colors in order to neutralize them.

As we can see from the chromatic circle (◘ Fig. 49.1):

- Green is the opposite color to red
- Yellow is the opposite color to purplish blue
- Coral is the opposite color to dark blue

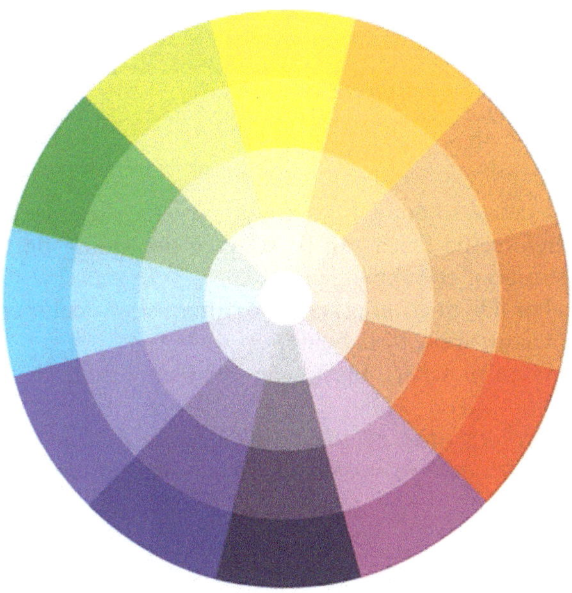

◘ Fig. Complementary color circle. Source: Eau Thermale Avène.

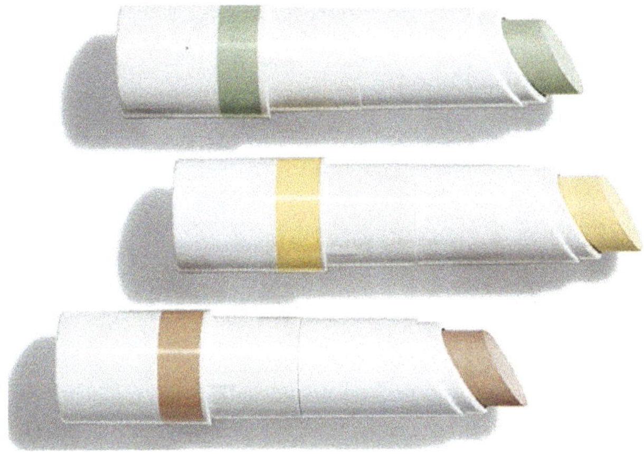

◘ Fig. Corrector sticks. Source: Eau Thermale Avène.

Therefore:

- A green corrector neutralizes imperfections that are predominantly red: inflammatory scars, rosacea, psoriasis, etc.
- A yellow corrector neutralizes imperfections that are predominantly purplish: ecchymosis, angioma, blue-toned dark circles, varicose veins, etc.
- A coral corrector neutralizes imperfections that are predominantly dark-blue: tattoos, nevus of Ota, etc. (◘ Fig. 49.2)

After having applied a corrector, the imperfection becomes slightly grey; therefore, it is not necessary to apply as much foundation.

The Value of Colors

The light amplitude of a color is known as its "value," from the lightest to the darkest; adding white or black to a color is all that is required to change its intensity. For example, with orange, as we can see from the chromatic circle, its dark value is brown and its light value is beige [4] (◘ Fig. 49.3).

In practice, if we want to correct a brown imperfection, it is necessary to apply an orange-ish shade to obtain a bright, light beige color, before applying foundation.

Therefore:

- A coral corrector neutralizes imperfections that are predominantly brown: hyperpigmented scars, melasma, brown-toned dark circles, lentigos, etc.

After having corrected the colored lesions using the complementary colors or the value of colors, we simply need to cover this with a little foundation to even out the complexion.

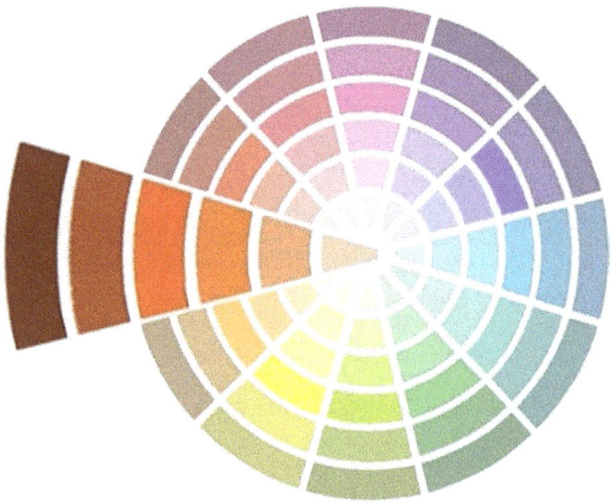

◘ Fig. Color value circle. Source: Eau Thermale Avène.

49.4.4.1 Corrective Foundations

Corrective foundations offer several advantages for medical makeup.

- Their high pigment concentration allows for correction using less product.
- Their excellent resistance means that there is no need to reapply the product during the day.
- Their resistance to water and sweat means they can be used in any situation, both on the face and body.
- They have a high sun protection factor.

There are two types of corrective foundations:

- Fluid for mild imperfections
- Compact for severe imperfections

Compact Foundation Creams

These are the most suitable for concealing severe imperfections and particularly for a long-lasting effect and a water, sweat resistance finish.

- For post-surgery patients: it is better to use a "comfort" texture with a supple formula that is easily applied, even on the most sensitive skin.
- For remote post-surgery patients: we select a "comfort" texture for the face and a "matt-finish" texture for the body as there is no transfer and excellent resistance [5] (◘ Figs. 49.4 and 49.5).

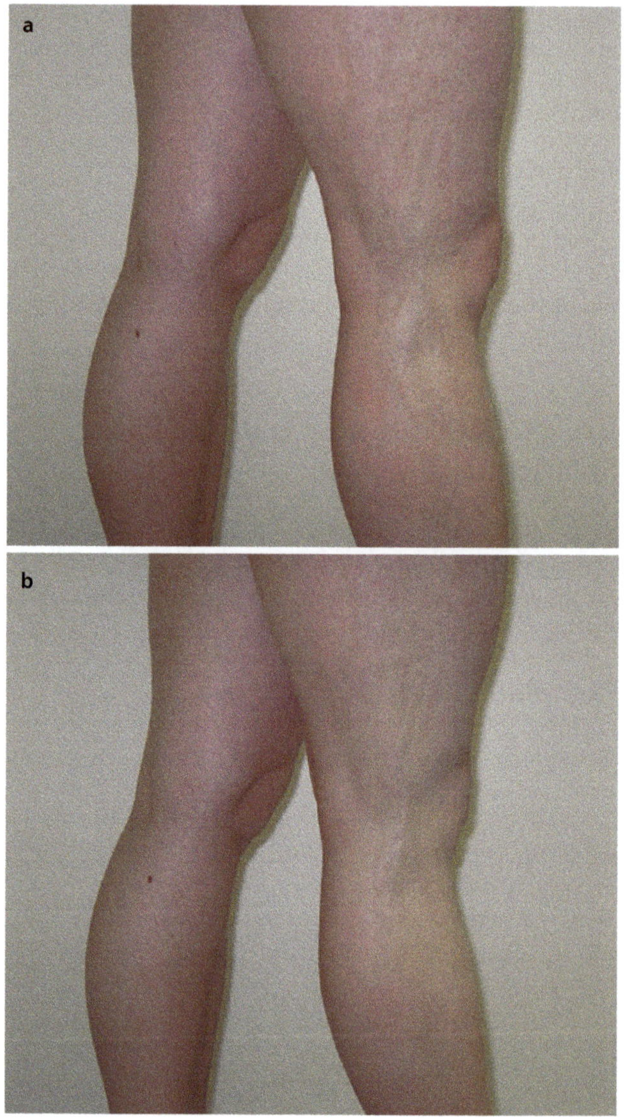

◘ Fig. Legs before (**a**) after (**b**) make up Source: Eau Ther-male Avène.

It is better to apply these products with a sponge and therefore the finish can be adapted depending on the intensity of the imperfection.

- For a high-coverage result or after using a color corrector, apply by dabbing.
- For a transparent result, apply by smoothing.

Do not forget to regularly clean the sponge with soap and water, or simply by washing it in the washing machine.

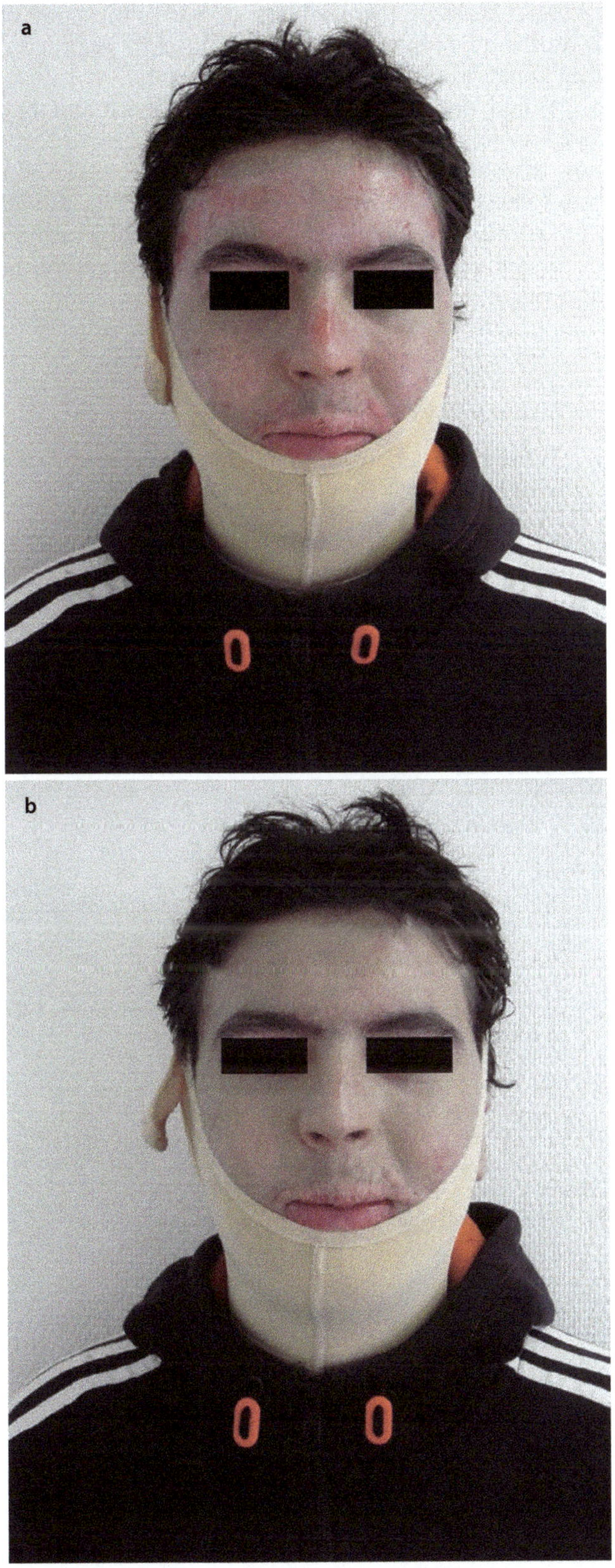

■ **Fig.** Face make up: before (**a**) and after (**b**). Source Eau Thermale Avène.

Fluid Foundation Correctors

These are more suitable for mild to moderate imperfections and as they have a lower pigment concentration, they are ideal for scaly skin. They can be applied using the tips of the fingers, but if the skin is very dry or scaly, a sponge is more effective to "blur" the scales. As for foundation brushes, they are chosen for a more transparent finish and for men who really like this method of application.

How to Decide on a Shade of Foundation

People often select the color of their foundation according to the color on the inside of their wrist, but this body area is quite fair and therefore this rarely achieves a natural result. The most effective method is to test the product on the jawline to check that there is no demarcation between the face and neck. For the body, test the product next to the imperfection that you are going to apply makeup to. In case of hyperpigmentation, opt for a shade that is slightly darker than the skin tone; this will help with correction.

Powder

This is essential to set the makeup and to ensure long-lasting hold. Opt for a powder suited to the skin tone and apply it with a large brush for a more natural effect. When scars are very raised, finish by applying the powder in the opposite direction to get rid of excess product so that the makeup is less visible. If skin is very scaly, it is better to avoid applying powder as it accentuates the appearance of scales.

Corrector Pencils

Eyebrows

Eyebrow corrector pencils are extremely useful for concealing localized scars around the eyebrows or to completely redefine and rebalance the eye area. The eyebrows are so important in makeup that it is said they act as a "frame for the eyes."

Lips

In case of scarring around the mouth, a lip pencil is generally applied after having concealed the scar with foundation and a little bit of powder. The lip pencil is therefore used to define the contours of the mouth [6]. In the case of cheilitis, you can suggest using a lip balm before applying lipstick, which can be used instead of lip gloss to treat dry lips at the same time.

Ensure Makeup Lasts longer

Spray a fine mist of thermal water 20 cm away from the makeup and leaving it to evaporate, this dries the makeup and makes it last longer. This is a very useful technique for body makeup, which is more subject to friction than the face.

Makeup Removal

An essential step! Most of the time, makeup remover is put on a cotton pad and rubbed against the skin with varying levels of force. If the pressure from the cotton pad is not strong enough, the makeup is not removed and if it is too strong, this could cause an irritation. The most suitable method is to remove makeup with just the tips of your fingers. The makeup remover must contain gentle surfactants, be fragrance-free, and in the form of a lotion or gel-like lotion so that it can be applied using gentle massage with the tips of the fingers. After having loosened the makeup and impurities, gently remove the rest with paper tissues before rinsing with a thermal water spray to achieve perfectly cleansed skin.

In brief:

1. Evaluation of needs: to evaluate the needs and expectations of patients
2. Makeup base: to prepare the skin before the makeup
3. Color correction: to neutralize the color imperfection
4. Corrective foundation: to unify the tone of the skin
5. Powder: to set the makeup
6. Corrector pencil: to correct scars or depigmentation on eyebrows and lips
7. Fine mist of thermal water: ensure makeup lasts longer
8. Makeup removal: to remove the makeup without creating irritation

Medical Makeup Classes

Because each patient needs personnel advice, it is important for them to learn how to hide their imperfections from medical make-up specialists or nurses similarly trained. Usually, these classes or workshops are in hydrotherapy centers specializing (in skin disorders), functional rehabilitation centers, or hospitals.

At first, patients can have individual advice, and they can also join a workshop with other patients to learn how to do it by themselves. This last solution is the best way to become autonomous and generally men should opt for this more than women, because usually men do not use makeup and they need to be more careful in applying it.

Take-Home Message

Medical makeup can be applied to all imperfections, ranging from mild to severe. It can be applied to the face and body and should be offered to men as well as women. Various studies have highlighted the positive effects of medical makeup on the patient's quality of life [7]. It improves patients' personal relationships and daily activities and reduces esthetic prejudice [8].

References

1. McMichael L. Skin camouflage. BMJ. 2012:d7921.
2. Grognard C. Tatouage et maquillage réparateur, 2008. p. 25.
3. Delebecque-Eginer C, Ferrere R, Nonni J, Segard C, Encyclopédie Médico-Chirurgicale, Maquillage: Technique de camouflage. Cosmestologie et dermatologie. 2000; 50–170-E-10.
4. Delamar P. Le maquillage artistique. Editions Vigot. 2002:8.
5. Nel-Omeyer M, Ambonati M, Mengeaud V, Taieb C, Merial-Kieny C, Intérêt du maquillage correcteur médical chez les grands brûlés : impact sur la qualité de vie , tolérance et acceptabilité cosmétique. J Plaies et cicatrisation. 2007;58: tome XII.
6. Mérial-Kieny C, Nonni J. Maquillage de correction médicale pour les peaux brûlées. J Plaies et cicatrisation. 2006;53, tome XI.
7. Holmes SA, Beattie PE, Fleming CJ. Cosmetic camouflage advice improves quality of life. Br J Dermatol. 2002;147: 946–9.
8. Graham JA, Jouhar AJ. The importance of cosmetics in the psychological appearance. Int J Dermatol. 1983;22:153–6.

24

Effectiveness of Corticosteroid Tapes and Plasters for Keloids and Hypertrophic Scars

Rei Ogawa

Contents

Introduction

Difference Between Steroid Tapes/Plasters and Steroid Injection

Typical Usage of Steroid Tapes/Plasters

Difference Between Deprodone Propionate Plaster and Deprodone Propionate Ointment

Therapeutic Effect and Usage of Steroid Tape Preparations

Side Effects of Steroid Tapes and Plasters

References

Introduction

In Japan, corticosteroid tapes and plasters have long served as a first-line therapy for keloids and hypertrophic scars. Pediatric patients are particularly responsive to this type of treatment. This may reflect the fact that children have thinner skin than adults and the steroids are therefore more easily absorbed. The postoperative application of corticosteroid tapes/plasters also significantly prevents the development of keloids and hypertrophic scars after surgery.

External corticosteroid preparations are classified into five classes on the basis of their vasoconstrictor activity and their clinical effect, namely, Group I (Strongest), Group II (Very strong), Group III (Strong), Group IV (Mild), and Group V (Weak). Steroid tape is available in the following three countries in different preparations. In the UK, the commercially available formulation comprises a fludroxycortide-impregnated tape (4 μg/cm^2) [1]. Fludroxycortide tape is a Group III preparation. The USA has a steroid tape preparation that contains 4 μg/cm^2 flurandrenolide, which is also a Group III preparation [2]. In Japan, two steroid tape formulations are available, namely, the Group III preparation found in the UK (4 μg/cm^2 fludroxycortide tape) and a 20 μg/cm^2 deprodone propionate tape. Deprodone propionate tape is considered to be a Group I or II preparation [3] (◘ Fig. 56.1). In our experience, deprodone propionate tape (Eclar® plaster) is the most effective tape for the treatment and prevention of keloids.

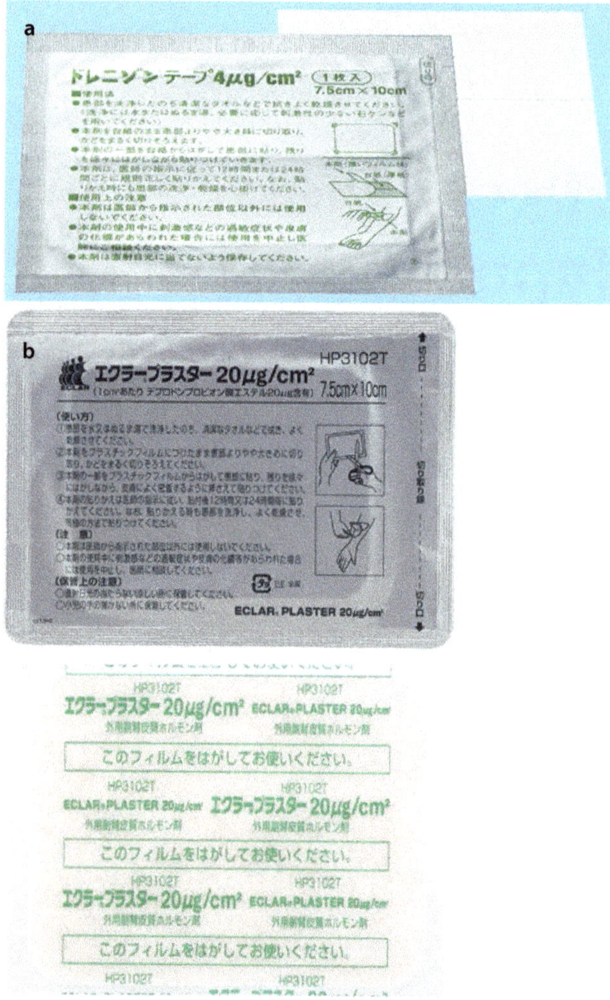

◘ **Fig.** The steroid tapes and plasters that are available in Japan. **a** Fludroxycortide tape (Teikoku Seiyaku CO., LTD., Kagawa, Japan). **b** Deprodone propionate plaster (Hisamitsu Pharmaceutical CO., LTD., Saga, Japan)

Difference Between Steroid Tapes/Plasters and Steroid Injection

Corticosteroid injections rapidly reduce the volume of keloids and hypertrophic scars. However, the downsides of corticosteroid injections include pain (caused by the injection itself) and difficulties associated with contraindications such as pregnancy, glaucoma, or Cushing's disease [4]. These problems can be overcome by using steroid tapes/plasters. Most pediatric and older patients can be treated by steroid tapes/plaster alone due to their thinner skin, which means that the steroids are easily absorbed.

Corticosteroid tapes/plasters can also be used in combination with other therapies such as corticosteroid injection. This is particularly suitable for adults with keloids and hypertrophic scars. The patients can apply the steroid tape/plaster every day in their homes and undergo the injection when they can go to the hospital. In our hospital, we succeeded in reducing the number of hospital visits of patients with pathological scars by adopting this approach. Indeed, many patients now only come to our hospital every 3–4 months.

Typical Usage of Steroid Tapes/Plasters

Steroid tapes/plasters should be changed every day. Important tips regarding the treatment of keloids and hypertrophic scars with steroid tapes/plasters are as follows. First, the patient should continue to use the tapes/plasters until the elevated mass becomes flat and soft. The patient must also cut the tape according to the shape of the keloid or hypertrophic scar. Second, once the mass has become flat and soft, the use of steroid tape/plaster should be stopped, even if the scar is still red. This reflects the fact that if the patient continues to use the tape just because the scar is still red, capillarectasia will occur. This is because the steroid treatment thins the structures supporting the blood vessels.

Difference Between Deprodone Propionate Plaster and Deprodone Propionate Ointment

At this stage, deprodone propionate plaster is the strongest steroid tape/plaster in the world. Deprodone propionate plaster was launched by Hisamitsu Pharmaceutical Co., Ltd., Saga, Japan in July 2001. Since the deprodone propionate in this plaster is at a concentration of 20 μg/cm^2, each 7.5 cm × 10 cm sheet contains 1500 μg of the steroid. The product sheet states that of the 910 cases, 24 (2.64%) exhibited side effects to this plaster. The main side effects were capillary dilation (nine cases, 0.99%), contact dermatitis (five cases, 0.55%), skin atrophy (four cases, 0.44%), and hair folliculitis (four cases, 0.44%).

Deprodone propionate ointment is considered to be a Group III preparation: thus, it is 1–2 ranks weaker than deprodone propionate tape. This is because of differences in the action time and how much steroid is absorbed. When choosing between deprodone propionate ointment or deprodone propionate plaster, it should be noted that to cover the 75 cm^2 area of one deprodone propionate plaster, one must apply 0.125 g of deprodone propionate ointment. This is because the product sheet states that 0.5 g of the ointment can coat an area of 300 cm^2. However, since the ointment consists of 0.3% of the active ingredient, 0.125 g of ointment will only contain 375 μg of deprodone propionate. This is one-quarter of the amount of one tape (1500 μg). Therefore, deprodone propionate ointment will only have the same effect as 24-hr/day deprodone propionate plaster if the ointment is applied to the affected area 4 times a day and is covered with an occlusive dressing technique (ODT) using, for example, a polyurethane film.

Therapeutic Effect and Usage of Steroid Tape Preparations

In adults, deprodone propionate plaster is a more effective therapy for pathological scars than other steroid tapes. However, in pediatric patients, the therapeutic effect of the other tapes is sufficient (◘ Fig. 56.2). This is indicated by our observational study [3] on the use of fludroxycortide tape in 30 adults and 30 pediatric patients with hypertrophic and keloid scars. The adults were, on average, 37 years old (range 23–67 years), while the pediatric patients were, on average, 7.2 years old (range 2–15 years). Each patient had one scar that was treated with the tape. The scars were on various body sites, including the trunk and extremities. The scars were over 1 year old and the tape was used for at least 1 year for 24 hr/day. The results after 1 year of treatment were judged by using the Japan Scar Workshop Scar Scale 2015 (JSS) [5]. The results suggest that the fludroxycortide tape improved the scars of 20% of the adult patients and 80% of the pediatric patients. After 1 year of fludroxycortide tape usage, the 24 unresponsive adults were switched to 24 hr/day deprodone propionate plaster treatment. Of these 24 cases, 17 (70.8%) exhibited scar improvements 1 year later. Thus, we conclude that adults require a stronger tape to obtain similar responses as children in terms of scar maturation. Thus, deprodone propionate plaster is better for adults, while fludroxycortide tape is sufficient

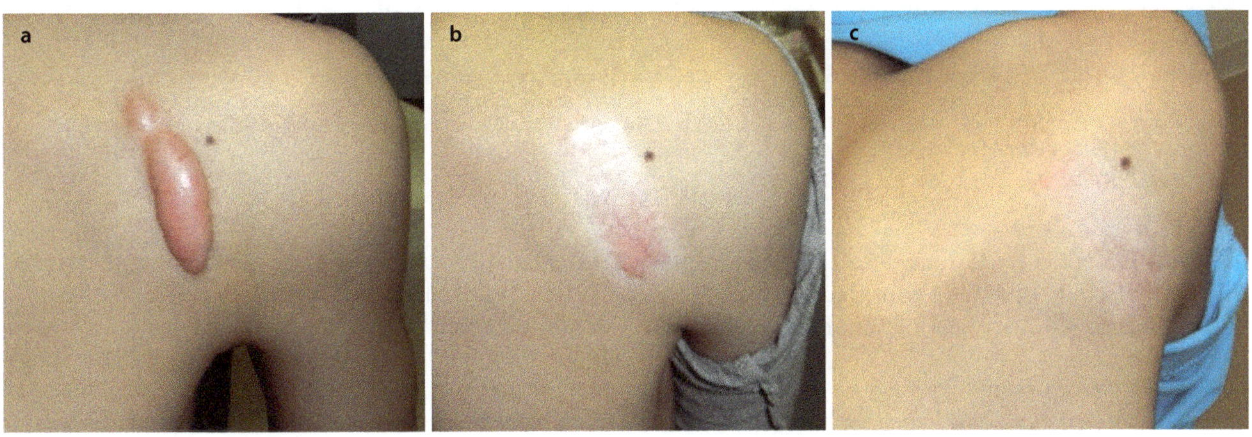

◘ **Fig.** Effect of fludroxycortide tape on a scapular keloid of a 9-year-old boy. **a** Before treatment commenced. **b** Sixteen months after starting treatment. **c** Twenty-six months after starting treatment

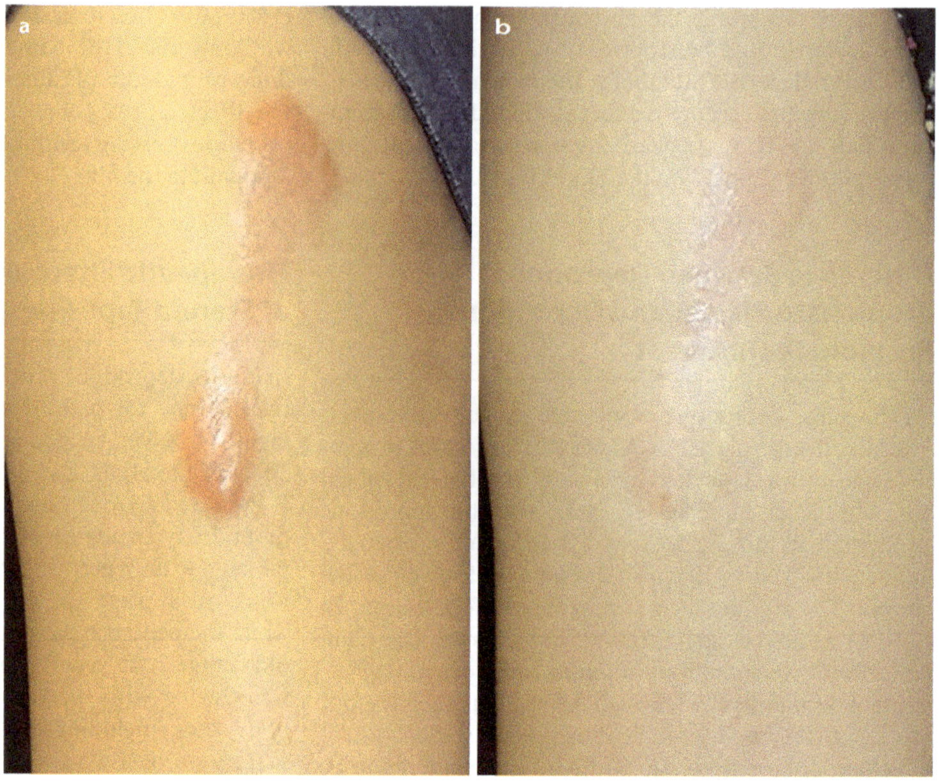

■ **Fig.** Effect of depro-done propionate plaster on an upper arm keloid of a 25-year-old female patient. **a** Before treatment commenced. **b** Twelve months after starting treatment

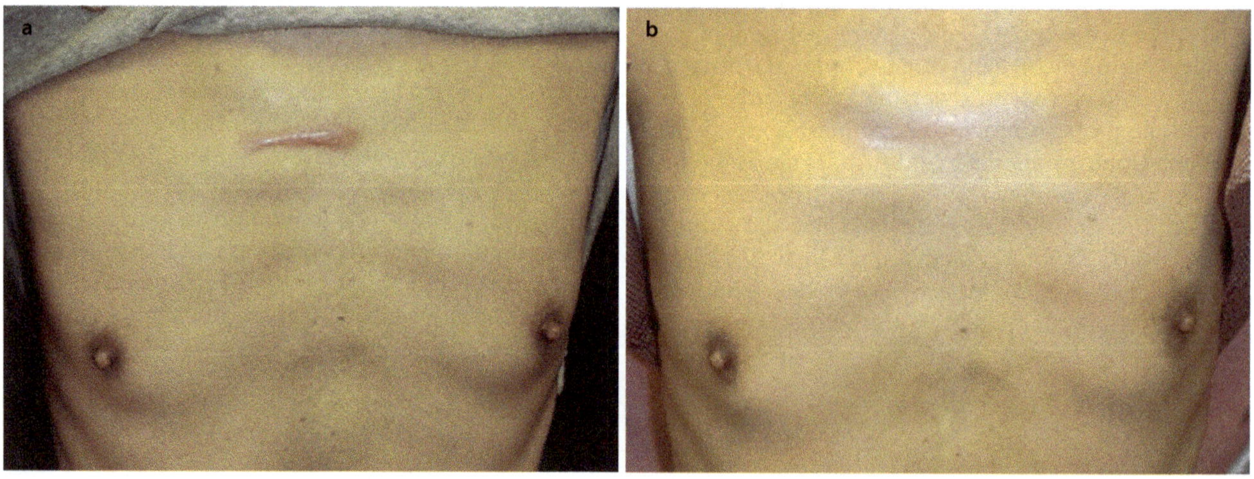

■ **Fig.** Effect of deprodone propionate plaster on an anterior chest wall keloid of a 68-year-old male patient. **a** Before treatment commenced. **b** Twelve months after starting treatment

for pediatric patients (■ Figs. 56.3, 56.4, and 56.5). The side effects in our study consisted of contact dermatitis in three adults. None of the children exhibited any side effects.

Steroid tapes/plasters can also be used to prevent recurrence after keloid and hypertrophic scar resection (■ Fig. 56.6). My empirical experience is that starting 24 hr/day deprodone propionate plaster treatment 1 month after surgery appears to suppress recurrence. Further research is needed to test this hypothesis. It should be noted that we currently routinely use deprodone propionate tape combined with radiotherapy as a postoperative adjunct in surgically treated keloid cases to reduce the recurrence rate. In our experience, this combination reduces the postoperative keloid recurrence rate to less than 10% [6].

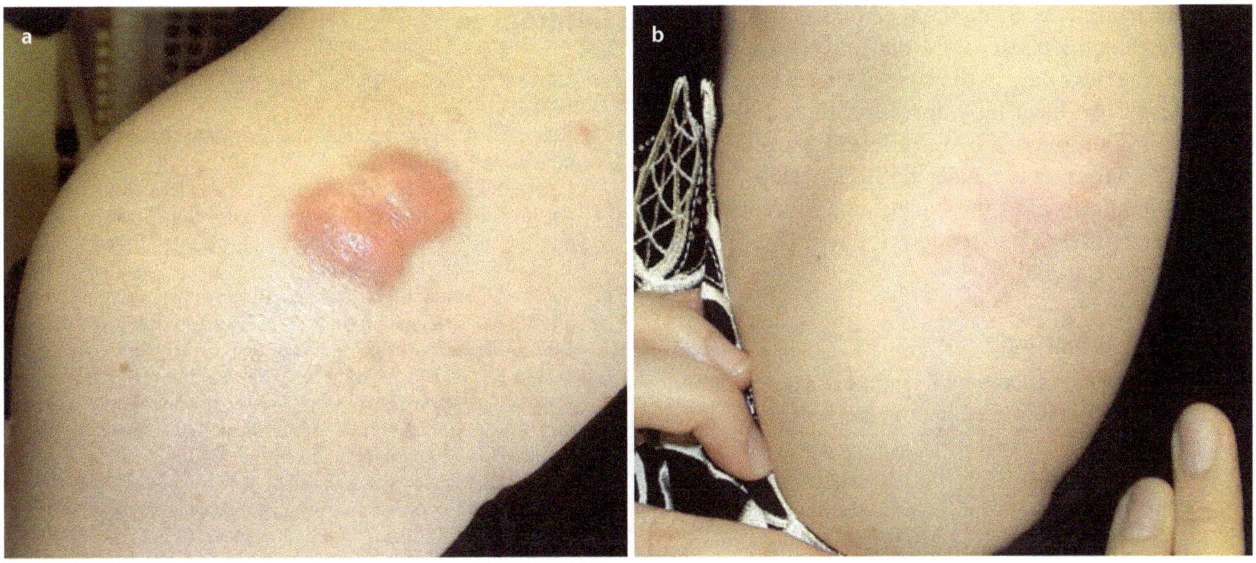

Fig. Effect of deprodone propionate plaster on a shoulder keloid of a 49-year-old female patient. **a** Before treatment commenced. **b** Thirty-six months after starting treatment

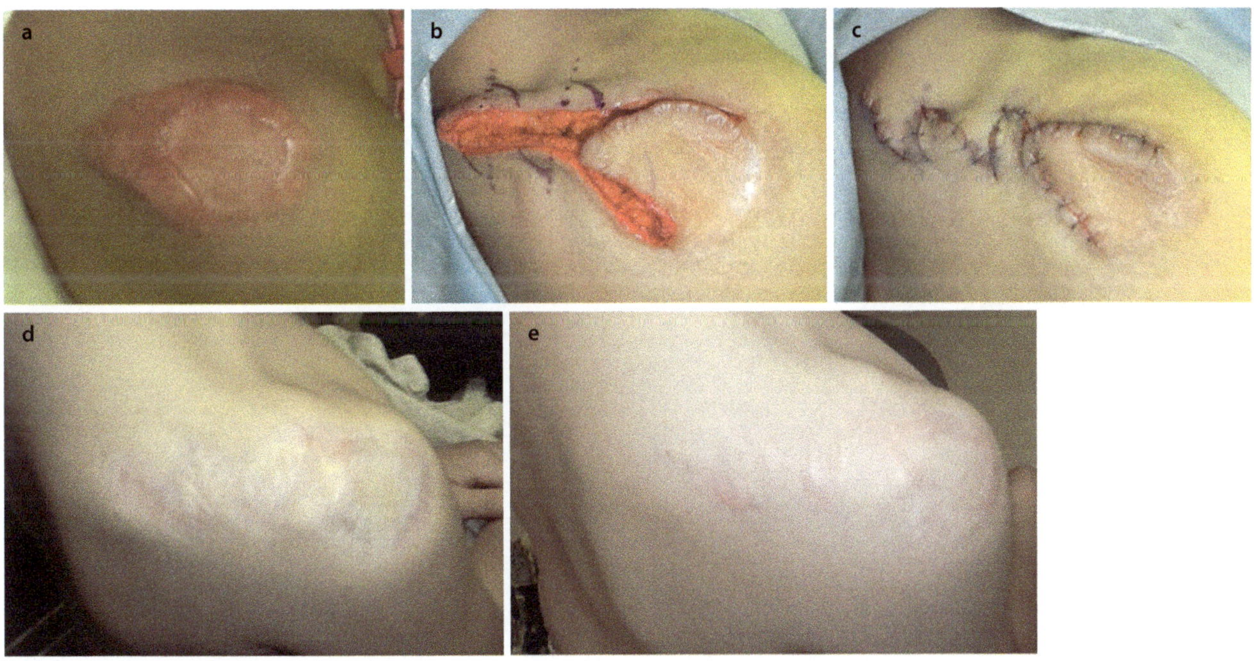

Fig. Effect of surgery and postoperative deprodone propio-nate plaster treatment on a shoulder keloid of a 9-year-old boy. **a** Before treatment commenced. **b** Intraoperative view. **c** View immediately after surgery. **d** Twenty months after surgery. **e** Thirty-six months after surgery

Side Effects of Steroid Tapes and Plasters

Contact dermatitis is the most common problem associated with the use of steroid tapes/plasters. According to the product sheets, the frequencies of contact dermatitis during fludroxycortide tape and deprodone propionate plaster treatment are 16.7% and 0.55%, respectively. This is consistent with our impression in clinical practice. Thus, deprodone propionate plaster associates with a lower incidence of contact dermatitis. There are two types of contact dermatitis, namely, irritant contact dermatitis and allergic contact dermatitis. One can reduce the possibility of the former by decreasing the frequency with which the tape/plaster is replaced and by reducing the duration of application. Thus, the risk of irritant contact dermatitis may be decreased by various strategies, including replacing the tape/plaster every

24–48 hours, only wearing the tape/plaster overnight, or applying the tape/plaster for 1 day and then using ointment on the next day. In the case of deprodone propionate plaster, we have the impression that mild contact dermatitis is suppressed by the effect of steroid itself. If, however, allergic contact dermatitis develops, it often arises 1–3 months after the start of use. Since it can produce strong pruritus and reddens the skin, it can hamper the continuous use of the tape.

Take Home Messages

- In Japan, corticosteroid tapes and plasters have long served as a first-line therapy for keloids and hypertrophic scars.
- Pediatric patients are particularly responsive to this type of treatment, because children have thinner skin than adults and the steroids are therefore more easily absorbed.
- The postoperative application of corticosteroid tapes/plasters also significantly prevents the development of keloids and hypertrophic scars after surgery.
- Deprodone propionate tape is the most effective tape for the treatment and prevention of keloids.

References

1. Nurse DS. Letter: Haelan tape. Australasian J Dermatol. 1974;15(3):152.
2. Kestel JL Jr. Hypopigmentation following the use of Cordran tape. Arch Dermatol. 1971;103(4):460.
3. Ogawa R, Akashi S. Effectiveness of corticosteroid tape/plaster for keloids and hypertrophic scars-comparative study of fludroxycortide and deprodone tape/plasters. Scar Manag. 2016;10:55–60. (Japanese).
4. Sukhumthammarat W, Putthapiban P, Sriphrapradang C. Local injection of triamcinolone acetonide: a forgotten aetiology of Cushing's syndrome. J Clin Diagn Res. 2017;11(6):OR01–2.
5. Ogawa R, Akaishi S, Akita S, Okabe K, Shimizu T, Sunaga A, Tosa Y, Nagao M, Yamawaki S. JSW Scar Scale Working Group. Japan Scar Workshop (JSW) Scar Scale 2015. Available online at: http://www.scar-keloid.com/en/index.html
6. Ogawa R, Akaishi S, Kuribayashi S, Miyashita T. Keloids and hypertrophic scars can now be cured completely: recent progress in our understanding of the pathogenesis of keloids and hypertrophic scars and the most promising current therapeutic strategy. J Nippon Med Sch. 2016;83(2):46–53.

25

Burn Hypertrophic Scar in Pediatric Patients: Clinical Case

Roohi Vinaik, Joel Fish, and Marc G. Jeschke

Contents

Background
Incidence of Hypertrophic Scars
Prevention
Burn Depth
Chapter Objectives

References

Background

Incidence of Hypertrophic Scars

Hypertrophic scarring has a greater incidence in darker skinned individuals and predominately occurs in American Indian/Alaskan Natives, followed by African Americans and Asians [1]. The highest risk of pruritus occurs in the latter population. Additional risk factors include young age, female gender, and those with wounds in particular anatomic locations such as shoulders, anterior chest, neck, upper arms, and cheeks. In the total patient population, hypertrophic scarring occurs in between 30% and 90% of burn patients, with a majority of these cases occurring in children [1]. The incidence rate of burn hypertrophic scars increases proportionally with the time to healing, with a recent study demonstrating that scarring risk is multiplied by 1.138 for every additional day needed for wound healing in pediatric patients, highlighting the need for rapid healing in scar prevention [2].

Prevention

Patients have a higher risk of development of hypertrophic scars in wounds that take longer than 3 weeks to heal. A study of 500 pediatric scald burns demonstrated that time to healing is a strong predictor of scarring, with similar results seen in a retrospective review of 59 pediatric patients and 41 adults [3]. Therefore, acute wound care is critical in ensuring rapid healing. Care for burn wounds includes early tangential excision and coverage with a split-thickness autografts, skin substitutes, or temporary xenografts or allografts. Since delayed healing may result from infection, topical application of antimicrobials may help prevent wound colonization. While time to healing is a strong predictor of scarring, patients can still develop hypertrophic scars despite healing earlier [2]. This highlights the importance of improving therapeutic strategies in addition to prevention.

Burn Depth

One of the ways to accurately treat burn scars is to reliably treat them in a timely fashion and determine burn depth accurately. Many modes of burn depth assessment have been used, including biopsy, thermography, and vital dyes, among other examples. The most widely used method for scald burns is the laser Doppler scanner, which was shown to improve prediction of the level of burns that will or will not heal by reepithelialization at 3 weeks.

Chapter Objectives

In this chapter, we discuss management options for pediatric hypertrophic scars. In addition, we provide a palmar hypertrophic scar case with a 5-year follow-up and list the interventions, which consist of laser therapy in combination with serial casting, grafts, and local flaps for treatment of scar tension. Objectives of this chapter include understanding risk factors for hypertrophic scar development, therapeutic options available, and rationale for particular treatment options in pediatric patients.

Clinical Case

A 3-year-old Filipino male initially presented to the clinic with a palm burn from a fireplace contact injury. The care of this wound consisted of once weekly dressings with a closed dressing technique to minimize pain and allow for undisturbed wound healing. The child remained as an outpatient for the entire course of acute care. The deep wound took a full 3 weeks to heal and the patient developed a right palmar contracted hypertrophic scar (◘ Fig. 60.1). The patient presented with a raised, pruritic scar that remained confined within the boundaries of the wound area, as indicated in ◘ Fig. 60.1.

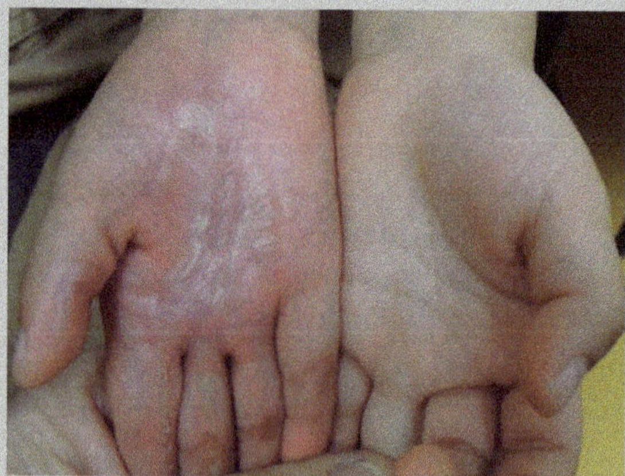

◘ **Fig.** Right palmar hypertrophic scar

Questions to the Medical History

- What are the primary risk factors for hypertrophic scarring in this patient?
- Is ethnicity a primary predetermining factor for development of hypertrophic scars?
- What are the features indicating that this is a hypertrophic scar as opposed to a keloid?
- Is this scar likely to progress over time?

Immediate Postintervention Situation

The patient presented with a scar contracture, which is one of the major detrimental effects of hypertrophic scars. Contractures of nonmatured scars can result in significant functional and developmental impairment and are frequently seen with scar hypertrophy. Conservative approaches guided by physical or occupational therapists have proven to be beneficial in these patients. Initially, scar massage in conjunction with moisturizers is commonly employed [3]. This may decrease pain, pruritus, scar thickness, and erythema, and moisturizers themselves decrease transepidermal water loss. Currently, scar massage and moisturizing with water-based lotions are the mainstay treatment for burn hypertrophic scars in children. Another approach is serial casting, which is used in burn patients to increase range of motion and prevent patient interference with the wound, an important concern in pediatric patients. With these considerations in mind, the patient was treated with conservative measures, including serial casting and scar massage three times a day. This treatment commenced immediately after the skin had healed in a verified burn center with rehabilitation specialists trained to treat this condition.

Contractures particularly in pediatric patients are challenging to treat. Distraction techniques and training of parents are challenges, along with the fact that the treatments are repeated multiple times daily, making this a difficult task for the children and their caregivers. In addition to treatment by serial casting/splinting to maintain the position, surgical correction may be indicated to restore function, especially if the patient has a persistent hypertrophic scar (>1 year). Techniques include scar-lengthening flaps and skin grafts, which are often delayed until the scar has matured unless the contracture interferes with the normal development of the child (use of the hand).

Intralesional corticosteroids such as triamcinolone acetonide are an option for treatment of hypertrophic scars and keloids [1, 3]. Corticosteroids can reduce pruritus and are effective in combination with cryotherapy in older hypertrophic scars and large keloids. In general, the corticosteroid is injected into the papillary dermis every 2–4 weeks until the scar is flattened. Although intralesional steroids are a common treatment for hypertrophic scars, they are rarely used for pediatric burn hypertrophic scars. They have limited utility due to the small dose that can be administered. In addition, the child needs to be sedated for the procedure in many cases. So, intralesional injections are usually reserved for small areas that are slow to settle after the majority of the burn hypertrophic scars have been treated.

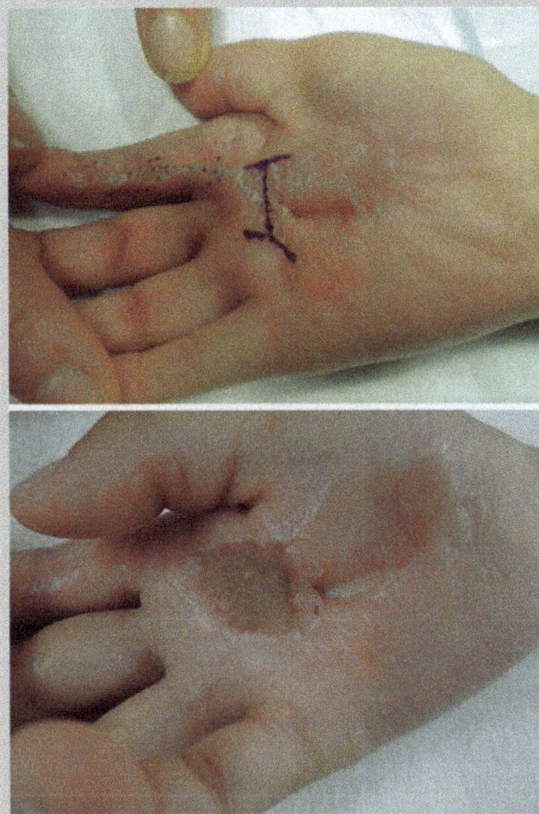

■ **Fig.** Surgical revision and grafting of the scar

At this point of treatment, the patient's palmar contracture had stabilized. However, therapists were noting difficulty with grasping objects in the affected hand and significantly reduced palmar measurements compared with the other hand. As a result, the patient's scar was treated by surgical revision and grafting after the initial conservative measures (■ Fig. 60.2).

Questions for Intervention

- What is the advantage of serial casting in this patient?
- Are there any alternative conservative rehabilitative strategies?
- Are these conservative strategies effective?
- In addition to the points mentioned earlier, what are other potential detrimental effects of intralesional injections?

Late Postintervention Situation

Surgical revision is necessary in such refractory cases, and correction of linear hypertrophic scars can be done by tension-releasing techniques. Typical surgical techniques for hypertrophic scar contractures include Z- and W-plasties. Z-plasties are a scar-lengthening technique that can relieve tension and mitigate contracture, improving range of motion, while W-plasties can minimize the appearance of prominent linear scars [4]. Several rounds of surgical releases, especially when combined with other techniques such as laser therapy, can facilitate successful rehabilitation of scars without excision. Lasers initiate an inflammatory response and induce moderate damage to local vasculature, resulting in local hypoxia and remodeling [3, 4]. This, in turn, results in reduced scar erythema, pruritus, pain, and scar texture and stiffness [5]. Lasers can be further subdivided into ablative or nonablative types. Ablative lasers reach their dermal targets by ablating the epidermis, which increases the risk of further scarring and other complications. As a result, traditional ablative lasers are no longer used. However, an exception is the fractional carbon dioxide (fCO_2) laser, which is regarded as an ablative laser but can be considered as an alternative to the conventional ablative CO_2 laser [5]. Alternatively, nonablative lasers can target dermal chromophores while preserving the epidermis, minimizing complications. There are several types of lasers that are used in the treatment of hypertrophic scars. These include pulsed dye laser (PDL), alexandrite and diode lasers, intense pulsed light (IPL), erbium:glass (er:glass), infrared neodymium:yttrium aluminum garnet (Nd:YAG), and nonablative fractional lasers 1550 or 1565 nm (NAFL). However, these nonablative lasers have a relatively shallow penetration depth, limiting their use to certain anatomical locations or shallow scars in the case of Nd:YAG and NAFL. Decision for which type of laser to use is dependent on scar characteristics, pain, and scar texture and stiffness [5]. The procedure itself is short and requires minimal additional rehabilitation, an advantage over surgical interventions, especially in younger patients.

A year after the initial surgical revision and grafting, the patient had laser treatments combined with Z-plasties (■ Fig. 60.3). This was followed by additional Z-plasties 5 years later. Several rounds of surgical releases combined with laser therapy facilitated successful rehabilitation of the patient's scar.

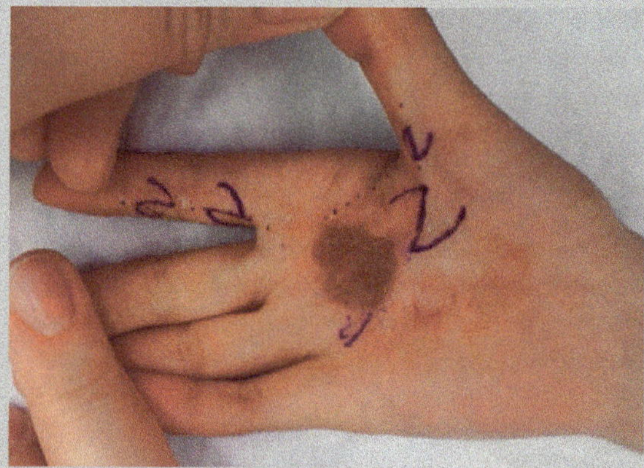

■ **Fig.** Treatment with Z-plasties and laser therapy

Questions for Intervention

- Why was this surgical management of this patient delayed?
- What are the reasons for a surgical intervention at this point in treatment?
- What is the purpose of Z-plasties?
- What are the potential consequences of laser treatment in this patient?

Answers

The primary risk factors for burn hypertrophic scars determined from the patient's clinical history are young age and increased time to wound healing (>3 weeks). While there is a higher incidence in Asians compared to Caucasians, hypertrophic scarring in general primarily occurs in darker skinned individuals and American Indian/Alaskan Natives [1]. Although hypertrophic scars and keloids have similar underlying mechanisms, they can be distinguished by certain clinical features. Hypertrophic scars are erythematous, pruritic, raised lesions that remain confined within the boundaries of the wound area, as indicated in ■ Fig. 60.1. In addition, the scar did not progress, unlike keloids, which continue to evolve over time.

The patient has limited range of motion and use of his hand due to scar contracture. Initial management with serial casting is beneficial in improving range of motion and softening the scar due to pressure. Casting provides pressure and stretch for an entire week giving caregivers a break, after which the cast is split and massage and stretching are resumed. The hand is placed back in the splint in between stretches, and the therapy is stopped after 2 or 3 weeks. Alternate options like compression therapy are used to reduce scarring by decreasing blood flow and collagen remodeling at the site of injury, and few studies have shown that it can possibly increase scar pliability and thickness. However, there is minimal evidence regarding effectiveness of these strategies [3]. In addition, they may be difficult to attain due to the poor patient compliance. Techniques such as intralesional injections are avoided in these patients due to the need for repeated painful injections and side effects such as lipoatrophy, altered pigmentation, and blistering.

Surgical management was necessary to allow for normal developmental use of the hand. This was dictated by review with a skilled rehabilitation team that followed the child's developmental needs. Surgery is typically delayed until the scar has matured since early intervention is associated with high recurrence rates and morbidity [4]. Here, rounds of Z-plasties combined with other treatment modalities (e.g., lasers) help relieve tension and improve range of motion. Potential consequences of laser therapy in this patient are hyperpigmentation and discomfort, the latter can be managed with topical anesthetics, oral or intravenous sedation, or nerve blocks to improve treatment tolerance [4].

Take-Home Message

- Burn hypertrophic scars in children are challenging, with multiple modalities of treatment. Children pose special considerations and, in addition to the scars, developmental stages and growth often dictate the treatments.

References

1. Gauglitz GG. Management of keloids and hypertrophic scars: current and emerging options. Clin Cosmet Investig Dermatol. 2013;6:103–14.
2. Chipp E, Charles L, Thomas C, Whitnig K, Moieman N, Wilson Y. A prospective study of time to healing and hypertrophic scarring in paediatric burns: every day counts. Burns Trauma. 2017;5(3)
3. Finnerty CC, Jeschke MG, Branski LK, Barret JP, Dziewulski P, Herndon DN. Hypertrophic scarring: the greatest unmet challenge following burn injury. Lancet. 2016;388(10052):1427–36.
4. Krakowski AC, Totri CR, Donelan MB, Shumaker PR. Scar Management in the Pediatric and Adolescent Population. Pediatrics. 2016;137(2):e20142065.
5. Zuccaro J, Muser I, Singh M, Yu J, Kelly C, Fish J. Laser therapy for pediatric scars: focusing on a combined treatment approach. J Burn Care Res. 2018;39(3)

26

Emerging Technologies in Scar Management: Laser-Assisted Delivery of Therapeutic Agents

Juhee Lee and Jihee Kim

Contents

Background

Laser Systems Used for Laser-Assisted Delivery

Carbon Dioxide (CO2) Laser and Erbium:Yttrim-Aluminum-Garnet (Er:YAG) Laser

Mechanism of Ablative Fractional Laser-Assisted Drug Delivery

Technique and Parameters
Main Parameters: MTZ Density and Depth
Clinical Application in Scar Treatment: Drugs and Bioactive Molecules
Other Modalities to Enhance the Effect of Laser-Assisted Delivery –

Conclusion

References

Background

Scars can cause significant impact on patients' quality life. Let alone cosmetic aspect, scars can result in functional and structural comorbidity. However, the treatment of scars is often challenging due to heterogeneity of etiologies and clinical presentations. Traditionally, surgical revision had been a mainstay for scars requiring structural remodeling to release the contracture of underlying tissue and relieve restricted range of motion. Nowadays, varieties of therapeutic options have been successfully introduced including physical therapy, silicon sheet, cryotherapy, corticosteroids, and laser modalities. Corticosteroids are often referred to as first-line treatment but its topical application is often ineffective. The major rate-limiting step for drug absorption is passage through the stratum corneum, which serves as the physiological barrier. Considering the pathogenic foci in scars are usually deep seated in the dermis, intralesional injection is considered as the best treatment option to bypass the thick stratum corneum barrier and deliver higher concentration of corticosteroids at the site. Yet the procedure inevitably accompanies excruciating pain. Corticosteroid is often associated with localized adverse events on repeated sessions causing skin atrophy, hyper or hypopigmentation, and telangiectasia. Treatment of keloid is even intriguing with varying success rates, and recurrence rates are high with conventional measures.

Target site for topically applied drug is the viable epidermis or dermis and the clinical response to a formulation is directly proportional to the concentration of the drug achieved at the target site. Transcutaneous absorption is limited by inherent skin barrier properties, minimizing the absorption to only 1–5% [1]. The innate barrier function of the skin, in particular the stratum corneum, provides the rate-limiting step in percutaneous penetration of drugs and other agents. Many different strategies have been developed to increase the permeability of the skin transiently for drug delivery. In skin with intact stratum corneum, only small (<500 Da in molecular weight) and lipophilic drugs succeed in partitioning into and diffusing through this dense lipid-rich layer. Transdermal patches have been used since 1970s but it is limited to drugs with low molecular mass. Accordingly, there is considerable interest in developing novel drug delivery methods. To enhance topical delivery of drug, currently available physical techniques include stripping, microneedling or sonophoresis, or iontophoresis to overcome the skin barrier.

The advent of lasers, particularly fractional laser systems, significantly advanced scar treatments in past decades [2]. Laser-assisted drug delivery was first described in 1987 and initially practiced with fully ablative lasers [3]. Laser-assisted delivery has been reported and evaluated in animal models for variety of skin diseases including premalignant lesions to inflammatory conditions. Ablative lasers can be effectively used to induce absorption of medications beyond the epidermal barrier. In precancerous skin lesions such as actinic keratosis, ablative fractional laser (AFL) is used to induce penetration of photosensitizer prior to photodynamic therapy. Chemotherapeutic agents and immunomodulators like 5-fluorouracil (5-FU) or imiquimod have been successfully used. Laser-assisted drug delivery has also shown to enhance absorption of topical anesthetics, nonsteroidal anti-inflammatory drugs, and corticosteroids [4].

Laser Systems Used for Laser-Assisted Delivery

Ablative lasers system has been employed to improve skin penetration of active molecules. Laser devices have traditionally been used in continuous mode, in which the entirety of the water-containing epidermis is completely ablated. Elimination of the physical barrier of stratum corneum allows transcutaneous delivery of large molecules, although it requires significant recovery time after removing large areas of stratum corneum. To overcome significant drawbacks from ablative fractional resurfacing, the concept of fractional photothermolysis (FP) was proposed in 2004 [5]. Fractional photothermolysis (FP) is a technique whereby an ablative laser is administered in a fractionated pattern instead of full ablation. Fractionated systems create discreet columns of ablated tissue, known as microthermal zones (MTZs), sparing intact portion of skin. The untreated skin surrounding MTZs serves as a reservoir of growth factors and stem cells promoting tissue regeneration and wound-healing response. Accordingly, ablative fractional lasers (AFLs) have provided an emerging option with a lower side-effect profile. AFL emerged as a promising tool in the treatment of scars with minimal pain and rapid wound healing in few days [2]. Moreover, fractional laser-assisted drug delivery is employed with high precision by controlling the area and degree of ablation through laser settings. MTZs facilitate penetration of topical molecules from the surface to the layer of interest (◘ Fig. 50.1). Due to its predictable tissue response, it can be an effective alternative to injection or topical formulations of drugs targeting cutaneous diseases.

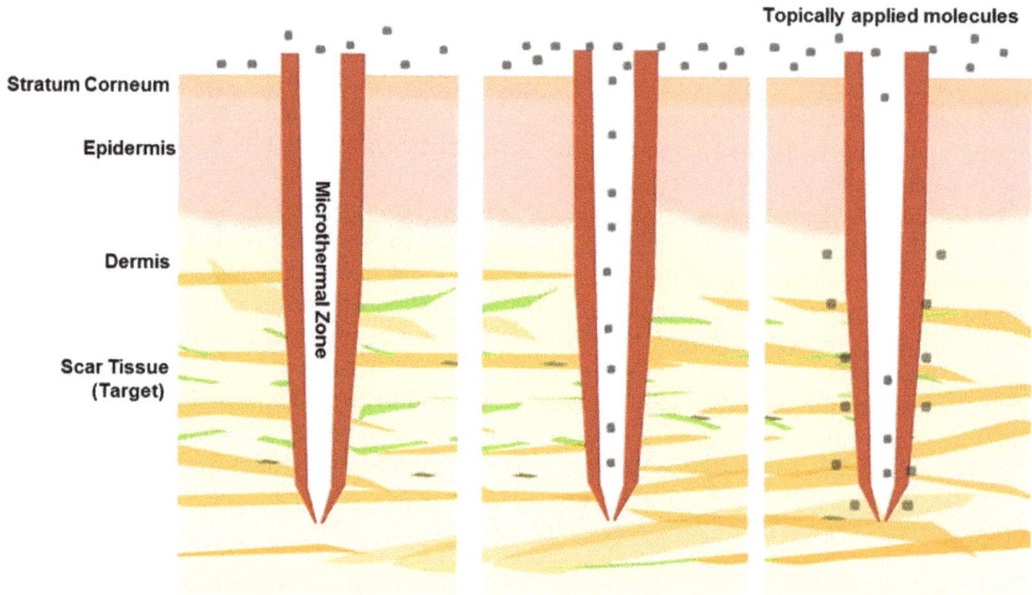

Fig. Schematic diagram of ablative fractional laser (AFL)-assisted drug delivery. AFL irradiation creates microchannels extending from the skin surface to the dermis. Microthermal zones (MTZs) vaporize accumulated scar tissue (orange) and influence collagen remodeling (green). Microchannels transverse stratum corneum and topically applied molecules can reach target tissue in the dermis and permeate into the skin

Carbon Dioxide (CO_2) Laser and Erbium:Yttrim-Aluminum-Garnet (Er:YAG) Laser

Carbon dioxide (CO_2) laser and erbium:yttrim-aluminum-garnet (Er:YAG) laser are the two types of laser devices most commonly studied in regard to laser-assisted drug delivery. CO_2 laser (10,600 nm) heats cells instantly, resulting in vaporization and coagulation of irradiated cells. Subsequently, denaturation of extracellular proteins and heat-induced shrinkage of collagen is noted in a subjacent residual layer. Histologic studies of scar tissue after ablative fractional CO_2 laser treatment demonstrated complete re-epithelization within 48 hours. Er:YAG laser (2940 nm) system delivers energy more precisely without extensive thermal damage to the surrounding tissue, permitting quicker wound healing and recovery of dermis. CO_2 devices generate larger degrees of heat diffusion to the surrounding tissue while Er:YAG system exerts less hemostatic effect. Differences between fractional CO_2 laser and fractional Er:YAG laser are similar to their full-field counterparts in that the CO_2 systems cause more residual thermal damage. Studies have reported that fractional Er:YAG laser causes significantly less residual thermal dermal damage, with a faster healing time and less post-procedure erythema compared to fractional CO_2 laser [4]. When applicable, the combined-mode Er:YAG/CO_2 laser system can offer synergistic benefit of ablative and coagulation effect. Both lasers have been successfully applied for scar treatment with favorable clinical outcomes. Fractional CO_2 and Er:YAG provided comparable outcome, yet fractional CO_2 system was associated with a higher degree of procedural pain in few studies [6]. However, it is difficult to determine superiority between the two modalities due to clinical heterogeneity and lack of comparative study design.

Mechanism of Ablative Fractional Laser-Assisted Drug Delivery

Ablative fractional lasers irradiate high-fluence laser beam forming multiple, discrete columns of thermal damage. Ablative fractional photothermolysis (AFP) systems generate MTZs by vaporizing full thickness zones of scar tissue that may extend to deep dermis. Surrounding the denatured columns created by MTZs is a collateral area of thermal denaturation that is sufficient to coagulate collagen. Moreover, thermal irradiation stimulates neocollagenesis for collagen remodeling. Studies have demonstrated that the increased expression of heat shock proteins (HSPs) induces anti-inflammatory effect after ablative laser treatment for scars. Additionally, the altered expressions of matrix metalloproteinases (MMPs) and tissue inhibitors of metalloproteinases (TIMPs) are noted along with increased expression of growth factors. Collectively, the differential expression of anti-inflammatory mediators and cytokines attribute to improvement in clinical appearance of scars.

MTZs facilitate penetration of topically applied drugs and other bioactive agents by acting as an alternative pathway for cutaneous drug delivery. Increased penetration of molecule can be explained by Fick's first law of diffusion. The diffusive flux of molecule goes from regions of high concentration to lower concentration, with a magnitude that is proportional to the concentration gradient. The degree of flux (J) is described as a product of partition coefficient (K), diffusion coefficient (D), and concentration difference across the barrier (ΔC) divided by the diffusion distance (L). Partition coefficient (K) indicates the equilibrium solubility of the drug molecules available for diffusion across a membrane.

$$J = \frac{K \times D \times \Delta C}{L}$$

The diffusion coefficient reflects the measure of inherent diffusivity of a molecule and determines the diffusion rate once the molecule permeates the membrane. The diffusion distance represents the length of a path for the diffusion. MTZs generated by AFL impact flux in various aspects of Fick's first-law variables. Firstly, increased permeability via MTZs enables increase in K compared to intact skin. Secondly, larger molecules with higher diffusivity can permeate directly into epidermis. Lastly, the distance of the diffusion is decreased from the skin surface and enables delivery to deeper layer. As a result, pretreatment with AFL facilitates traditionally challenging uptake of large hydrophilic molecules. The use of AFL increases the transdermal drug delivery of large molecules by 8- to 15-fold [4].

Technique and Parameters

Main Parameters: MTZ Density and Depth

AFL system irradiates target scar tissue with high precision by controlling the area and degree of ablation through laser settings such as power, pulse duration, percentage of skin coverage, and ablation pattern. For AFL-assisted drug delivery, the density and depth of microablative columns should be determined by operator for the given clinical characteristics of the scars. MTZs formed by AFP system can be adjusted to target specific depth and diameter by increasing the fluence and induce regulated disruption of epidermal barrier. In general, relatively modest energy fluence and density are considered applicable for laser-assisted delivery. Low energy levels are classically all that are needed to impair the physical barrier of stratum corneum. By calibrating laser settings, it is possible to influence the delivery rate and drug biodistribution, which may lead to improved clinical efficacy with shortened incubation time. Studies of the effect of laser parameters on the transdermally absorbed molecules are limited.

MTZ Density and Coverage

The MTZs consist of sharply confined tissue denaturation with a diameter of about 100 μm at intervals of about 200 μm. In animal models, increased density of MTZs achieved overall drug delivery, yet there was threshold density to achieve maximum diffusion. Fluorescent labeling demonstrated that the absorption of topically applied photosensitizers, immunomodulators, and lidocaine reached maximum biodistributions of 5%, 10%, and up to 20%, respectively, while further increase only resulted in deposition to stratum corneum [3]. More importantly, complications, such as scarring and hypopigmentation, have been observed at coverages in excess of 45%.

MTZ Depth and Energy

The depth of ablation represents how deep the MTZs extend into the skin and for a given laser beam diameter is mainly controlled by laser pulse energy. Microbeams of AFL irradiation typically induce MTZs ranging from 100 to 300 μm in diameter and it can extend down to the deep reticular dermis. The optimal depth threshold is yet undetermined as studies report drug deposition as both dependent on and independent of laser channel depth. It is expected that increase in the laser fluence and irradiation time increases the cellular uptake of large molecules across the skin in a dose-dependent manner. The usual threshold in the literature is approximately 200–250 μm in diameter. Hydrophilic or semi-lipophilic molecules (methotrexate, prednisone, and diclofenac) are generally dependent on MTZ depth while lipophilic molecules (lidocaine, ingenol mebutate, and imiquimod) do not show obvious depth-dependent uptake [6]. The variation between optimal depths for penetration can be related to the location of vascular plexus in different types of skin used for evaluation.

Clinical Application in Scar Treatment: Drugs and Bioactive Molecules

Delivery of every molecule will vary based on its inherent properties such as size, diffusion coefficient, and individuals' predisposed skin barrier conditions. In stratum corneum, corneocytes are embedded in a lipid matrix and bioavailability of hydrophilic drugs is low. While lipophilic or semi-lipophilic molecules can penetrate lipid barrier of the outmost layer of the epidermis, large or hydrophilic molecules are able to transverse the stratum corneum after AFL pretreatment.

Corticosteroid

Corticosteroid has been a mainstay in the scar treatment. It is mostly known to inhibit inflammatory mediators and promotes remodeling of extracellular matrix. To exert its clinical effect, corticosteroid should penetrate cell membrane to bind the nuclear receptor. Sustained release of corticosteroid can be beneficial because wound regeneration of the inflammatory stages is known to persist for several days after laser irradiation. Triamcinolone acetonide is the most widely used and available as micronized suspensions of corticosteroid crystals. Currently, intralesional injection of corticosteroid has been well advocated in the treatment of both hypertrophic scars and keloids. After its administration, micronized crystals of corticosteroids persist in skin and are released over a period of weeks. However, local injection of triamcinolone actinide is often painful and consistent dosing is difficult to achieve throughout the scar.

Combination treatment of AFL and topically applied corticosteroids demonstrate encouraging results. Application of triamcinolone immediately after AFL can induce synergistic effect of deep penetration into the scar tissue to induce collagen remodeling. Use of relatively low-dose triamcinolone (10 mg/mL) is sufficient to induce clinical improvement in various types of scars including burn, trauma, or surgical scars. AFL-assisted delivery of topical triamcinolone potentially offers an efficient, safe, and effective adjunctive treatment. Corticosteroids available as topically applied formulations demonstrated mediocre effect in scar treatment. There are only few reports used to alleviate symptoms or appearance of hypertrophic scars immediately after surgical procedure [7]. Nevertheless, the combination of AFL and topical corticosteroid application yields successful result for the treatment of keloid without any adverse event [8]. AFL-assisted corticosteroid application is a promising tool with minimal pain and rapid wound healing in few days. Beyond the specific action of the lasers on scar remodeling, the channels that they create can be used to deliver active molecules to potentiate its efficacy (◘ Fig. 50.2). On the other hand, the presence of MTZ-induced channels is transient mostly at presence for 3 to 7 days. Accordingly, disrupted physical barrier of stratum corneum is restored within a week after AFL. Thus, further study is required to determine the optimal dosage of triamcinolone suspension and potency of topically applied formulations.

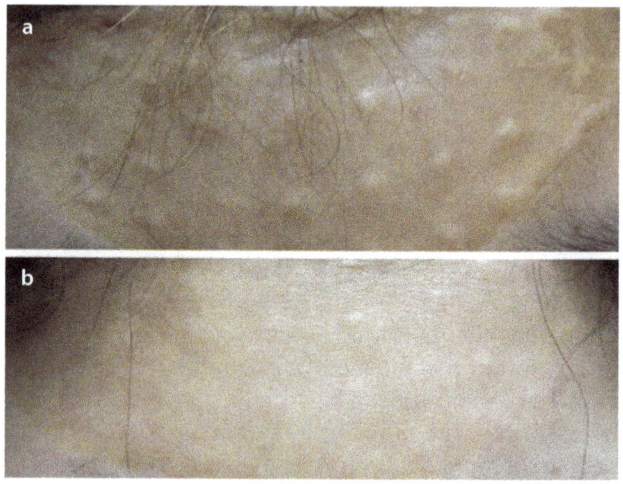

◘ **Fig. 50.2** **a** A 16-year-old woman with Fitzpatrick skin type IV with hypertrophic scars after facial reconstruction surgery. **b** Patient underwent five sessions of fractional CO_2 laser (eCO_2 Lutronic, Goyang, Korea. 60 mJ, 10% density) combined with topical application of triamcinolone acetonide suspension of 10 mg/mL

Other Agents for Scar Treatment

When routinely applied, topical corticosteroids do have risk to cause localized adverse effects such as skin atrophy, pigmentary changes, or telangiectasia. To spare such undesired skin reaction, drugs with immunomodulatory function has been applied in various skin conditions.

5-Fluorouracil (5-FU) is a pyrimidine analog antimetabolite that results in an irreversible inhibition of thymidylate synthase, commonly used for premalignant skin lesions. Laser-assisted delivery of 5-FU has been tested in animal models using various types of laser systems. Pretreatment with AFL resulted in more than 50-fold and 30-fold increase in penetration using Er:YAG and CO_2 system, respectively. In a study comparing the effect of 5-FU and triamcinolone to treat hypertrophic scars, lesions subjected to 5-FU demonstrated comparable results in terms of scar texture and height [9]. Appropriate dosing of 5-FU should be evaluated due to concern for increased systemic absorption with laser-assisted drug delivery, which can expand the adverse effect profile unlike bland topical application.

Atrophic scars result from loss of dermal or subcutaneous tissue during the wound-healing process. Fillers are high-molecular-weight biopolymer developed to provide structural support for volume restoration of skin. On this account, it is unable to permeate through intact epidermis and employed by injection. Laser systems, AFL in particular, can improve atrophic scars by promoting new collagen synthesis after irradiation. Concomitant use of AFL and topically applied poly-L-lactic acid (PLLA) fillers proved to be successful in treating patients with atrophic scars from various etiologies including acne and trauma. Histologic evaluation on cadaveric skin demonstrated the penetration of PLLA to the dermis, albeit large molecular size [10]. Additionally, sustained release by prednisolone encapsulated in PLLA microsphere provided continuous delivery enough to suppress prolonged inflammatory response [6]. Likewise, several bioactive molecules and peptides such as polydeoxyribonucleotide (PDRN) are evaluated for potential application for scar treatment. Recently, enhanced percutaneous delivery of adipocyte and hematopoietic stem cells by AFL systems has been evaluated in scar management.

Other Modalities to Enhance the Effect of Laser-Assisted Delivery

Emerging Devices

AFL-assisted drug delivery of therapeutic agents emerging devices is one of the latest strategies to enhance cutaneous bioavailability of topically applied molecules. Notwithstanding that MTZs can empower to bypass the skin barrier, passive uptake through MTZs can be inadequate as the channels are rapidly restored within few days. Furthermore, within few hours after ablation, the depth of columns is gradually shortened by accumulated fibrin and interstitial granulation tissue. Therefore, several physical maneuvers have been suggested to enhance the delivery of active molecules. Ultrasound may temporarily reduce the intact biding of stratum corneum. Acoustic waves by ultrasound may induce cavitation, which increases the penetration of molecules. In animal model, active filling of MTZs was observed by altering the pressure during the topical application of test molecule [6]. Similarly, combination of sonophoresis and iontophoresis with AFL-assisted drug delivery can induce favorable results.

Radiofrequency (RF) devices locally generate heat depending on the local electrical resistance and current density. RF devices deliver thermal energy to the dermis and subdermal tissue, which induces collagen contraction and remodeling by disrupting its structural bond, thereby most commonly applied to the treatment of facial rhytides and skin tightening. Advances in laser and energy-based devices expanded clinical indications of RF devices. Fractionated RF systems are used to improve scar texture, and bipolar fractional microneedle RF systems have shown the resolution of atrophic acne scars. Furthermore, ablative fractional RF associated with acoustic pressure generated by ultrasound was used to increase the delivery of triamcinolone into hypertrophic scars [8].

The use of non-ablative fractional lasers (NAFL) needs to be examined as a less invasive method of laser-assisted drug delivery. NAFL systems create a similar array of microablative columns as does AFLs; the MTZs consist of columns of thermal injury with intact overlying stratum corneum. NAFL systems heat tissue without vaporization, thus being less associated with patient discomfort. Although the epidermis is not fully vaporized, barrier function of the skin in the treated area is transiently impaired allowing for enhanced drug delivery. NAFLs applied alone have confirmed its therapeutic efficacy in skin rejuvenation and various types of scars. NAFL-assisted drug delivery of minoxidil or corticosteroids can be applied to treat alopecia areata. Fractional erbium glass laser (1550 nm) was reported to effectively enhance percutaneous delivery of photosensitizers [4].

Limitations

Further investigations are required to establish the safety and efficacy of laser-assisted delivery of molecules as a transcutaneous drug delivery system. The majority of the existing studies have been performed on animal models and additional human studies are needed. Drug permeation through AFL-generated MTZs inevitably raises concern about systemic absorption and potential systemic toxicity. Transdermal delivery is considered relatively safe as the dosage required for the therapeutic effect of a drug is lower than the oral dose and avoids the drug metabolism in the liver. Although most applications of laser-assisted drug delivery have been intended for local effects in the skin, some reports have demonstrated that systemic absorption does occur. Along with increased transcutaneous absorption, a decreased dose should be considered to minimize side-effects that could be local or systemic. Further clinical studies are needed to fully evaluate the safety and efficacy of laser-assisted drug delivery for scar treatment.

Conclusion

Laser-assisted drug delivery is an evolving technology with many possible applications as a highly targeted customizable method for distribution of drugs within the skin. Current studies have demonstrated that laser pretreatment of the skin can increase the permeability and depth of penetration of topically applied drug molecules. Fractional laser systems can be successfully utilized in the treatment of various forms of scarring with a very favorable safety profile. Fractional photothermolysis, both ablative and non-ablative, can improve the texture of various scars by promoting collagen remodeling. AFL-assisted drug delivery systems offer distinct advantage by enabling the topical medication to penetrate deeper and reach target pathogenic site even for the systemic drug administration. Corroborative efforts with multidisciplinary measure and novel combinations of existing treatments can help ensure optimal clinical and cosmetic results.

Take-Home Message

- Lasers are safe and effective means of enhancing the delivery of topically applied agents through the skin.
- Ablative fractional laser-assisted drug delivery is increasingly used to enhance percutaneous uptake.
- Microthermal zones generated by fractional laser create precise, uniform columns of tissue vaporization, which facilitates delivery of various drugs.
- Ablative fractional laser-assisted corticosteroid delivery may take advantage of the newly formed channels to penetrate uniformly and deeply into the scar tissue. Combination of valuable scar treatment options can create synergistic therapeutic response.
- Laser-assisted drug delivery provides a new opportunity for a minimally invasive modality in scar treatment.

References

1. Sandberg C, Halldin CB, Ericson MB, Larko O, Krogstad AL, Wennberg AM. Bioavailability of aminolaevulinic acid and methylaminolaevulinate in basal cell carcinomas: a perfusion study using microdialysis in vivo. Brit J Dermatol. 2008;159(5):1170–6. https://doi.org/10.1111/j.1365-2133.2008.08795.x.
2. Anderson RR, Donelan MB, Hivnor C, Greeson E, Ross EV, Shumaker PR, et al. Laser treatment of traumatic scars with an emphasis on ablative fractional laser resurfacing consensus report. JAMA Dermatol. 2014;150(2):187–93. https://doi.org/10.1001/jamadermatol.2013.7761.
3. Haedersdal M, Erlendsson AM, Paasch U, Anderson RR. Translational medicine in the field of ablative fractional laser (AFXL)-assisted drug delivery: a critical review from basics to current clinical status. J Am Acad Dermatol. 2016;74(5):981–1004. https://doi.org/10.1016/j.jaad.2015.12.008.
4. Sklar LR, Burnett CT, Waibel JS, Moy RL, Ozog DM. Laser assisted drug delivery: a review of an evolving technology. Laser Surg Med. 2014;46(4):249–62. https://doi.org/10.1002/lsm.22227.
5. Manstein D, Herron GS, Sink RK, Tanner H, Anderson RR. Fractional photothermolysis: a new concept for cutaneous remodeling using microscopic patterns of thermal injury. Laser Surg Med. 2004;34(5):426–38. https://doi.org/10.1002/lsm.20048.
6. Ali FR, Al-Niaimi F. Laser-assisted drug delivery in dermatology: from animal models to clinical practice. Laser Med Sci. 2016;31(2):373–81. https://doi.org/10.1007/s10103-015-1853-z.
7. Park JH, Chun JY, Lee JH. Laser-assisted topical corticosteroid delivery for the treatment of keloids. Laser Med Sci. 2017;32(3):601–8. https://doi.org/10.1007/s10103-017-2154-5.
8. Cavalie M, Sillard L, Montaudie H, Bahadoran P, Lacour JP, Passeron T. Treatment of keloids with laser-assisted topical steroid delivery: a retrospective study of 23 cases. Dermatol Ther. 2015;28(2):74–8. https://doi.org/10.1111/dth.12187.
9. Waibel J, Wulkan A. Treatment of hypertrophic scars using laser assisted corticosteroids vs laser assisted 5-fluoruracil delivery. Laser Surg Med. 2013;45:14.
10. Rkein A, Ozog D, Waibel JS. Treatment of atrophic scars with fractionated CO2 laser facilitating delivery of topically applied poly-L-lactic acid. Dermatol Surg. 2014;40(6):624–31. https://doi.org/10.1111/dsu.0000000000000010.

27

Minimally Invasive Technologies for Treatment of HTS and Keloids: Fractional Laser

M. Tretti Clementoni and E. Azzopardi

Contents

Introduction

Method of Action

Fractioned Laser Platforms

Fractioned CO_2 Laser

Settings for Ablative Fractional CO_2 Laser

Fractioned Erbium:YAG

Fractional Non-ablative Laser

Picosecond, Fractioned, 1064 nm Nd:YAG

Cautions and Contraindications

Preoperative and Postoperative Regimes

Expected Outcomes

Potential Complications

Fractioned CO_2 Laser as a Method for Potentiating Transdermal Laser-Assisted Drug Delivery (LADD)

Consensus Practice

References

Introduction

Hypertrophic fractional laser and keloid scars present a spectrum of disorders that are difficult to treat. Multiple treatments have been tried, to ameliorate the clinical sequelae of scarring, such as erythema, pruritus, functional limitation, reduced range of movement, dyschromias, hyper and/or hypopigmentation. Early international clinical recommendations on scar management first recognized the importance of laser therapy in this armamentarium [1]. Within the years that followed, laser technology and the understanding of how it modulates the underlying processes that leads to hypertrophic and keloid scarring have experienced a quantum leap [2] and are still evolving. Lasers also present a considerable financial commitent, and it is possible, in the authors' experience, that limited early results partially stemmed from limited availability of multiple lasers with consequent attempts to overstretch the indications for what was available.

This chapter presents a state-of-the-art insight into the use of fractional laser for the management of this complex problem. In particular, we focus on the management of complex scars such as those occurring post-burn injury and split-thickness skin grafting.

Method of Action

Light energy can be used to modulate or ablate specific targets in the skin through selective absorption of energy and specific heat energy dissipation properties [3]. The theory of selective photothermolysis, first described in 1983, laid the foundations for subsequent developments and standard practices [3]. When used to induce a controlled thermal injury, lasers initiate information processes to increase vascular permeability and modulate matrix metalloproteinase production of collagen fiber deposition and tissue hypoxia caused by targeted vascular ablation [4]. Through these processes, wound healing specifically in the remodeling phase may be manipulated, resulting in scar maturation and obviation of symptoms [5]. Different types of lasers are useful in targeting the different components of this disease scar tissue and it is important that the laser practitioner has the essential range of appropriately powered tools required to produce an optimal effect.

The choice of fractional laser in the management of a hypertrophic spectrum scar depends upon whether an ablative or non-ablative effect is desired, the target chromophore, the background skin type, the thickness of scarring, requirement for laser-assisted drug delivery (LADD), and the patient's compliance with postoperative downtime and regimes. The Azzopardi classification of chromophores also helps the practitioner rationalize the likely target and downstream metabolic effects [6]. Fractionated lasers with established effectiveness include CO_2 and Er YAG (nanosecond modality). More recently, fractioned, picosecond Nd: YAG has emerged as a potent platform in this context.

Fractioned Laser Platforms

Fraction laser resurfacing creates microscopic columns of ablation in epidermis and dermis, termed microscopic treatment zones. The relationship of these zones to intervening blocks of normal tissue permit rapid heat dissipation yet deliver enough energy to allow immediate changes in scar pliability, and instigate scar remodeling and neocollagenesis. The use of non-fractioned platforms such as pulsed dye and KTP (532 nm) are well documented and discussed elsewhere.

Fractioned CO_2 (10,600 nm) and Er:YAG (2940 nm) are the two main ablative modalities in use, targeting water and collagen to produce mass transfer zones (MTZs) of defined diameter (70–100 μm) and depth, tissue vaporization, and coagulation.

At the molecular level, fractional ablative laser treatment induces upregulation of heat shock protein, upregulation of matrix metalloproteinase, fibroblast apoptosis, downregulation of transforming growth factors and basic fibroblast growth factors, and modulation of collagen-type ratios. These changes are evident beyond the microscopic treatment zones, yet the spared tissues contribute to rapid, normalized wound healing. A major difference however between CO_2 and Er:YAG laser is the potential to achieve immediate coagulation and hemostasis: CO_2 laser is 10 times more effective in this regard. This is critically important when considering resurfacing of extensive areas and when considering LADD, as in our experience, bleeding results in plugging and reduced LADD efficacy. Moreover, the waveform characteristics of a CO_2 laser have a significant bearing on the potential for side effects.

Fractioned CO_2 Laser

Indications and timing: The latest version of consensus international guidelines for prevention and treatment of pathological scarring (2014) reserve the use of fractional laser therapy for scars refractory to pulsed dye laser; widespread hypertrophic burn scars that failed to improve with treatment with silicone gel or sheeting, pressure garments, and/or onion extract preparations for 8–12 weeks; minor keloids that failed to improve within 8–12 weeks with silicone gel sheeting and intralesional corticosteroids; and major keloids resistant to improvement with intralesional corticosteroids and 5-FU may be treated with ablative fractional laser or PDL therapy. This philosophy has been challenged by recent literature.

First, the use of fractioned CO_2 has since been successfully used (to date, off-license) with extensive and well-documented success, as an adjunct facilitating transdermal delivery (see below) [7]. Pulsed dye is less effective in scars more than 1.2 mm depth, and do not allow for effective scar pliability that may substantially facilitate post-procedure physical therapy. From a basic sciences perspective, once it has been established that fractioned ablative laser may re-instigate appropriate scar remodeling, it would be more useful to target the scar during the remodeling phase once epidermal integrity is well established. Recent literature supports earlier intervention than the previous 6 months to a year postinjury dogma, in concordance with our experience. In our experience, a treatment interval of 4–6 weeks is acceptable. Further, given the tendency of corticosteroid to exacerbate telangiectasias, use of fractioned CO_2 first (±LADD) followed by vascular-type laser to correct any resulting telangiectasia may also be an acceptable and more time-efficient approach.

Settings for Ablative Fractional CO_2 Laser

Utmost caution is advised when deciding clinical settings as these will vary between platforms. Many superpulsed lasers can only produce a shark tooth–type waveform. This results in the need to impart substantially more energy for the therapeutic threshold to be achieved. This additional energy may be responsible for the increased risk of complications seen in the literature (both medical and legal) with these laser platforms. In contrast, lasers imparting a "top hat pattern" waveform impart only enough energy for the therapeutic threshold to be achieved. Further safety considerations include maintaining an inverse ratio of power to density, and ideally to avoid imparting a fluence that is above TRT, density sets the number of MTZs per unit area, which should not be above 10%. Ideally, for purposes of safety, pre- and post-cooling regime should also be considered. A cold-air blower provides excellent pre-and post-cooling as well as being an effective analgesic.

Further settings include the size, shape, pulse stacking, and depth. Shape and size of the fractioned beam can be changed according to prevailing need. Whether the beam should penetrate beyond the scar thickness is still being investigated; however, injuries beyond the dermis may well lead to scarring and should be avoided [8].

Fractioned Erbium:YAG

The clinical efficacy of Er:YAG in keloid scars is limited. Cavale et al. combined Er:YAG with twice daily topical betamethasone under occlusion until therapeutic maximum was achieved, resulting in 50% improvement (median, $n = 70$), but recurrences also occurred in 22% of lesions [9]. One factor which may explain this disappointing result is the limited ability of current Er:YAG technology to penetrated deeply, and lower hemostasis.

Fractional Non-ablative Laser

Fractional 1550 nm Erbium-doped fiber laser reported overall improvement in scar texture after four treatments spaced 2 weeks apart, compared to the non-treated part of this split-scar study [10]. Literature reports that the response is mediated by heat shock protein, fibroblast proliferation, and consequent neocollagenesis [10].

A recent comparative RCT reports 1550 nm Er-doped fiber (70 mJ/23% coverage) to be superior to pulsed dye laser (7.5 mJ/10 mm/0.45 ms), with a 75% compared to 53% improvement reported [11, 12].

Picosecond, Fractioned, 1064 nm Nd:YAG

Management of hypertrophic and keloid scarring in darker skin types is a formidable challenge. Longer wavelengths, cooling devices, and lower treatment fluences have been shown to minimize complications [13, 14]. Recently, fractional picosecond 1064 lasers have reported good outcomes with very few side effects [15]. Compared to the conventional nanosecond domain QS Nd:YAG laser, the ps-Nd:YAG can produce significantly higher peak powers at the same energy level [16]. It is therefore expected that such technology works principally through photomechanical rather than photothermal effects [17]. The inhibitory effect of the 1064-nm Nd:YAG laser against dermal collagen formation is documented in the literature [18–20]. More recently, the use of fractioned 755 nm picosecond laser has been reported to be effective and safe in patients with Fitzpatrick skin types 4–6 [20].

Cautions and Contraindications

Caution is advised with any underlying process that impedes wound healing. History of herpes simplex virus, especially if lasering is to be attempted in the peroral area, should prompt prophylactic management. Oral antivirals or more recently bromelain should be considered [12, 21, 22]. Current depth of penetration for ablative fractional devices is approximately 4 mm, and therefore management of deeper scars is less likely to be as effective [22].

Preoperative and Postoperative Regimes

No consensus exists with regard to preoperative preparation. Some prepare skin with chlorhexidine solution and moistening hair-bearing areas prior to treatment [23]. Others, including the authors, are content with cleansed, dry skin [24]. It is important to note that whatever preparation method is favored, that moist and humid surfaces result in reduced ablation, and increased heat latency since the primary target, water, is now in increased abundance.

Several factors influence the choice of anesthesia, depending on the age of the patients, available equipment, and extent of surface area treated. However, overarching principles governing the practice of both authors include the use of the safest, least-invasive modality first, pre-optimization, and dual effect of skin cooling in increasing safety as well as providing an analgesic effect. Within this context, pretreatment with topical anesthetics of increasing strength coupled with cold-air blowers may provide the mainstay of analgesia requirements [25].

Where general anesthesia is required, it is possible to apply topical anesthesia immediately after fractioned CO_2 lasering. However, the facilitation of transdermal delivery will facilitate increased absorption (see below), and therefore it important to consider the maximum safe dose to avoid anesthesia-related toxicity. Use of ice-water packs immediately following treatment provides additional modalities for heat dissipation and analgesia [26].

Again, postoperative regimes vary widely, depending on resource, patient compliance, and experience. Use of antiseptic moisturizers, followed by a regime of moisturization is strongly advised, along with hydrocortisone for pruritus. Sun protection is mandatory. Patients may resume normal activity almost immediately, including physical or occupational therapy. Showering is permitted, with the exception of full immersion in standing (bath) water where ablative laser has been used. Some degree of edema is expected. Depending on the patient's tolerance, compressive garments may be worn immediately after, but they may cause shear of treated tissue, and therefore it is sensible to recommend waiting for 24–48 h before use.

Expected Outcomes

Benefits associated with CO_2 laser treatment include increased scar pliability and reduced tightness, but it is important to impress on the patient that laser treatment creates the *potential* for increased scar pliability which is *accomplished only* by compliance with aggressive physical therapy postoperatively. Appropriate patient selection is therefore paramount, as is the availability of experienced and motivating physical therapists. Further benefits include reduced scar height and thickness. Pruritus has been observed to decrease in several studies presumably because nerve endings are no longer encased in tight scar tissues.

Similarly, fractioned CO_2 laser may directly address the source of keloid formation, when this occurs in hair-bearing skin. Here, the hair follicle is encapsulated in the scar, which subsequently inflames, infects, and results in perpetuation of the insult-driving keloid growth. Scar remodeling results in amelioration of pliability, and in the authors' experience it is not uncommon to result in resolution of the insult-driving keloidal growth as well as regrowth of hair in the site.

By inversely relating density to energy settings, it is also possible to attenuate relative scar height, resulting in flattening.

Potential Complications

The principal complications reported in the literature include burns, infection (viral, bacterial, mycotic) postoperative pain, and abnormal pigmentation: Post-inflammatory hyperpigmentation as well as hypopigmentation have been reported. In those being treated for burn injury memory flashbacks to the original incident have been reported in the literature, therefore it is essential that patients are forewarned. It is of course important to discuss the potential of multiple treatments. A large prospective study performed by Hultmann and colleagues puts the overall complication rate at 3.9% of all treatments: in decreasing order of incidence, hypopigmentation, blistering, hyperpigmentation, infection, cellulitis of the adjacent skin, superficial mycoses, and oral herpes simplex [27].

Practical recommendations for improving patient safety are judicious use of fluence (especially in darker skin types), use of pre- and post-cooling regimes, single pass, and avoiding stacking pulses, intentionally or otherwise [8]. Multimodality treatment to one area within the same sitting is indeed possible, given the mastery of the underlying principles, correct understanding of the disease extent, the background skin type, and the patient's potential for healing. However, it significantly increases the risk for adverse events and therefore best avoided, except where mandated by individual risk–benefit considerations and availability of experts with appropriate experience. The use of test-patching and initiation of treatment in non-cosmetically conspicuous areas are advocated. In addition, a readily available database of previous patient-specific settings allows setting optimization to be delivered based on previous successes or complications.

Fractioned CO_2 Laser as a Method for Potentiating Transdermal Laser-Assisted Drug Delivery (LADD)

Ablative fractional laser breaches epidermal integrity, producing newly formed, uniform, and deep channels into hard dermal scars. It is well established (but at time of publishing as yet off license) to harness this phenomenon as an effective method for trans-dermal drug delivery (◘ Fig. 33.1). The two-fold advantages may be summarized as follows: less pain and more even distribution. First, traditional injection of volume into tight dermal scarring produces uneven distribution, creating blebs of volume while no treatment to adjacent areas. Volume injection into a tight scar also increases pain and discomfort [28]. Recent literature also points to various aspect of improvement this technique addresses, including pain tolerance, texture, dyschromia, and hypertrophy [26, 28, 29].

Pain relief: Intra-scar injection is often poorly tolerated pain-wise, especially when larger surface areas are being considered. Several studies have established that fractional Er:YAG pretreatment reduces up to twelve-fold the time required for topical anesthesia to take effect. However, within these studies, it is impossible to assess whether mild adverse events reported (including residual pain, redness, or mild-moderate swelling) was due to the needle or laser, as the effect was measured only after the needle was inserted. Typical settings for this indication are fluence of 250 mJ/pulse, a pulse width of 300 microseconds, and an estimated pore depth of less than 20 mm [30–32].

More importantly, this data demonstrates that application of local anesthesia post-procedure is likely to be more efficiently absorbed. While care needs to be taken with maximum dose due to altered absorption, post-procedure topical anesthesia may provide valuable pain relief, and is the standard practice of one of the authors (EA) when treating larger areas of sheet hypertrophic scarring post burns, with no side effects noted to date.

LADD has been used to potentiate transdermal delivery of both corticosteroid [33–37] as well as 5-fluorouracil [38] as well as combination treatment [38]. More recent evidence suggests that both are equally effective, but 5-FU does not lead to dermal atrophy or telangiectasia seen with corticosteroid delivery [39].

Consensus Practice

Established clinical consensus is that ablative lasers are significantly more effective per treatment for scar improvement than their non-ablative counterparts, especially for keloid and hypertrophic contracted scars, with significant gain in pruritus, pain, and physical mobility within days and up to 2 weeks posttreatment. Usually, rapid improvement in dyspigmentation is followed by slower improvement in texture and range of movement [22].

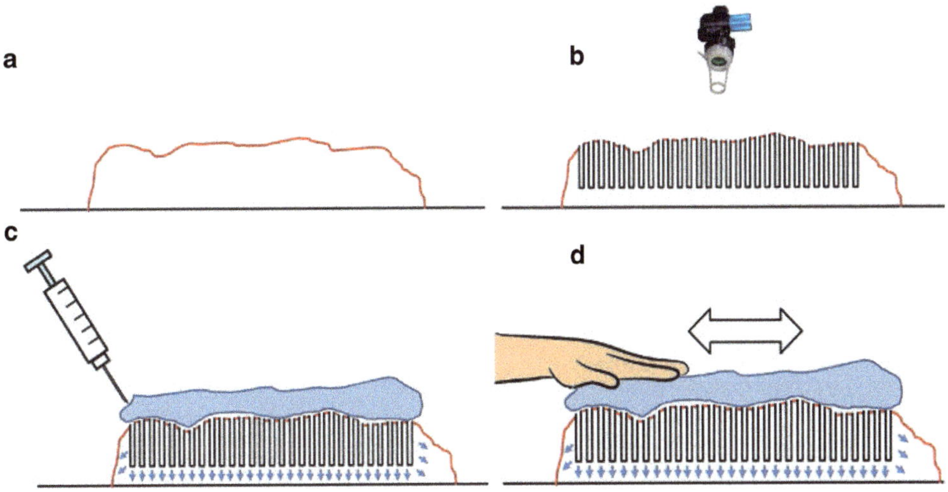

◘ **Fig.** In Laser Assisted Drug Delivery, is a recent advancement where laser energy is used to enhance trans-dermal drug delivery. For scarring **a**, typically, a fractioned ablative laser beam is used to create channels within the scar **b**. This is followed expeditiously with topical application **c**. The topical application is massaged in to the lasered area to enhance absorbtion **d**

Take-Home Messages

- Hypertrophic and keloid scars present a spectrum of difficult to treat disorders, and different types of lasers are useful in targeting the different components of this disease scar tissue.
- The choice of fractional laser in the management of a hypertrophic spectrum scar depends upon whether an ablative or non-ablative effect is desired, the target chromophore, the background skin type, the thickness of scarring, requirement for laser-assisted drug delivery (LADD), and the patient's compliance with postoperative downtime and regimes.
- Fraction laser resurfacing creates microscopic columns of ablation in epidermis and dermis, termed microscopic treatment zones.
- The relationship of these zones to intervening blocks of normal tissue permit rapid heat dissipation yet deliver enough energy to allow immediate changes in scar pliability and instigate scar remodelling and neo-collagenesis.
- Fractional ablative laser treatment induces remodelling changes that are evident beyond the microscopic treatment zones, yet the spared tissues contribute to rapid, normalized wound healing.
- The main modalities in use are CO_2 and Er:YAG laser. CO_2 has the potential to achieve 10-fold more immediate coagulation and hemostasis. This is critically important when considering resurfacing of extensive areas and for LADD.
- Picosecond systems act principally through photomechanical rather than photothermal effects and may be useful in darker skin types.
- Ablative fractional laser breaches epidermal integrity, producing newly formed, uniform, and deep channels into hard dermal scars. It is well established (but at time of publishing as yet off license) to harness this phenomenon as an effective method for trans-dermal drug delivery.
- There is no universally accepted skin prep regime, however moist surfaces result in reduced ablation, and increased heat latency.

References

1. Mustoe, Thomas A., et al. "International clinical recommendations on scar management." Plastic and reconstructive surgery 110.2 (2002):560–71.
2. Gold MH, et al. Updated international clinical recommendations on scar management: part 2—algorithms for scar prevention and treatment. Dermatol Surg. 2014;40:825–31. https://doi.org/10.1111/dsu.0000000000000050.
3. Manstein D, Herron GS, Sink RK, Tanner H, Anderson RR. Fractional photothermolysis: a new concept for cutaneous remodeling using microscopic patterns of thermal injury. Lasers Surg Med. 2004;34:426–38.
4. Jih MH, Kimyai-Asadi A. Seminars in cutaneous medicine and surgery. Philadelphia: WB Saunders. 2008. p. 63–71.
5. Laubach HJ, Tannous Z, Anderson RR, Manstein D. Skin responses to fractional photothermolysis. Lasers Surg Med. 2006;38:142–9.
6. Azzopardi EA, et al. Chromophores in operative surgery: current practice and rationalized development. J Control Release. 2017;249:123–30.
7. Zaleski-Larsen LA, Fabi SG. Laser-assisted drug delivery. Dermatol Surg. 2016;42:919–31.
8. Tredget EE, Levi B, Donelan MB. Biology and principles of scar management and burn reconstruction. Surg Clin. 2014;94:793–815.
9. Cavalié M, et al. Treatment of keloids with laser-assisted topical steroid delivery: a retrospective study of 23 cases. Dermatol Ther. 2015;28:74–8.
10. Hantash BM, et al. In vivo histological evaluation of a novel ablative fractional resurfacing device. Lasers Surg Med. 2007;39:96–107.
11. Tierney E, Mahmoud BH, Srivastava D, Ozog D, Kouba DJ. Treatment of surgical scars with nonablative fractional laser versus pulsed dye laser: a randomized controlled trial. Dermatol Surg. 2009;35:1172–80.
12. Graber EM, Tanzi EL, Alster TS. Side effects and complications of fractional laser photothermolysis: experience with 961 treatments. Dermatol Surg. 2008;34:301–7.
13. Alexis A. Lasers and light-based therapies in ethnic skin: treatment options and recommendations for Fitzpatrick skin types V and VI. Br J Dermatol. 2013;169:91–7.
14. Ross EV, et al. Treatment of pseudofolliculitis barbae in skin types IV, V, and VI with a long-pulsed neodymium: yttrium aluminum garnet laser. J Am Acad Dermatol. 2002;47:263–70.
15. Cho S, et al. Efficacy and safety of 1064-nm Q-switched Nd: YAG laser with low fluence for keloids and hypertrophic scars. J Eur Acad Dermatol Venereol. 2010;24:1070–4.
16. Abergel RP, et al. Control of connective tissue metabolism by lasers: recent developments and future prospects. J Am Acad Dermatol. 1984;11:1142–50.
17. Koike S, et al. Nd: YAG laser treatment for keloids and hypertrophic scars: an analysis of 102 cases. Plast Reconstr Surg Glob Open. 2014;2(12):e272.
18. Dang Y, Ye X, Weng Y, Tong Z, Ren Q. Effects of the 532-nm and 1,064-nm Q-switched Nd: YAG lasers on collagen turnover of cultured human skin fibroblasts: a comparative study. Lasers Med Sci. 2010;25:719–26.
19. Abergel RP, Meeker CA, Dwyer RM, Lesavoy MA, Uitto J. Nonthermal effects of Nd: YAG laser on biological functions of human skin fibroblasts in culture. Lasers Surg Med. 1984;3:279–84.
20. Haimovic A, Brauer JA, Bae Y-SC, Geronemus RG. Safety of a picosecond laser with diffractive lens array (DLA) in the treatment of Fitzpatrick skin types IV to VI: a retrospective review. J Am Acad Dermatol. 2016;74:931–6.
21. Hassouneh B, Newman JP. Lasers, fillers, and neurotoxins: avoiding complications in the cosmetic facial practice. Facial Plast Surg Clin. 2013;21:585–98.
22. Anderson RR, et al. Laser treatment of traumatic scars with an emphasis on ablative fractional laser resurfacing: consensus report. JAMA Dermatol. 2014;150:187–93.
23. Khandelwal A, Yelvington M, Tang X, Brown S. Ablative fractional photothermolysis for the treatment of hypertrophic burn scars in adult and pediatric patients: a single surgeon's experience. J Burn Care Res. 2014;35:455–63.
24. McGoldrick RB, Theodorakopoulou E, Azzopardi EA, Murison M. Lasers and ancillary treatments for scar management part 2: keloid, hypertrophic, pigmented and acne scars. Scars Burns Heal. 2017;3:2059513116689805.
25. Edkins RE, et al. Improving comfort and throughput for patients undergoing fractionated laser ablation of symptomatic burn scars. Ann Plast Surg. 2015;74:293–9.

26. Hædersdal M, et al. Fractional CO_2 laser-assisted drug delivery. Lasers Surg Med. 2010;42:113–22.
27. Hultman CS, Friedstat JS, Edkins RE, Cairns BA, Meyer AA. Laser resurfacing and remodeling of hypertrophic burn scars: the results of a large, prospective, before-after cohort study, with long-term follow-up. Ann Surg. 2014;260: 519–32.
28. Waibel JS, Wulkan AJ, Shumaker PR. Treatment of hypertrophic scars using laser and laser assisted corticosteroid delivery. Lasers Surg Med. 2013;45:135–40. https://doi.org/10.1002/lsm.22120.
29. Lee W-R, et al. Laser-assisted topical drug delivery by using a low-fluence fractional laser: imiquimod and macromolecules. J Control Release. 2011;153:240–8.
30. Baron ED, et al. Laser-assisted penetration of topical anesthetic in adults. Arch Dermatol. 2003;139:1288–90.
31. Bachhav Y, et al. Effect of controlled laser microporation on drug transport kinetics into and across the skin. J Control Release. 2010;146:31–6.
32. Shapiro H, Harris L, Hetzel FW, Bar-Or D. Laser assisted delivery of topical anesthesia for intramuscular needle insertion in adults. Lasers Surg Med. 2002;31:252–6.
33. Majid I, Imran S. Fractional carbon dioxide laser resurfacing in combination with potent topical corticosteroids for hypertrophic burn scars in the pediatric age group: an open label study. Dermatol Surg.2018;44:1102–8.https://doi.org/10.1097/dss.0000000000001413.
34. Park JH, Chun JY, Lee JH. Laser-assisted topical corticosteroid delivery for the treatment of keloids. Lasers Med Sci. 2017;32:601–8. https://doi.org/10.1007/s10103-017-2154-5.
35. Sobhi RM, et al. Comparative study of fractional CO_2 laser and fractional CO_2 laser-assisted drug delivery of topical steroid and topical vitamin C in macular amyloidosis. Lasers Med Sci. 2018;33:909–16. https://doi.org/10.1007/s10103-018-2457-1.
36. Tu JH, Udkoff JA, Eichenfield LF. Treatment of pediatric treadmill burn contractures with ablative fractional laser and topical triamcinolone suspension. Dermatol Surg. 2018;44:1656–9. https://doi.org/10.1097/dss.0000000000001553.
37. Willows BM, Ilyas M, Sharma A. Laser in the management of burn scars. Burns: J Int Soc Burn Inj. 2017;43:1379–89. https://doi.org/10.1016/j.burns.2017.07.001.
38. Lee BW, et al. Ablative fractional laser resurfacing with laser-assisted delivery of 5-fluorouracil for the treatment of cicatricial ectropion and periocular scarring. Ophthal Plast Reconstr Surg. 2018;34:274–9. https://doi.org/10.1097/iop.0000000000000948.
39. Waibel JS, Wulkan AJ, Rudnick A, Daoud A. Treatment of hypertrophic scars using laser-assisted corticosteroid versus laser-assisted 5-fluorouracil delivery. Dermatol Surg. 2019;45: 423–30. https://doi.org/10.1097/dss.0000000000001678.

28

New Drugs for Scar Treatment

Sun Hyung Kwon, Jagannath Padmanabhan, Dominic Henn, Kellen Chen, and Geoffrey C. Gurtner

Contents

Background

Objectives of the Proposed Chapter

Description of the State-of-the-Art Historical Evolution: Recent Data

Transforming Growth Factor-β (TGF-β)

Interleukins (IL)

Mechanotransduction Pathway Inhibitors

Supportive Articles in the EBM Literature

Clinical Relevance

Conclusion

References

Background

Cutaneous wound healing following injury is a complex biological process involving the orchestration of the immune system, inflammatory pathways, mechanotransduction pathways, and various types of participating cells. In adult humans, the wound repair process results in the replacement of the damaged functional tissue with a patch of cells (i.e., mostly fibroblasts) and disorganized collagen-rich extracellular matrix that is commonly defined as a scar [1]. While scarring occurs in almost all tissues, it is most apparent in the skin. Cutaneous scarring poses a significant psychological and physiological burden on patients, and an estimated $12 billion are spent annually on scar treatments in the USA alone [2]. Additionally, dysfunctional healing and hypertrophic scarring often causes lifelong disability, which has a significant additional economic impact [1, 2]. Over 40 million patients undergo surgical procedures annually, which often lead to the formation of hypertrophic scars (HTSs) resulting in substantial morbidity and disfigurement of the skin. Similarly, scar formation occurring as a result of burns and other forms of trauma leads to severe functional disabilities costing the economy over $4 billion per year [2]. Keloidal scars, which are characterized by excessive fibrosis in areas of the skin with acne or other minor injuries, represent another major fibrotic skin disorder. Several other skin fibrotic diseases such as Dupuytren's disease, psoriasis, and scleroderma lead to cutaneous scarring as well [2].

In current practice, cutaneous scars are treated using corticosteroid injections or cryotherapy, surgical revisions, topical silicone gels, sheets and pressure garments, radiation, and laser treatments [3]. These traditional treatment modalities have shown mixed success and most methods lead only to partial alleviation of scar formation. Further, many of these treatment modalities are associated with other practical issues such as patient discomfort and pain, multiple and frequent visits to the doctor's office, or even higher recurrence of scars [3]. Recent progress in the identification of key signaling pathways involved in fibrosis and scar formation has led to the emergence of new therapeutic agents for scar treatment, with promising results in animal studies. Agents targeting collagen synthesis pathways, cytokines, growth factors, and cytotoxic agents are under investigation for scar therapy. Of these, drugs that inhibit expression of transforming growth factor (TGF)-β1/TGF-β2 or augment TGF-β3 had shown initial promise, but have been shown to be ineffective in later clinical trials as discussed below [3, 4]. Similarly, treatment of scars with interleukin-10 (IL-10), an interleukin that is involved in regulating inflammatory pathways, has shown some promise in treating psoriasis, but has failed to show any significant benefit for other types of scars [5].

A paradigm shift in our understanding of the scar pathophysiology emerged when the role of mechanotransduction in fibrosis was explored. The role of mechanical stress in scar formation had been described as early as in the 1800s, with the description of Langer's lines of skin tension used for surgical incisions to minimize scarring. But recent work elucidating the role of mechanical cues activating inflammatory pathways and scar-promoting cells highlighted mechanotransduction as a central focus of scar pathophysiology [6]. In the past decade, aberrant activation of mechanosensitive skin cells have been shown to underlie abnormal wound healing and scar formation in various skin diseases including hypertrophic and keloidal scars, Dupuytren's disease, and scleroderma [6]. Offloading of mechanical forces during healing of human skin incisions following abdominal surgeries has been shown to be effective in reducing scar formation in Phase I clinical trials [7]. In particular, focal adhesion kinase (FAK), a molecular mediator of mechanotransduction, has been identified to play a key role in fibrosis and scar formation (◘ Fig. 52.1) [8]. Animal studies have shown that pharmacological inhibition of FAK can lead to significantly reduced scar formation and accelerated wound healing [9].

In this chapter, we will review the latest pharmacological therapies that are being evaluated for scar management in the currently available literature. This includes agents that have recently completed clinical trials and drugs that target cellular mechanotransduction pathways.

Objectives of the Proposed Chapter

This chapter describes the evidence-based new drug therapies introduced in recent scientific literature for scar mitigation and prevention. Although the underlying pathophysiology of hypertrophic scar formation following injury is far from completely understood, over the past decade, advances in our understanding of the cellular and molecular mechanisms by which fibrotic scars develop have paved the way for devising new approaches in scar therapies.

Description of the State-of-the-Art Historical Evolution: Recent Data

Traditional scar revision technologies include surgical treatment, topical silicone gels, sheets and pressure garments, radiation, and laser treatments [3]. In current practice, intralesional corticosteroidal therapies and antiproliferative 5-fluorouracil therapy are also commonly used to pharmacologically mitigate hypertrophic scars, although their effectiveness is mainly supported

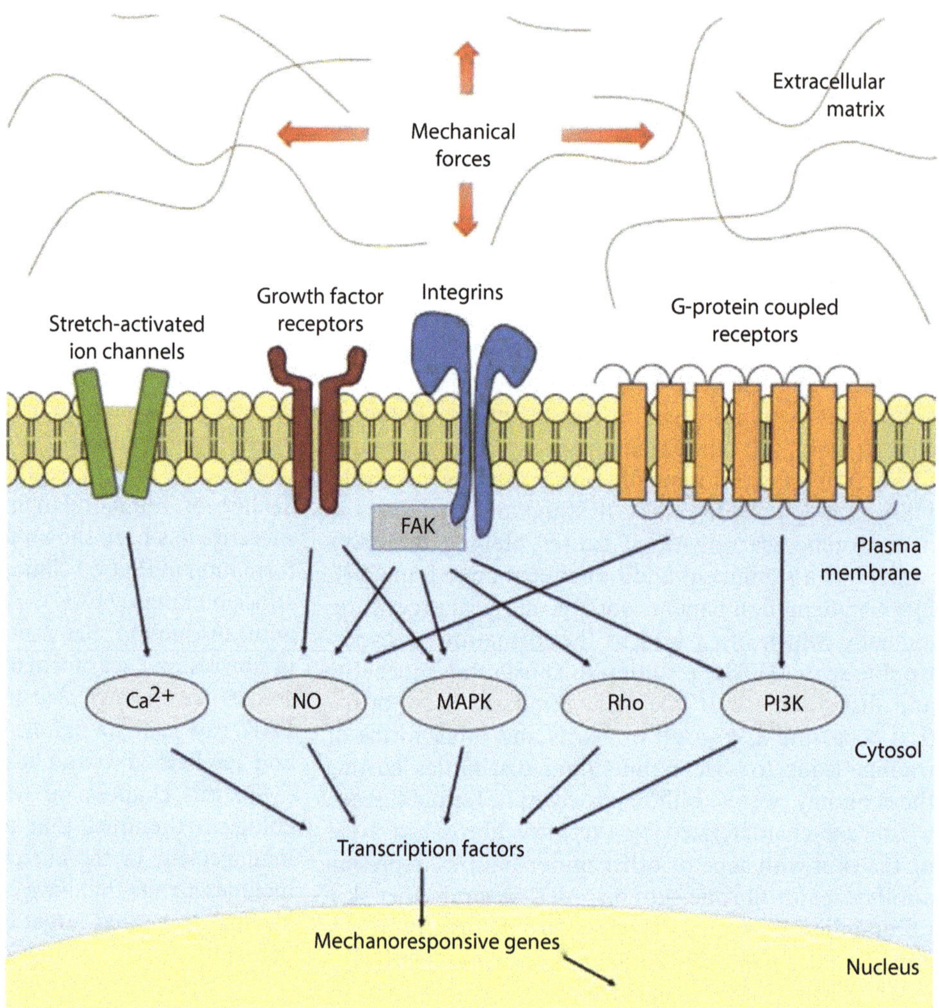

Fig. Focal adhe-sion kinase (FAK)-mediated mechanotransduction. Mechanical forces activate FAK, which activates several downstream effectors and transcriptional factors that mediate cellular mechanotransduction [6]. Source: Mechanobiology in Health and Disease, 1st Edition. Elsevier.

by case studies and preliminary clinical studies [3]. These treatments are often associated with adverse reactions, such as dermal atrophy or hypopigmentation, leading many patients to seek alternative treatment modalities after prolonged use. Recent studies have investigated new pathways to reveal drug targets such as modulators of wound inflammatory cytokines, growth factors, and mechanomodulatory mediators as potential targets for scar-mitigating therapies [6].

Transforming Growth Factor-β (TGF-β)

TGF-β expression is involved in almost all stages of the wound-healing process, including wound inflammation, angiogenesis, extracellular matrix synthesis, and tissue remodeling. Various studies have established the important role this wound-growth factor plays in dermal fibroblast differentiation into myofibroblasts and subsequent scar formation across a range of fibrotic diseases [3, 4]. Studies exploring the scarless and regenerative ability of the fetus have pointed toward the possibility that different isoforms of TGF-β could contribute to different stages of wound healing. While TGF-β1 and TGF-β2 are expressed highly in postnatal adults, TGF-β3 is the dominant isoform in fetal wound healing, leading many researchers to identify either TGF-β3 as a therapeutic target to upregulate or TGF-β1/GF-β2 as targets to inhibit for scarless wound healing [3, 4].

Despite strong preclinical outcomes, current TGF-β clinical trials have had disappointing results. Juvista, a new recombinant TGF-β3 product developed by Renovo, had shown promise in early phase efficacy trials but failed to meet primary endpoints in Phase III trials [3, 4]. Renovo also pursued a trial with Juvidex (mannose-6 phosphate), an inhibitor of TGF-β1/TGF-β2 [3]. Juvidex failed to meet its primary goal in a Phase II trial but it did meet a number of secondary endpoints [3]. Other researchers have also explored the clinical potential for a recombinant human antibody to neutralize TGF-β1 to combat systemic sclerosis, but their clinical studies did not prove any difference in efficacy from control during their Phase I/II trials [3]. TGF-β therapy could potentially have confounding results due to its dual importance in both normal wound healing and also in excessive fibro-proliferation during scar formation. TGF-β receptors are upregulated during fibrosis, and while blocking TGF-β expression seems to prevent fibrosis, it can also lead to chronic, nonhealing wounds. Albeit, TGF-β continues to be an attractive pharmacological target for a wide variety of fibrotic diseases, and newer strategies modulating TGF-β pathophysiology await further investigation.

Interleukins (IL)

Neutrophils and macrophages, two of the major cell types during the inflammatory phase of wound healing, secrete cytokines such as interleukins (ILs). IL-10 has been shown to regulate inflammatory cell function during wound healing by sequestering pro-inflammatory IL-6 or IL-8 and by regulating the Th1 cell cytokine production [3, 5], leading some research groups to explore the therapeutic effect of administering IL-10 to the wound bed during early wound healing. The previously mentioned Renovo also demonstrated the ability of IL-10 to potentially improve scar healing in human patients during Phase I/II trials administering Prevascar, their recombinant human IL-10 (rhIL-10) product [3]. However, they were unable to pursue Phase III trials after failing the aforementioned Juvidex and Juvista trials. Treatment with rhIL-10 has also been explored in several other clinical trials to potentially combat various inflammatory diseases such as Crohn's diseases and rheumatoid arthritis with disappointing results, but has shown promise in treating psoriasis.

Mechanotransduction Pathway Inhibitors

During wound healing, mechanical stress plays an essential role in promoting pro-fibrotic cellular events through mechanisms that stimulate inflammatory pathway components leading to exuberant fibro-proliferation. Manipulation of the wound mechanoenvironment with new medical devices that can modulate local biomechanics, therefore, has gained a rapidly growing market for scar reduction of surgical wounds [6–8]. Based on long-standing surgical principles clinically used to minimize scar development, these polymer-based medical devices offload mechanical force to release tension imposed upon healing surgical incisions. In particular, incisions created at high-tension body locations such as the central chest, shoulders, knees, ankles, and/or the back are prone to forming HTS than other body sites. For example, abdominoplasty wounds can develop into wide scars due to their natural high-tension closure, and application of a stress-shielding device on these wounds has demonstrated clear efficacy in mitigating scar formation [6]. This technology successfully led polymer stress-shielding devices to the market, and numerous patients have seen benefits in the clinic.

Despite success on surgical incisions, polymer mechanomodulatory devices are difficult to use on large-sized excisional wounds, burn injuries, and wounds that formed in contoured body areas. Alternatively, noninvasive therapeutics that pharmacologically target key mechanotransduction (cellular machinery that transduces mechanical stimuli to biochemical signals) pathways have also received highlight in recent literature. Currently, a prototype of such therapeutic agents is at the early preclinical development stage with translational potential.

Small molecule-mediated suppressors of pivotal mechanomodulatory proteins have been studied as anticancer agents for many decades. A non-receptor protein tyrosine kinase, focal adhesion kinase (FAK), is a key upstream mediator of the Integrin mechanotransduction pathway and an important inducer of cell adhesion, proliferation, migration, and angiogenesis [8, 9]. FAK is known to be deregulated in cancer and is thought to be a rational target to block tumorigenic activities using pharmacological inhibitors [10]. Because emerging studies have shown that FAK transduces mechanical stress signals to stimulate the activation of the FAK–ERK–MCP-1 signaling pathway and is an important regulator of cancer-promoting pathways [6–8], many pharmaceutical companies have taken effort to develop later-generation FAK inhibitors that display improved pharmacodynamic and pharmacokinetic properties. Clinical trials are ongoing in human cancer subjects, and the therapeutic potential to antagonize stromal solid tumors seems promising to date [10].

In currently available literature, small molecule-mediated inhibition of the kinase activity of FAK has been successfully used to prevent experimental bleomycin-induced lung fibrosis and mechanically induced skin HTS formation [6, 9]. FAK inhibition significantly reduced scar-forming fibroblast migration, myofibroblast production of α-smooth muscle actin, and aberrant collagen extracellular matrix deposition in these studies (◘ Fig. 52.2) [9]. Because wound healing and cancer development share similarities in terms of overlapping mechanisms that promote transformation, proliferation, and survival of cells, FAK inhibitor therapy that can be safely delivered to wound sites would be a new and promising approach to wound and scar management. In most circumstances, cutaneous scar development is a localized event; therefore, this provides rationale and support to develop targeted FAK inhibitor delivery modalities in attenuating scar formation. Localized drug delivery has the advantage of circum-

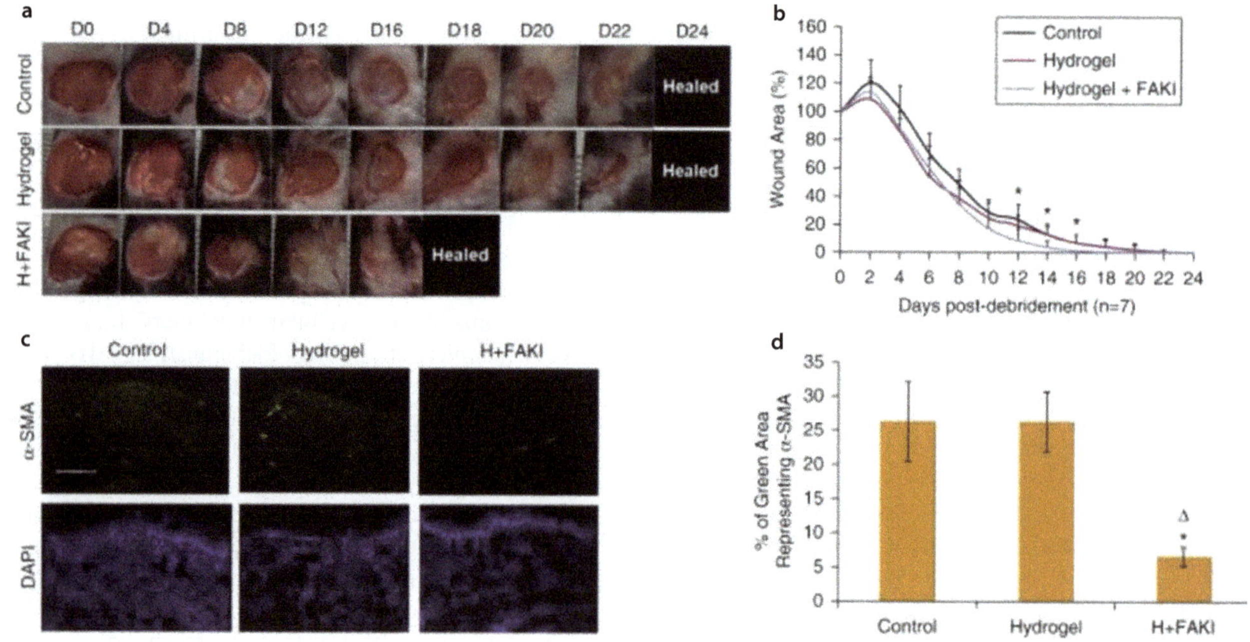

▪ Fig. Pharmacological blockade of focal adhesion kinase (FAK) improves wound healing and reduces scarring of murine burn wounds. (**a**, **b**) Mouse contact burn wound healing was accel-erated with FAK-I hydrogel treatment. (**c**, **d**) Wound expression of α-smooth muscle actin (SMA) was significantly reduced with FAK-I hydrogel treatment [9]. Source: *Journal of Investigative Dermatology* (2018), Volume 138. Elsevier.

venting systemic toxicity while maximizing bioavailability and local drug efficiency. Localized topical FAK inhibitor therapy ideally requires drug delivery vehicles that are biocompatible, eliciting no or low immunogenicity. Medicated self-adhesive patches that release therapeutic molecules upon dermal contact may not be suitable for large-sized open wounds, and other topical formulations in the form of topical cream, lotion, or ointment are easily subject to over- or under-dosing if application amount per treatment is not accurately measured. The latter is also problematic especially for therapeutic compounds with potential toxicological effects at the systemic level. Therefore, it is scientifically reasonable to devise a dermal delivery vehicle that can deliver topical FAK inhibitor to wounds and/or scars in a controlled manner. Biopolymers have strong advantages as drug delivery carriers because of their ability to carry bioactive compounds to target tissues and cells and to release compounds over a prolonged duration. Recent studies have used collagen-based bioscaffolds to develop biodegradable hydrogels that release FAK inhibitors in a regulated manner upon direct contact with the skin, which has proven preclinical efficacy in rodent wound models for HTS reduction [9]. Development of relevant drug delivery systems and extensive safety studies on potential adverse effects of each agent will be imperative to successful development of pharmaceutical therapies against fibrotic scar formation.

Supportive Articles in the EBM Literature

To date, currently available scar treatment modalities, especially for large-sized excisions and burn-related injuries, have not led to successful clinical outcomes, and the future market for new wound healing and scar mitigation therapies remains strongly promising. Recent progress in the identification of new signaling pathways and cellular components implicated in fibrotic scar formation has advanced our knowledge toward developing nontraditional therapies for scar treatment. Promising results in preclinical studies have resulted in many publications from multiple research groups with some therapies already completing human clinical trials. Scientific rationale for these newer therapies is strong; however, clinical development of some of these agents have faced failure during clinical trial phases. TGF-β-based therapies, Juvista and Juvidex, both displayed strong preclinical effects but failed during multiple human trials. IL-10 products also showed disappointing clinical outcomes. A mechanomodulatory agent, specifically localized FAK inhibitor therapy, is in its early preclinical development stage with promising animal data recently published. The more we understand the cellular and molecular mechanisms underlying fibrosis and scar formation, the more therapeutic opportunities will be revealed for scar mitigation.

Clinical Relevance

Cutaneous scar development of the skin, particularly the formation of HTS and keloidal scars following wound healing, constitutes a major clinical challenge for health care, both in terms of individual suffering and economic burden.

Scar formation can occur at any site of dermal lesion resulting from burn-related trauma, or surgical wounds. Burn patients are particularly prone to severe disfigurement and functional impairment through often extensive scarring, and affected children are the most vulnerable patient group in regard to long-term suffering. HTS formation affects a variety of life quality determinants. Cosmetic disfigurement by scar appearance may strongly diminish a person's self-consciousness, as well as their ability to participate in social activities and professional life, and is often associated with serious physical impairments, especially in the context of scar-induced contractures. Moreover, scars frequently cause secondary illnesses requiring complex multidisciplinary treatment not only by plastic surgeons but also by dermatologists, physical therapists, and psychotherapists. In children, abnormal scars can profoundly limit the potential of physical as well as emotional and psychosocial development during childhood. Therefore, effective scar treatment approaches can critically determine a person's long-term ability to lead a self-determined life.

From the perspective of health care professionals, researchers, and health economists, and for the society as a whole, scar formation is perhaps still an underestimated yet growing burden for the public health. In the United States alone, about 500,000 patients are treated for burn injuries each year, resulting in expenses of about \$7.5 billion. Conversely, treatment of scarring is a considerable economic factor, generating a \$12 billion annual market with further potential to grow [1, 2, 6].

It is a long-standing clinical observation that the proneness to HTS formation and keloids is considerably influenced by individual genetic traits as well as ethnic risk profiles [6]. Studies showed that about 16% of patients with Hispanic or African ancestry are affected from keloidal scarring, as patients with darker skin color are approximately 15 times more likely to be affected than light-skinned individuals. As the individual recurrence risk of keloids also strongly depends on constitutional determinants, progress in research toward their identification and, ultimately, targeted modulation can immediately affect therapeutic strategies of scar formation in the future. Consequently, scarring is a promising as well as challenging field of translational research into personalized medicine in the field of plastic and reconstructive surgery. Beyond that, the search for novel pharmacological treatments addressing molecular targets in the pathways of wound healing and fibrosis has the potential to improve the lives of numerous patients, and also to generate new products for health care of major economic value.

Conclusion

Wound healing and repair following injury is a complex and poorly understood process that leads to cutaneous scar formation, which constitutes a significant health care burden. Despite spending billions of dollars every year on scar management, traditional scar treatment modalities have not proved to be effective. Treatment modalities such as corticosteroid injections and radiation can be largely uncomfortable for the patients. Surgical revisions, which are targeted at reducing the wide base of the scar, are associated with high recurrence rates in the absence of other therapeutic strategies. Identification of key signaling pathways that are dysregulated during abnormal wound healing has led to the emergence of a range of new pharmacological interventions that target growth factors, cytokines, and collagen biosynthesis, and have showed promising results initially but have not led to successful outcomes in later clinical trials.

The clarification of the role of mechanotransduction in fibrosis has opened up a new avenue for scar therapy research. Offloading of mechanical forces of surgical incisions during healing has been shown to be effective in reducing scar formation, which further underscores the importance of mechanical signaling in scar development. Specifically, inhibition of focal adhesion kinase, a key regulator of mechanotransduction has been shown to be effective in attenuating scars and accelerating wound healing. Small molecule inhibition of FAK blocks the activation of inflammatory signaling pathways, thus uncoupling mechanical force from pathologic scar formation. This strategy has been employed to reduce scar formation in burn wounds as well as excisional wounds in mice. Taken together, recent findings indicate that molecular strategies targeting mechanotransduction pathways in general and specifically FAK pathway can effectively reduce fibrosis and show promise as an effective and versatile strategy for scar management.

Take-Home Messages

- The underlying pathophysiology of cutaneous hypertrophic scar formation following injury is incompletely understood; however, improved understanding of the molecular mechanisms by which fibrotic scars develop has paved the way for devising new approaches in scar therapies.
- Traditional scar management modalities include surgical revision, corticosteroid injections, and radiation treatment methods. These conventional therapies are often associated with practical issues and higher recurrence rates.
- Recent scientific evidence suggests that mechanical stress plays a crucial role in promoting pro-fibrotic cellular events via pro-inflammatory pathways leading to exuberant cutaneous scar formation and fibrosis.
- New medical devices that can modulate local biomechanics has gained a rapidly growing market for scar reduction of surgical wounds.
- Pharmacological inhibitors of the mechanotransduction pathways are promising evidence-based new scar therapies that block inflammation and pathologic scar formation.

References

1. Gurtner GC, Werner S, Barrandon Y, Longaker MT. Wound repair and regeneration. Nature. 2008;453:314–21.
2. Padnnanabhan J, et al. In vivo models for the study of fibrosis. Adv Wound Care. 2019; https://doi.org/10.1089/wound.2018.0909.
3. Meier K, Nanney LB. Emerging new drugs for scar reduction. Expert Opin Emerg Drugs. 2006;11:39–47.
4. So K, et al. Avotermin for scar improvement following scar revision surgery: a randomized, double-blind, within-patient, placebo-controlled, phase II clinical trial. Plast Reconstr Surg. 2011;128:163–72.
5. Asadullah K, Sterry W, Volk HD. Interleukin-10 therapy–review of a new approach. Pharmacol Rev. 2003;55:241–69.
6. Kwon SH, Padmanabhan J, Gurtner GC. Chapter 14 - Mechanobiology of skin diseases and wound healing, Editor(s): Stefaan W. Verbruggen, Mechanobiology in Health and Disease, Academic Press, Cambridge, MA. 2018;415–448.
7. Gurtner GC, et al. Improving cutaneous scar formation by controlling the mechanical environment: large animal and phase I studies. Ann Surg. 2011;254:217–2250.
8. Wong VW, et al. Focal adhesion kinase links mechanical force to skin fibrosis via inflammatory signaling. Nat Med. 2011;18:148–52.
9. Ma K, et al. Controlled delivery of a focal adhesion kinase inhibitor results in accelerated wound closure with decreased scar formation. J Invest Dermatol. 2018;138:2452–60.
10. Infante JR, et al. Safety, pharmacokinetic, and pharmacodynamic phase I dose-escalation trial of PF-00562271, an inhibitor of focal adhesion kinase, in advanced solid tumors. J Clin Oncol. 2012;30:1527–33.

29

Emerging Technologies in Scar Management: Remodeling of Post-surgical Linear Scar Using Microplasma Radiofrequency

Wei Liu

Contents

Introduction
Fractional Microplasma Radiofrequency Technology

Procedures: Clinical Protocol for Microplasma-Based Tissue Remodeling
Pre-therapy Preparation
Microplasma Treatment
Post-therapy Wound Care

Application Areas for FMRT-Mediated Tissue Remodeling
Microplasma Therapy for Post-scar Revision Skin to Enhance Cosmetic Result
Microplasma for Early Wound Intervention to Prevent Scar Formation
Microplasma Remodeling for an Existing Linear Scar

References

Introduction

A strategy of remodeling of an existed scar is by changing its tissue architecture that can eventually lead to a grossly non-visible or minimally visible scar. Since some years, mechanical or energetic manipulation of scarred skin has received considerable attention in attempts to improve scar quality. Next to techniques as dermabrasia, CO_2 laser, or microneedling, microplasma technology might represent a new technique in this field [1].

Fractional Microplasma Radiofrequency Technology

There are four formats of matter: solid, liquid, gas, and plasma. With energy, solid can be converted into liquid and liquid into gas. Similarly, gas can also be transformed into plasma with energy input. The fractional microplasma radiofrequency technology (FMRT) employs the energy of radiofrequency to act on nitrogen of the air in the narrow space between the therapy tip and the treated skin, and thus to form a grid of high-energy focal-led plasma sparks, which result in ionization of a portion of the atoms. With this physical effect, the FMRT can cause mild ablation of the epidermis with the formation of micro-channels in a fractional way (◘ Fig. 53.1).

The device we used in the past 13 years for patient treatment was a product from Alma Lasers (Caesarea, Israel) called Pixel^{RF} with both roller and stationary tips. ◘ Figure 53.1 demonstrates its working mechanism of the device. In general, this device creates the depth of ablative point in 100–150 μm, and the size of ablative point 80–120 μm in diameter, and heating effect with a unipolar can reach the depth of 1000 μm, depending on the radiofrequency power and pulse duration. However, the ablative depth could reach to the upper part of the dermis with increasing energy, and thus to remodel a superficial layer of dermis. By this way, the FMRT can remodel tissue structure via ablative microchannel of epidermis and controlled thermal modification of the underlying dermis, with new collagen synthesis and collagen remodeling [2, 3]. With this type of working mechanism, the created micropore wound can be healed in 7 days (◘ Fig. 53.2) and thus repeated treatments can be applied.

Although this particular device was used because of its availability to the author at that time, the effect of wound/scar remodeling is also likely to be achieved by other devices such as CO_2 fractional laser or others made by Lumenis, Cynosure, Alma, or Syneron, depending on physicians' clinical expertise (◘ Fig. 53.3).

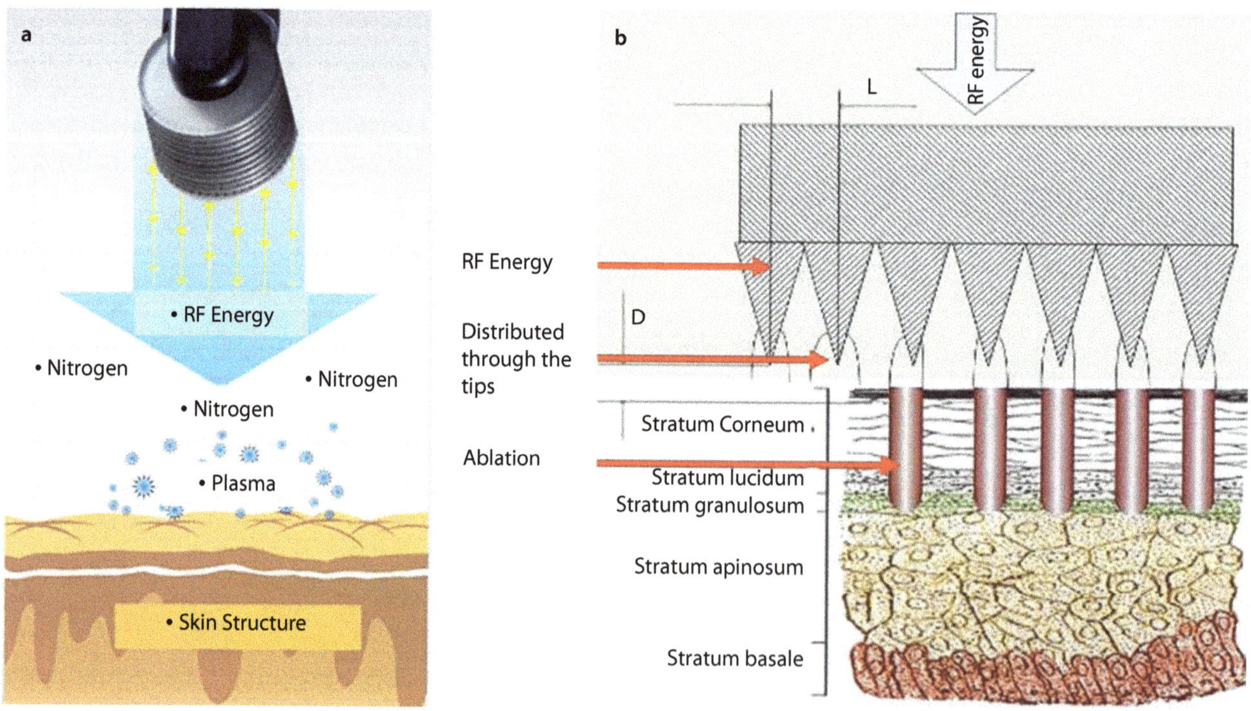

◘ **Fig.** The schematic picture of FMRT working mechanism. **a** Radiofrequency energy acts on nitrogen to create plasma particles. **b** Plasma particles penetrate epidermis in a fractional way. (*Photo courtesy from Alma Lasers.*)

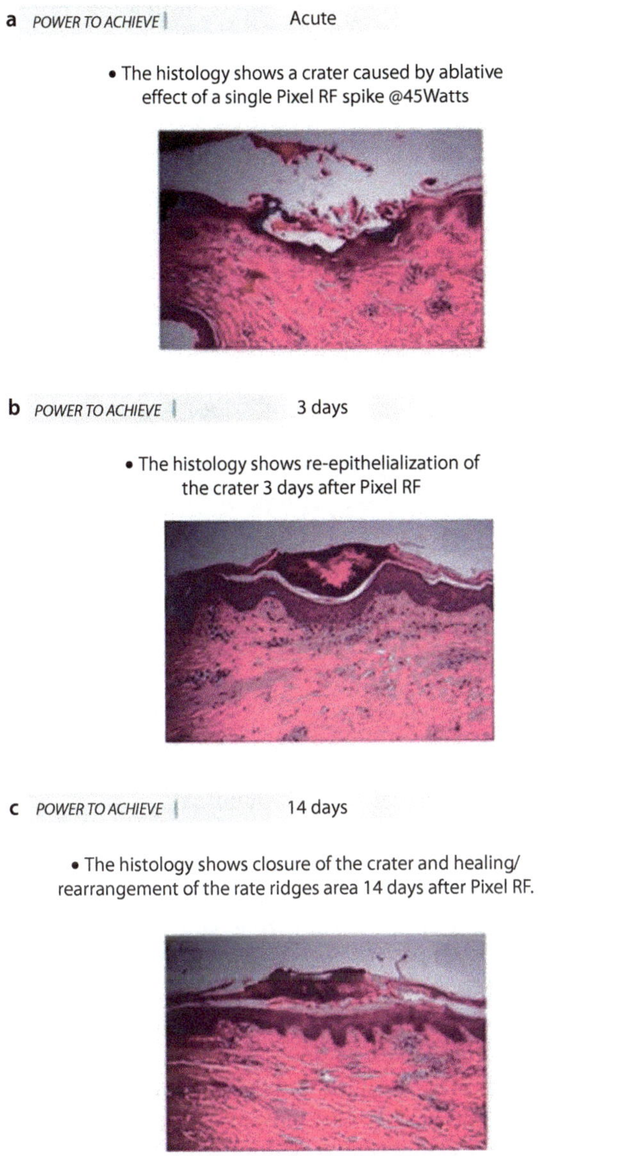

◘ Fig. Histological demonstration of microplasma working depth and healing process. **a** Acute wound immediately after microplasma. **b** Healing at day 3. **c** Healing at day 14. (*Photo courtesy from Alma Lasers*.)

Procedures: Clinical Protocol for Microplasma-Based Tissue Remodeling (◘ Fig. 53.3)

Pre-therapy Preparation

1. Patients with skin lesions at the treating area should be advised not to receive the treatment before the cure of these lesions, including infectious skin lesions caused by both virus and bacteria, dermatitis, psoriasis, eczema, and urticaria.
2. Patients should be advised for proper management of the micropore wound post-therapy and potential side effects with signed written informed consent.
3. Photography before the treatment. Be sure that it is taken before topical anesthesia and it is in the same conditions of environment such as light, focus, and positions.
4. Topical application of 5% lidocaine hydrochloric gel under plastic wrap for 60–90 minutes before the treatment followed by thorough cleaning and sterilization with 70% alcohol.
5. Non-treated skin should be protected with paper tape surrounding the treated skin if the tip is larger than the area to be treated.

Microplasma Treatment

1. Fractional microplasma radiofrequency treatment was performed with the device of Pixel RF (Alma Lasers, Caesarea, Israel).
2. A roller tip was used with the power setting at 60–90 watts, and 3–4 passes were usually made in different directions.

Post-therapy Wound Care

1. Patients are advised for comprehensive instructions of post-procedure care.
2. Sterile saline cleaning and erythromycin eye ointment were topically applied daily for 6 days to prevent infection.
3. Patients are advised not to be exposed to sunlight to avoid post-therapy pigmentation.
4. Patients are advised to protect the treating area by avoiding scratching or rubbing.

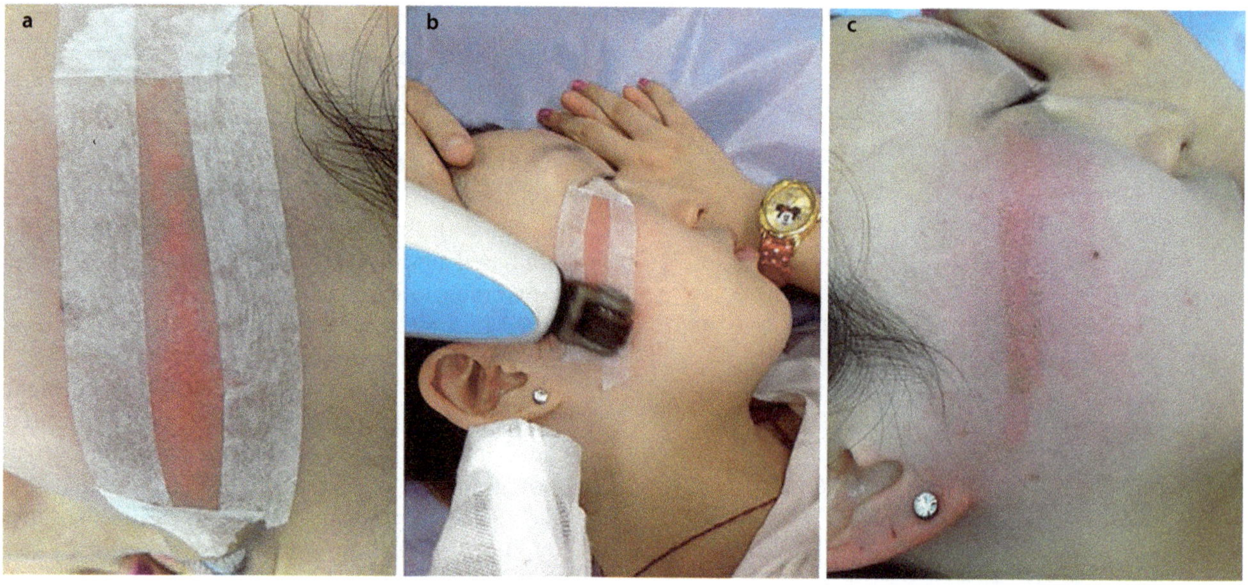

■ **Fig.** Microplasma procedure. **a** Paper taping is applied to protect untreated skin and 2–3 mm skin surrounding the healed wound tissue is also included in the procedure. **b** A roller tip is applied to perform the procedure. **c** The gross view of the treated wound/skin tissue immediately after the procedure

5. Patients are advised to have the follow-up regularly.
6. In the case of early wound remodeling, anti-tension type or device should be applied before and after the treatment.

Application Areas for FMRT-Mediated Tissue Remodeling

Microplasma Therapy for Post-scar Revision Skin to Enhance Cosmetic Result

Brief descriptions of the procedures for treating a linear scar for cosmetic reasons are as follows:

1. In general, a patient will visit our clinics and seek a consultation through discussing what a patient is expected and what can be achieved from the procedures. Then the patient will make an appointment for a scar revision surgical procedure.
2. In the surgical procedure, the patient is given a local injection of 1–2% lidocaine for anesthesia. In most cases, a w-plasty procedure will be applied along with the surgical excision of a linear scar to prevent linear tension, which usually causes observable scarring after the scar revision. To reduce wound tension, wound edge flap should be freed before wound closure. In addition, suturing of wound tissue at various levels also helps reducing wound tension, including subcutaneous, dermal, and epidermal tissues. For patients who are prone to scarring, wound irrigation with triamcinolone acetonide (5 mg/mL) or 5-fluorouracil (2–4 mg/mL) or both combined should be applied before wound closure to prevent scar formation.
3. After the surgical procedure, tension-reduction tape (such as 3 M tape) should be applied to keep the wound in a tension-free state. Patients are advised to have the tape changed every 2–3 days and maintained for at least 6 months post-surgery. The stiches are removed at day 5 or 6 post-surgery for head and neck regions, and stich removal can be postponed for 1 or 2 days at other regions. In case of the scar-prone patients who were treated for hypertrophic scar or keloid, an injection of triamcinolone acetonide (5 mg/mL) or 5-fluorouracil (2–4 mg/mL) or both combined with lidocaine into the healed wound can be administered at 1 or 2 months post-suturing.
4. In most cases, Pixel RF microplasma is applied to the healed incisional wound at 8 weeks post-surgery. Generally, the therapy should include 2–3 mm normal skin on both sides of the linear wound. The procedure is usually applied with a roller tip at 60–70 watts with 3–4 passes (■ Fig. 53.2).
5. Pixel RF microplasma therapy should be repeated for 3–5 times with 8–12 weeks' interval in general and patients should be closely followed up every 4–8 weeks until a linear wound mark and stich marks are completely removed. By this procedure, the linear scar resulting from scar revision procedure can be largely removed and the fine linear scar becomes grossly less visible or non-visible.

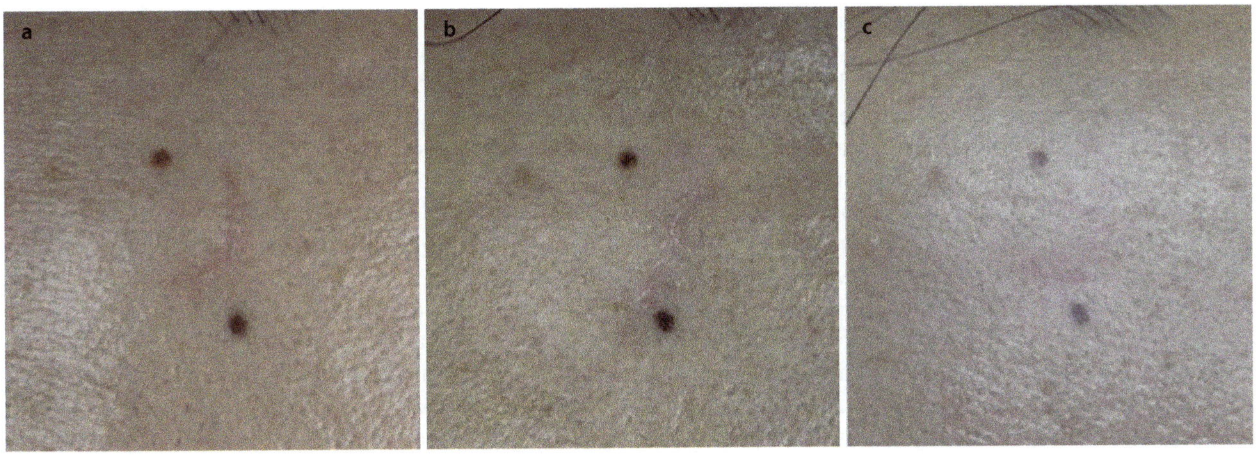

▪ **Fig.** Case presentation of microplasma remodeling of a linear scar resulting from surgical scar revision procedure. **a** Before surgery. **b** The gross view of a linear scar at 8 weeks after the first microplasma remodeling on a post-scar revision scar. **c** After 3 microplasma remodeling, the gross view reveals complete scar remodeling and no visible linear scar at the time points of 8 weeks after the third remodeling

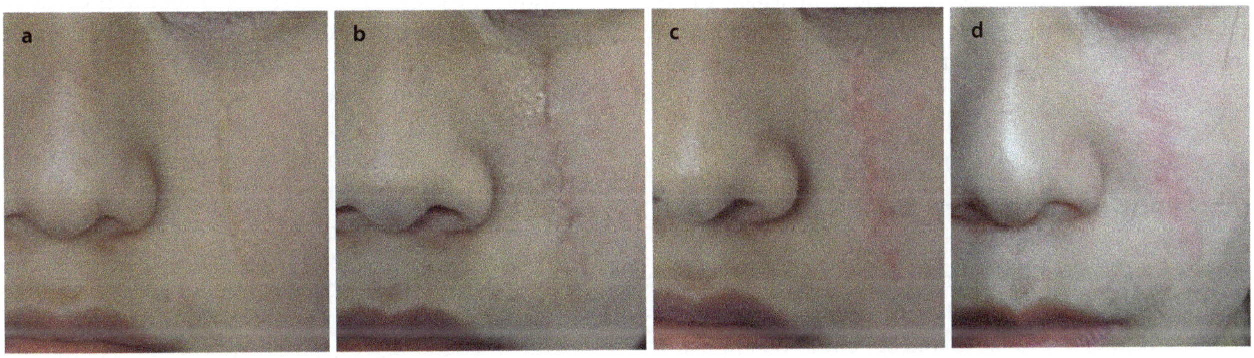

▪ **Fig.** Case presentation of microplasma remodeling of a linear scar resulting from surgical scar revision procedure. **a** Before surgery. **b** The gross view of a linear scar at 8 weeks post-surgical scar revision. **c** Gross view of a remodeled linear scar at 8 weeks after the first microplasma remodeling. **d** After 3 microplasma remodeling, the gross view reveals complete scar remodeling and no visible linear scar at the time points of 8 weeks after the third remodeling. However, erythema resulting from tissue remodeling remains visible

The following are the case presentations.

▪▪ Case 1

A 32-year–old female patient visited our clinic to request for forehead scar treatment solely for cosmetic reason. Physical examination showed a red-colored linear scar with a length of 2 cm and a width of 0.2 cm. In addition, the linear scar was also a bit elevated and with a few stich marks scar on both sides (▪ Fig. 53.4a). The patient received a scar revision surgery along with w-plasty procedure. After the surgery, the patient wore 3 M anti-tension paper tape vertical to the incision line. Later, silicone gel was also applied topically on the incisional line, and then 3 M paper was used. At 8 weeks post-surgery, she received microplasma therapy with an energy of 65 watts and 4–6 passes of rolling therapy. At 8 weeks after the first treatment, the follow-up photo showed significant improvement of the gross view of her forehead scar, although a fine linear scar remains when observed closely (▪ Fig. 53.4b). Then, the patient received another two treatments with 8 weeks' interval between them. At 8 weeks after the third therapy, the follow-up photo shows no visible linear scar on her head (▪ Fig. 53.4c), and the patient was completely satisfied as the result match her original request of removing her forehead scar completely.

▪▪ Case 2

A 27-year-old female patient visited our clinic for cosmetic treatment of a linear scar on her left face. Physical examination showed a mature flatten linear scar with a length of 6 cm and a width of 0.5 cm as shown in ▪ Fig. 53.5a. The patient received a surgery of scar revision plus w-plasty. The follow-up photo at 8 weeks post-surgery showed an apparent linear scar resulting from scar surgical revision, with which the patient was significantly unsatisfied despite the fact that an original wide and flatten scar has been transformed into a fine linear scar (◻ Fig. 53.5b). At this time point, microplasma tissue remodeling procedure was applied to the patient with an energy of 70 watts and six passes using a roller tip. Interestingly, at 8 weeks after the first therapy, the linear scar has already been significantly remodeled with the previous linear scar obscured; however, the linear scar remained obviously visible (◻ Fig. 53.5c). Thereafter, the patient was given another two microplasma therapies with 8 weeks' interval between them. At 8 weeks after the third therapy, the follow-up photo showed that a linear scar resulting from scar revision surgery was almost completely remodeled with no apparently visible linear scar (◻ Fig. 53.5d). Due to the thorough tissue remodeling process, in which the tissue structure of a healed linear wound has been significantly changed along with a regenerative skin repair, angiogenesis apparently occurred with manifestation of skin redness (◻ Fig. 53.5d), which will disappear in 3–6 months after the discontinuation of the treatment. The patient was very satisfied with the end result, in which microplasma tissue remodeling played a role significantly more important than the surgical procedure.

Microplasma for Early Wound Intervention to Prevent Scar Formation

With the success of remodeling healed linear wound tissue, we wondered if such a concept could be applied to tissue remodeling of an early incisional wound to prevent scar formation. The scenario is that linear wounds of non-elected surgical procedures such as trauma and wounding are usually difficult to prepare an optimal condition for their healing, and thus these linear wounds are more likely to form an obvious linear scar than the wounds created by elected surgical procedure of scar revision.

Due to the non-optimal healing condition, the wound tissue remodeling procedure should be applied at an early-stage wound. In addition, improvement of wound healing conditions by other wound manipulation methods should also be applied comprehensively including anti-tension, silicone product, drug local injection, or even re-suturing of an already sutured wound. Following are the general principles:

1. When a patient with an acute linear skin wound visits the clinic, proper wound cleaning should be the first consideration. In case of severe wounds or appearance of early signs of wound infection, antibiotics should be applied either locally or systemically or both.
2. Anti-tension tape or device should be applied before and after stich removal, such as 3 M tape, Zipline™ or Neodyne™ or other tension reduction device in order to maximally reduce the tension-induced scarring during wound healing process.
3. Silicone product should be applied as early as possible, such as Dermatix™, Kelo-cote™ or other products. This should be applied along with taping or tension-reduction device and wound tension-free procedure should not be compromised by other procedures.
4. Proper surgical procedures for wound closing is important as a thick scar will be too difficult to be remodeled for achieving a desirable effect. When decided to perform, proper debridement, wound edge preparation as well as fine suturing should all be included.
5. The timing for microplasma procedure can be decided on the basis of the wound condition. If an injured wound is properly managed with a condition similar to that of elected surgical procedure, the remodeling procedure can be performed at time point about 8 weeks post-wound closure to give a wound sufficient time to heal as a very fine linear immature scar, which can be completely remodeled with microplasma procedure. If a wound is improperly closed with a thick linear wound mark and obvious other stich marks, then the procedure should be applied as early as 1–4 weeks post-wound closure.
6. The energy of microplasma remodeling can be adjusted according to the wound condition. For example, a wound of a child or a wound with fine closure technique, then the wound can be treated with a relative low energy; whereas a wound is closed unprofessionally or in a poor condition, a relatively high energy should be applied and the treatment should be repeated until a desirable result can be achieved.
7. The comprehensive scar-reduction management should be continually applied after the remodeling and maintained for at least for 6 months post-wound closure.

The following are the case presentations.

▪▪ Case 3

A 52-year-old male (◻ Fig. 53.6)was wounded on his left-side face 3 days before, and he came to our clinic for assistance of the wound management in order to prevent severe scarring. Physical examination showed that there was a linear wound on his left-side face with a length of 3 cm. The wound had been closed unprofessionally by single layer suturing with tight knots that would be bound to form a thick linear scar with obvious stich marks after the healing of the wound (◻ Fig. 53.6a). To better prepare the wound closure, the stiches were removed and the wound was re-opened. After thorough

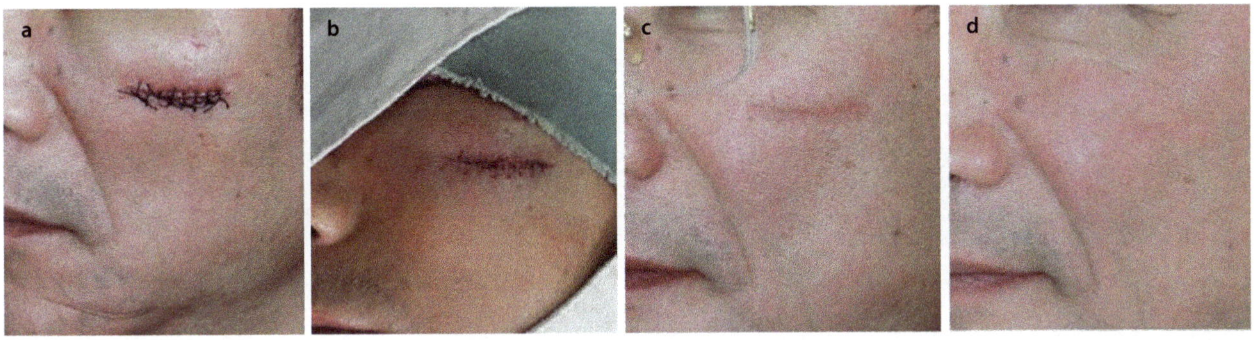

■ **Fig.** Case presentation of microplasma intervention of an early stage wound to prevent scar formation. **a** The patient has facial wound 3 days ago with unprofessional wound closure technique. **b** The stiches were removed and the wound was reopened. After wound debridement and proper position of wound tissues, the wound was properly closed with fine suturing technique, which paved the way for further tissue remodeling. **c** Gross view shows remodeling of a linear scar at 8 weeks after the first microplasma remodeling. **d** Gross view shows that post-wound linear scar is almost completely remodeled with no visible scar

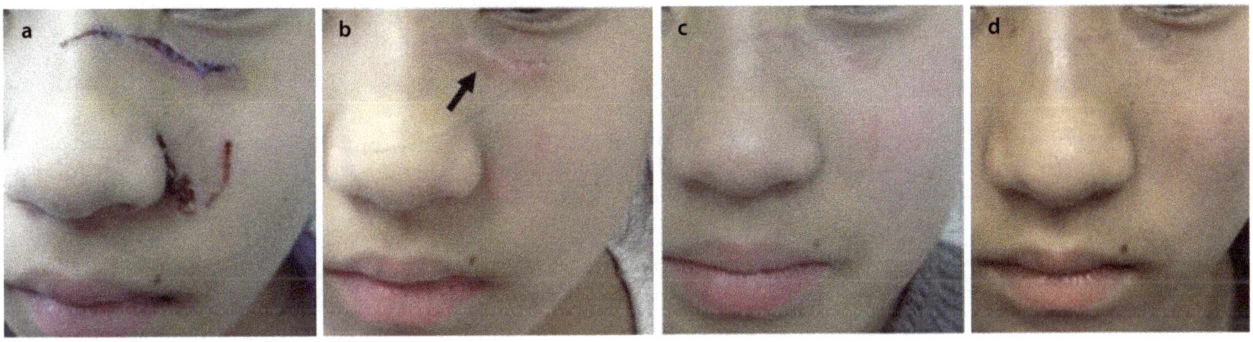

■ **Fig.** Case presentation of microplasma intervention of an early stage wound to prevent scar formation. **a** The patient has two wounds on her face for 5 days. **b** Early sign of scar formation was observed on her upper face scar at day 12 post-wounding. The arrow shows elevated tissue growth that would develop into hypertrophic scar, and thus a steroid injection was given. **c** Significant improvement of the linear scar was observed at 8 weeks after the first microplasma remodeling. **d** Gross view shows almost complete remodeling of the linear scar except for minor hyperpigmentation caused by microplasma treatment

wound debridement, wound dermal and epidermal layers were properly positioned and closed with fine suturing (■ Fig. 53.6b). The stiches were removed at day 5 post-surgery and 3 M tape was applied. At 4 weeks post-surgery (31 days after wounding), the patient received his first microplasma remodeling. Eight weeks later (87 days after wounding), the follow-up photo showed significant improved gross view of the healed linear wound (■ Fig. 53.6c). Then the patient was given the second microplasma remodeling. Eight weeks later (143 day after wounding), the patient was followed up with a photo demonstrating that linear wound mark was almost all removed via tissue remodeling (■ Fig. 53.6d). The patient was very satisfied with the wound remodeling result.

▪▪ Case 4

A 11-year-old female was injured on her left-side face and part of nose 5 days before she visited our clinic. She had concern of possible scar formation on her face after wound healing. Physical examination showed that there was a linear scar on her left-side face starting from suborbital region and extending to the left part of the upper region of the nose. In addition, she also had a curved linear wound at the left side of her left ala nasi as shown in ■ Fig. 53.7a. The patient was asked to remove her stiches and to apply 3 M tape for anti-tension purpose. The patient was given COX-2 inhibitor (oral medicine) for 2 weeks to reduce wound inflammatory process. At day 12 post-wounding, there was an early sign of scar formation as raised tissue was observed on the upper wound of her face (arrow, ■ Fig. 53.7b). The patient was thus given an injection of low concentration steroid to inhibit potential scar formation. Four weeks later, several more injections were given with 4 weeks' interval between them. During the time period, taping and silicone gel were consistently applied. At 3.5 months post-wounding, the patient was given the first microplasma remodeling. Eight weeks after the first therapy (5.5 months post-wounding), the scarring was significantly remodeled with obvious improvement of the gross view as shown in ■ Fig. 53.7c. Afterward,

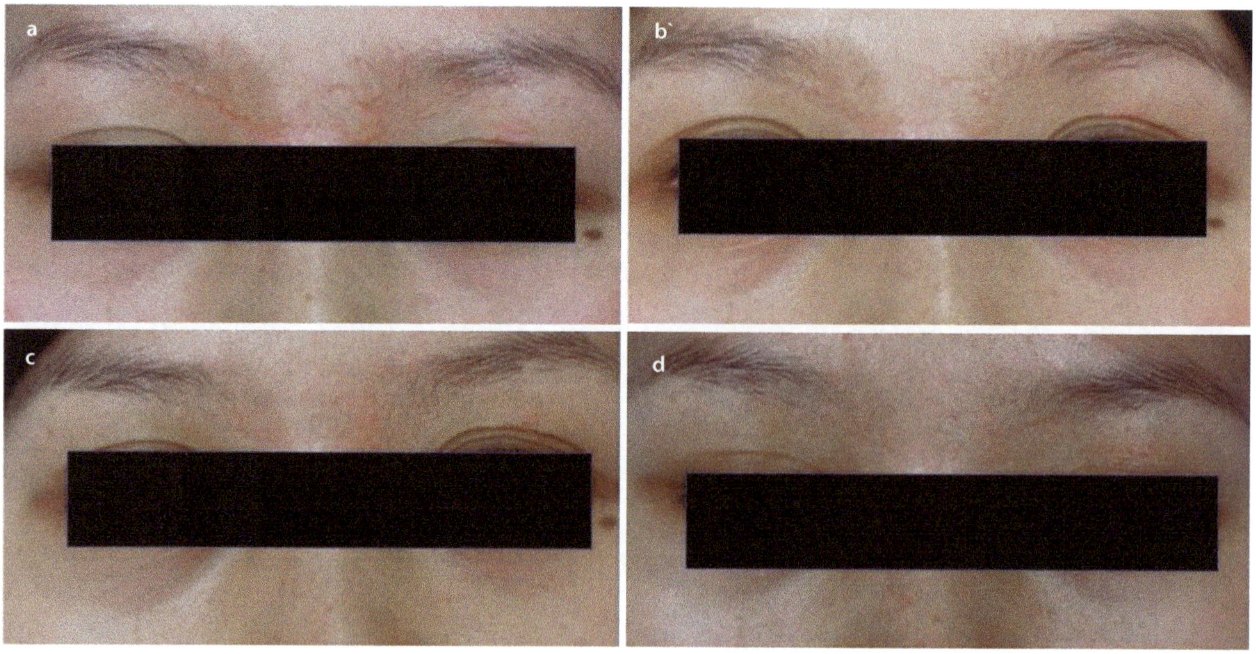

◘ Fig. Case presentation of microplasma remodeling of an existed linear scar. **a** Gross view of an existed linear scar at the region between forehead and nose. **b–d** Gross view of remodeling the scar at 8 weeks, respectively, after the first, third, and fourth microplasma remodeling. The end result shows almost no visible linear scar in the region

the patient was given three more procedures of microplasma remodeling. The final follow-up photo demonstrated that original scar was barely visible except for minor pigmentation. The patient was extremely satisfied with the results.

Microplasma Remodeling for an Existing Linear Scar

As described previously, scar revision surgery along with microplasma tissue remodeling is a preferred procedure to deal with the significant linear scars in majority cases. However, direct remodeling with microplasma is also a choice for linear scars under certain conditions. These include (1) a superficial linear scar; (2) an irregular shaped linear scar that is difficult to revise with surgical procedure; (3) a linear scar that formed in not too long time; and (4) the scar contains less dense collagen. These linear scars are more likely to be remodeled than other types of linear scars.

The following is a case presentation:

▪▪ Case 5

A 35-year–old female patient had an irregular linear scar caused by trauma in less than 1 year on the region between forehead and nose (◘ Fig. 53.8a). The linear scar was relatively irregular and superficial and was a bit raised above the skin. Microplasma remodeling procedure was applied using a roller tip with 70 watts for 4–6 passes. ◘ Figure 53.8 shows the tissue remodeling results after the first (◘ Fig. 53.8b), third (◘ Fig. 53.8c), and fourth (◘ Fig. 53.8d) microplasma treatments, which demonstrated gradual improvement of the gross view of the linear scar, and the scar was barely detectable at the end of the treatment. The patient was very happy with the end result.

References

1. Halachmi S, Orenstein A, Meneghel T, Lapidoth M. A novel fractional micro-plasma radio-frequency technology for the treatment of facial scars and rhytids: a pilot study. J Cosmet Laser Ther. 2010;12(5):208–12. https://doi.org/10.3109/14764172.2010.514921.
2. Xin F, Li-hong L, Alexiades-Armenakas M, Luebberding S, Cui-ping S, Yue H, Yu-xi A, Dan-xia Y, Rong-ya Y. Histological and electron microscopic analysis of fractional microplasma radio-frequency technology effects. J Drugs Dermatol. 2013;12(11):1210–4.
3. Wang S, Mi J, Li Q, Jin R, Dong J. Fractional microplasma radiofrequency technology for non-hypertrophic post-burn scars in Asians: A prospective study of 95 patients. Lasers Surg Med. 2017;49(6):563–69. https://doi.org/10.1002/lsm.22640.

30

Minimal Invasive Technologies for Treatment of HTS and Keloids: Medical Needling

Antigona Aliu and Matthias Aust

Contents

Background

Introduction

Method

Effects of Medical Needling

Needling Techniques

Postinterventional Treatment Measures

Induction of the Post-Needling Wound-Healing Cascade

Effects of Medical Needling Regarding Different Parameters

Dermal Remodeling

Improved Perfusion

Dermal Thickness and Erythema

Richness of Moisture

Conclusion

References

Background

HTS (hypertrophic scars) and keloids remain a serious and challenging issue regarding medical and therapeutic intervention. Clinical symptoms such as pain or pruritus are followed by psychological deficits of stigmatization or even discrimination for the affected people. Considering the multifactorial pathogenesis of these pathological scars, the injury to the skin reaches the reticular dermis and causes subsequent aberrant wound healing. A secondary intention of wound healing is characterized by inflammation by promoting various tissue and immune cells. Hence, the vulnerable skin layer of HTS and keloids contains inflammatory cells, increased numbers of fibroblasts producing collagen and endothelial cells for a nutritive angiogenesis. This may promote chronic inflammation, which in turn may cause the invasive growth of keloids and explains clinical symptoms. The situation becomes even more complex with bacterial superinfection or other inflammatory responses, as proinflammatory cells and cytokines are highly upregulated. Pathophysiological parameters create a complex profile of HTS and keloids, which demand therapeutic attention and medical intervention.

Introduction

In this chapter, we are going to present medical needling as an ideal therapy for the treatment of hypertrophic scars and keloids. The past has shown difficulties in treating these types of scars that are characterized by a complex anatomy and a progressive degradation of the scar texture. Serious challenges for various therapy approaches are a rapid and uncontrolled growth, a lack of moisture and a rigid structure. Affected people are confronted with dysfunctional and aesthetic deficits in their daily life or suffer from further harm through stigmatization. For this indication, medical treatment is required that replaces surgical interventions and other ablative treatments. HTS and keloids are prominent scars that frequently occur in combination with persistent erythema. Widespread and deep damage of the skin layers is often followed by secondary wound healing, which enhances the formation of either HTS or keloids. Keloid scars occur when the skin overreacts to the injury, after which they continue to grow and get dark in color. The histopathology of keloid demonstrates an extensive tissue proliferation beyond the margin of primary wound. Dark skin types are predisposed for the development of keloids that appear when a forced wound closure proceeds under tension. That is why keloids can cause great discomfort, tightness, or a limited range of mobility if they develop near a joint such as the knee or ankle. An excessive stretching of skin creates uncomfortable pressure over the fibrotic tissue, which can cause itching. Because of their typical larger size, they tend to rub on clothing, causing unbearable irritation.

Whereas the development of HTS is fairly manageable, keloids reveal specific features concerning the parameters of size and growth. Keloid scars develop uncontrolled or excessive fibrogenesis and are a tremendous source of collagen that still causes clinical problems until now. Thus, keloid is an active tissue that demonstrates signs of inflammation such as redness, itch, and mild pain. The permanent tendency to uncontrolled growth exceeds the original wound area and reaches massive proportions due to uncontrolled fibrosis. The last-mentioned issue is associated with a dysregulation of growth factors, which leads to an overproduction of scar tissue and an uncontrolled synthesis of the extracellular matrix. Hence, therapeutic treatment of keloids differs from those of normal hypertrophic scars. Keloid is often recurrent, although it has been treated with either pharmacological agents or surgery. Dermatological approaches of scar removal are not based on ablative treatment methods. They include compression therapy, intralesional corticosteroid injections, and excisions. When injected into the keloid, appropriate medication helps shrink the scar for a short time. The patient is due to receive a series of injections once every month, which means a constant therapy in order to prevent renewed scarring. Moreover, the use of radiation therapy instead of laser therapy is a common practice. However, this method also means a radiation exposure, which is always a health hazard. Ionizing radiation should only be implemented when medical indication is given or other alternatives are not reachable.

With regard to HTS, ablative treatments such as surgical interventions show temporary success by reducing the scar tissue to the level of the surrounding skin. These circumstances support the risk of recurrence and a continuous degradation of scar texture and healthy skin. The majority of conventional treatments are based on ablative and radical principles that provoke short-term responses and only suited for the removal of HTS. For this reason, conventional therapy approaches show little success and permit poor access to an efficient treatment of keloids or HTS.

Against this background, the demand for less invasive and effective functional and aesthetic treatments is steadily growing and remains a permanent issue in modern medicine. The focus is clearly defined by the patient's satisfaction with the aim of maximal outcome and minimal risk at the same time. Medical needling seems to be an ideal method for what is postulated in many fields of modern medicine. PCI displays a simple regenerative technique that affects skin-related indications and in particular scars. Its success is manifested in skin regeneration particularly for severe and widespread scars with hypertrophic and keloid features. The method of PCI requires neither expensive apparatus nor the need of complex instruments and sets a new trend in plastic and aesthetic medicine. By stimulating complex signal transduction pathways in the postneedling wound-healing cascade, the natural regeneration process is modified and, hence, is more efficient. According to that, medical needling improves the appearance and quality of scars with comparatively low risk and stress for the patient. The postneedling cascade induces gene expression and the proliferation of skin and stem cells that are important for dermal remodeling. The expression of specific proteins and reorganization of the extracellular matrix affect epidermal thickness and creates a stable and functioning skin barrier [1]. Furthermore, the PCI-induced synthesis of collagen and release of endogenous growth factors allow an association with scarless wound healing. Epidermal as well as dermal structures remain intact and histological findings show a complete re-epithelialization of the epidermis after treatment.

Current medical standards offer a diversity of noninvasive treatments (e.g., silicone patches) and minimal invasive procedures (e.g., cortisone injections) or surgical options such as scar excisions, tissue transfer, and W- and Z-plasties. Keloids show a limited therapy spectrum, which is mainly based on nonablative treatments (radiation, injections). Ablative methods such as laser resurfacing, dermabrasion, and deep chemical peels are all together defined by the same principle and find use in the treatment of HTS: they lighten the scar by destroying the skin structure and provoke an inflammatory response. As a result, the treated area is replaced by a thinner epidermis that shows flattened rete ridges and parallelly orientated scar collagen that is typical for fibrosis [2]. Furthermore, the skin is more vulnerable for bacterial or viral infections and external stress. These complications make a successful treatment of hypertrophic and keloid scars almost impossible, as they already have dysfunctional qualities. Complex structural and physical features of keloids have shown that common methods display temporary solutions that conceal the actual problem instead of improving the scar quality. In most instances, the scar quality of keloids or HTS would be much worse then. Compared to that, PCI has been proved to be a relatively simple, fast, and controlled method, which can be safely repeated and used in body regions where ablative or semi-ablative treatments have limited usage. Current studies on medical needling show a positive effect on hypertrophic scars regarding the parameters elasticity, moisture, transepidermal water loss, and erythema. In terms of dermal reorganization, high levels of structural proteins – glycosaminoglycans and proteoglycans – as well as an increased presence of physiological collagen are measurable after needling. PCI preserves dermal structures and promotes the formation of physiological collagen instead of scar collagen. For this reason, PCI overcomes shortcomings of other conventional methods that are available for treating problematic scars such as HTS or keloids. Study outcome has already shown the positive effect of medical needling on HTS in the past years and latest clinical data reveal similar results concerning keloids.

Method

Medical needling is based on a simple idea of puncturing the affected area repeatedly with a roller covered with needles of a specific length. Approximately 20 years ago, Camirand and Doucet had the experience that treating hypertrophic scars with a tattoo gun affects the scar texture and achieves significant improvements regarding clinical parameters [3]. Based on these ideas, Fernandes developed the technique of percutaneous collagen induction. In 1997, he realized this scientific discovery by establishing a roller equipped with needles in order to produce thousands of neighboring micro-wounds in the dermis, which cause intradermal bleeding. Thanks to targeted research within the last 15 years, scientific data have been provided by Aust et al. at first, and underline the efficacy as well as safety of medical needling.

In Germany, medical needling is now a licensed therapy for the treatment of scars and other related indications. The needling device is covered with needles of the desired length (0.5–3 mm) and needs to be rolled over the scar in three directions under constant pressure: vertically, horizontally, and diagonally. In the case of hypertrophic scars and keloids, surgical needling with a needle length of 3 mm is instructed in order to reach the scar collagen as deeply as possible. A straight guidance of the device is necessary in order to prevent shear forces and deeper damage. Relative to the extent of the scar size, this procedure requires 30–60 minutes of mechanical exposure. The penetration of the papillary dermis leads to thousands of micro-wounds and intradermal bleeding through the parenchymal canals. Minimal lesions of the epidermis do not impair basal layers containing stem cells with regenerative capacity. The increased expression of specific growth factors and release of structure proteins induce a modified wound-healing cascade with a great regenerative potential. The scar is sufficiently needled when multiple and confluent ecchymosis as well as skin swelling are clearly indicated. After 24 hours, epithelial cells close the channels and are reorganized into a natural protection barrier, which reduces the risk of potential postoperative complications such as infections. Therapy benefits are optimized by the application of nourishing products in first 24 hours. Swelling and local redness or edema of the treated area disappears after approximately 4–7 days. PCI is performed under general

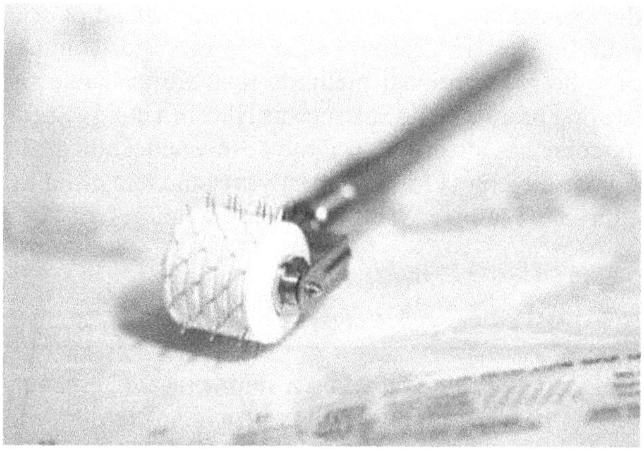

Fig. Roller device for medical needling

anesthesia in an operation theatre. When smaller areas are treated, the performance can be done under local anesthesia. Preoperative formalities include an informed consent form signed by informed patients or parents of patients younger than 18 years of age. Pre- and post-operative management is kept simple and includes the application of Vitamins A, C, and E as antioxidants [4]. According to latest research, maximal therapeutic outcome regarding epidermal thickness and a better prognosis for rapid healing can be expected. Postoperative monitoring is not substantially necessary. However, after surgical needling, a short down time of a few days needs to be considered, as the procedure requires general or local anesthesia. Therefore, a stay in hospital is only recommended, not obligated. Nevertheless, patients are able to get back to their daily life after a short time of recovery (Fig. 34.1).

Effects of Medical Needling

The intradermal bleeding caused by the mechanical procedure induces second-messenger substances of significant signal transduction pathways, which lead to a modified physiological regeneration of the skin. Specific features of both skin layers are not only preserved in their functional structure but also promoted in a positive qualitative way. Epidermis and dermis remain functionally intact and protect subcutaneous structures. Moreover, single layers of the epidermis become thicker, which guarantees great stability and a reduced vulnerability. Treated skin reacts less sensitively to damaging physical factors such as UV radiation that is associated with postinflammatory hyperpigmentation [5]. Furthermore, medical needling is also suited for all skin types. Treating dark skin is not followed by any dyspigmentation or even hypopigmentation, although dark skin is indeed predisposed for color shifts due to the naturally increased amount of melanin. Molecular and cellular processes induced by PCI affect neither the amount of melanocytes nor the mechanisms of synthesizing melanin. However, PCI specifically modifies the expression levels of the melanocyte-stimulating hormone (MSH) and Interleukin-10 (Il-10). MSH influences the activity of melanocytes and is downregulated within the postneedling cascade. On the other hand, high levels of Il-10 are evident, which is an antiinflammatory cytokine, and support immunological tolerance. As a targeted therapy, PCI concentrates especially on those areas that are aimed to be treated and also affects the surrounding healthy skin in a positive way. Due to the fact that needling does not create an open wound surface, there is a low risk for the development of viral or fungal infections, which could complicate a scar-free wound healing.

Needling Techniques

The needling treatment needs to be planned and prepared in advance. This includes the examination and categorization of the scars according to specific features. The selection of the appropriate length of needles depends on the type of scar, pain management, and expectation from the patient's side. From this perspective, downtime repetition capacities and aesthetic achievements are considered. Massive scars with intense deficits would be HTS and keloids that are predominantly treated by surgical needling. This means a longer downtime but also maximum results. Considering input and outcome, maximizing the patient's expected results is aimed to achieve.

In principle, medical needling can be classified into cosmetic, medical, and surgical needling. The difference depends on the length of the needles used and the intensity of the physiological effects as well as the post-operative regime they require. First mentioned types of needling play a minor role for the treatment of HTS or keloids, as the desired effects cannot be achieved.

Cosmetic needling is performed as a purely cosmetic treatment with needles 0.1–0.5 mm in length for structural and superficial skin modifications. The needling procedure does not cause any intradermal bleeding and hence any postinterventional reactions remain unnoticed. Using the minimal length of needles does not require any anesthesia and allows repeating the treatment daily. The patient does not experience any downtime and gets back to his daily routine without any complications. All together, the cosmetic needling is used as a penetration enhancer for topical skin care products.

Medical needling can be defined as PCI when the needles have a length between 1 and 2 mm. Needles of this length reach just beyond the basal membrane and lead to minimal petechial hemorrhages in the papillary dermis, which activate the TGF-ß signal cascade and give a skin-regenerating effect. The needle length is proportional to the provoked bleeding, as it gets more intense when longer needles are used. However, intradermal lesions are so small that there is a minimal downtime without obvious edemas or bruises. Moreover, effective topical anesthetics can be used to make the process nearly painless. Afterward, the treated area might be reddened and needs a few days to recover and normalize.

From the perspective of clinical efficacy, surgical needling proves to be more intense and impressive when the performance is done with a needle length of 3 mm. That is why HTS and keloids are indications for surgical needling. This procedure is carried out under general or local anesthesia and can also require a stay in hospital. The puncture depth does not only affect the epidermis and dermis but also the upper layers of the subcutis including the vascular system that is responsible for the desired and controlled bleeding after needling. This mechanical prodecure affects the skin structure and function by provoking stress and regenerative resources at the same time which is aimed to improve the natural skin barrier with intact skin layers. For this reason this step needs to be performed wisely and carefully observed. The relatively painful procedure under local anesthesia provokes primary inflammatory wound-healing reactions with temporary erythema, swelling, and bruising. The needling device needs to be rolled over the affected area until these signs of sufficient needling are apparent. The potential for aesthetic correction and reduction of the scar is on the highest level and provides maximal outcome. When selecting a needle length of 3 mm, the patient is expected to accept a protracted downtime in order to achieve maximal results in the phases of recovery. According to that, longer recovery periods of weeks should be taken into account (◘ Figs. 34.2 and 34.3).

The selection of the needle length varies relative to the indication and its intensity of cicatrization. Moreover, there are important differences notable: The

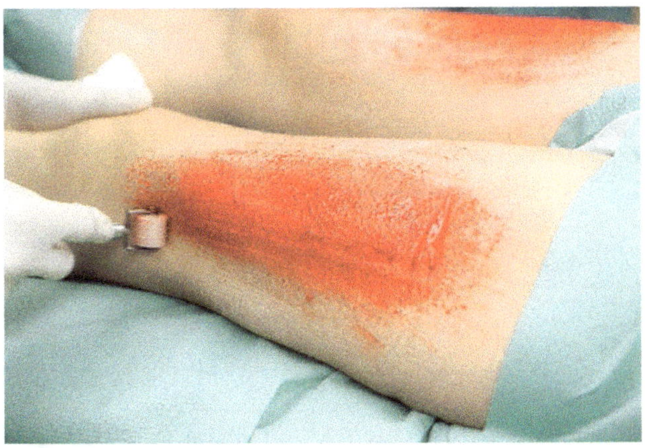

◘ **Fig.** Technique of surgical needling performed with a needle length of 3 mm. Desired bleeding and marked edema induce therapeutically effective collagen production during the postneedling wound-healing cascade

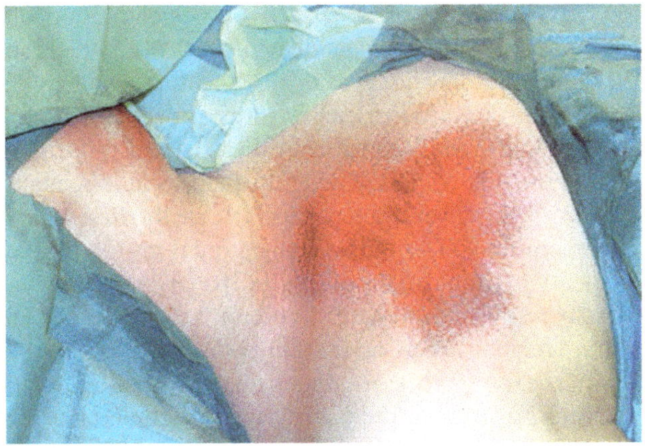

◘ **Fig.** A heavier bleeding caused by the 3 mm needling method

shorter the needles, the more often treatments need to be carried out in order to reach desired effects. Longer needles are indicated when treating prominent kind of scars such as HTS and keloids. Summing up, the combination of the patient's expectations and the desired result decides the amount of therapies and the selection of the three possible needle lengths.

Postinterventional Treatment Measures

Postoperative Wound Management – For optimizing and maximizing therapy outcome, it is instructed to treat the skin sufficiently and effectively under pre- and post-operative circumstances. The application of vitamin A and antioxidants such as vitamin E and C is necessary to achieve best results. A specific skincare that combines the above-mentioned vitamins with a strongly recommended gentle cleansing washing lotion containing tea tree oil should be performed every 2 hours as long as the needling canals are still open. While the skin remains bruised and swollen, direct exposure to sunlight should also be avoided. A moist wound-healing regime of vitamin-based creams prevents crust formation after the initial bleeding, which could eventually impair the final results. The loss of serous fluid through the puncture holes in the immediate postinterventional period can lead to crusting, which needs to be carefully averted by washing off any surface serum. In consequence, preventing crusting reduces the risk of bacterial superinfections. Moreover, inflammation and secondary wound healing associated with the development of HTS or keloids can be avoided.

Managing Complications – As needling does not produce open wounds, the postoperative complication rate is very low and postinterventional monitoring is not necessarily needed. However, local edema can develop with longer needles, especially done on large areas. It is recommended to keep the patient in the clinic for a few hours after treatment. It needs to be considered that after extensive surgical needling under general anesthesia, the patient may experience burning pain in the treated area. Therefore, pain should be managed with effective drugs particularly in the first hours postoperatively. The use of nonsteroidal antiphlogistic medication should be avoided, as the primary inflammatory response is desired. However, keloids and HTS require regular follow-up examinations in order observe wound-healing processes and to ensure that renewed scarring or proliferating tissue can be excluded. In the case of keloids, a further extension of the scarring is not that rare after treatment. Clinical data also reveal the formation of necrotic tissue when there is an inadequate blood supply. Special attention needs to be paid to patients with diabetes that shows difficulties in wound healing anyway.

The intradermal bleeding caused by PCI is the essential driving force in medical needling. In this context, the endogenous potential of natural wound healing induced by PCI differs from the conventional inflammatory response to traumatic incidences starting minutes after injury. Therefore, the difference between the postneedling regenerative cascade and the conventional wound-healing cascade becomes very clear. The PCI-induced regenerative process is based on completely different mechanisms that are associated with the desired bleeding, as plenty of blood vessels are pierced at the same time. However, an open wound surface is not created within this procedure that would need to be refilled by regenerative fibers in the course of conventional wound healing. Refilling can rapidly escalate into an overproduction of tissue fibers, which again supports the development of HTS and keloids. The extent of the initial bleeding and the excretion of serous fluids can appear in different intensities and mainly depend on the area treated as well as the needle length that has been specifically selected. In consequence, facial skin regions show a higher bleeding capacity, as they tend to react more sensitively to mechanical stress. Further, these regions are more affected by swelling and bruising because skin seems to be thinner and therefore reacts more intensely to operative interventions than the skin of other regions. Eventually, PCI-related results are achieved by replacing scar typical collagen with normal collagen of healthy skin [6].

Induction of the Post-Needling Wound-Healing Cascade

The intended trauma through the repetitive puncturing initiates a physiological wound-healing cascade. Platelets and neutrophils secrete growth factors such as the platelet-derived growth factor (PDGF), fibroblast growth factor (FGF), vascular endothelial growth factor (VEGF), tissue growth factor, and transforming growth factor-α and -ß (TGF-α, TGF-ß). The interactive cooperation of these factors provides blood coagulation, as well as the synthesis of dermal structures such as collagen, elastin, and fibronectin. Furthermore, the differentiation and migration of fibroblasts and keratinocytes contribute to regenerative processes. Fibroblasts have essential roles in synthesis of collagens I and III. Other cells that are represented in all tissues including the dermal layer are fibrocytes, dendrocytes, mast cells, and further immune cells secreting collagen I and collagen III protein. Seen from a dermatological view, TGF-ß has specific functions that have a key role in the postneedling wound-healing cascade. In general, wound healing can be divided into three phases interacting through numerous growth factors and other essential elements, into approximately month-long sequences: inflammation, proliferation, and regeneration (◘ Fig. 34.4).

◘ **Fig.** Wound-healing course schematic representation

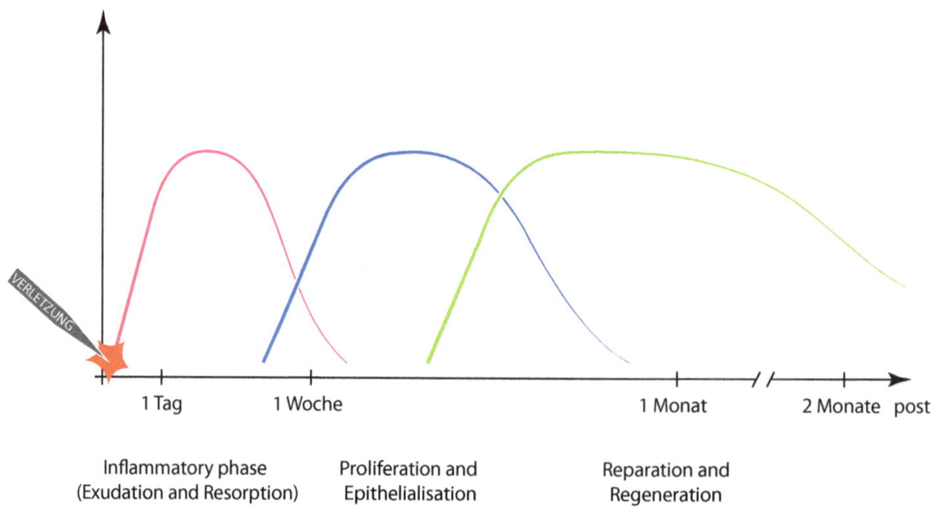

Right after the injury, the natural and typical reaction of inflammation starts by activating immune cells, blood coagulation, as well as vasoconstriction [7]. The following stage of proliferation is marked by growth factors, especially focused on TGF-ß, which is important for the regulation of growth processes. Dysregulated signal transduction pathways can lead to a malignant degeneration of cells, which can result in the development of cancer or malignant tumor in the worst case. Keloids have indeed characteristics that are similar to tumor cells. The persistent presence of TGF-ß1 and-ß2, as well as the absence of TGF-ß3 in the conventional wound-healing process, indicates the formation of typical rigid scar tissue. The activity of fibroblasts is necessary for the regeneration of the extracellular matrix and the synthesis of collagen. After the phase of regeneration, an intact skin barrier of renewed epithelial cells and a mechanically stable skin structure are evident. These are single steps described in a typical wound-healing procedure. On the contrary, the PCI-induced wound-healing mechanism is based on a modified principle of what is already known and described regarding wound healing. Special focus is manifested in the modified TGF-ß signal transduction pathway. Whereas TGF-ß1 and 2 are significantly downregulated in the postneedling cascade, TGF-ß3 shows a dominant activity 24 hours postinterventionally. Against this background, the traditional wound-healing paradigm is converted into a regenerative phase marked by the synthesis of structural collagen of healthy and vital skin instead of scar tissue. This is why there is a low risk for the development of hypertrophic or keloid scars where it usually comes to an uncontrolled hyperplasia of collagen fibers and an uncontrolled growth of the connective tissue. Very common consequences are rigid and difficult scars.

Effects of Medical Needling Regarding Different Parameters

Scarless Wound Healing – In order to avoid secondary wound healing, a controlled activity of growth factors is necessary. The close relation between TGF and the formation of collagen type I fibers represents a key role in repair and regeneration mechanisms. In this context, it needs to be considered that wounds healed by secondary intent tend toward an uncontrolled proliferation, which enhances the development of HTS or keloids. Type I collagen is the physiological desired collagen of lattice pattern structure in healthy and vital skin, whereas collagens type III shows parallelly orientated fibers that is typical for scars. TGF-ß1 and 2 are at their highest levels of activity when a dense collagen structure of type III in scars is built. Study results have proved that in keloids with excessive cell proliferation, the expression of procollagen I and III -mRNA as well as -protein is increased. In excessive cell proliferation of keloid tissue, there is a dominant presence of collagen III, although both collagen I and collagen III seem to be increased. Significant differences to normal skin are manifested in the shift of the collagen I and III ratio toward collagen III. However, a significant downregulation of TGF-ß1 and 2 is evident in scar-free, embryonal wound healing determined by TGF-ß3. Second kind of wound healing is still active in juvenile tissue to a lesser extent, but not present in adult tissue that is rather predisposed for the development of scars. High levels of TGF-ß3 in the postneedling cascade do not only induce the synthesis of collagen type I, but also manage the conversion from collagen type III to the desired type I collagen (◘ Fig. 34.5).

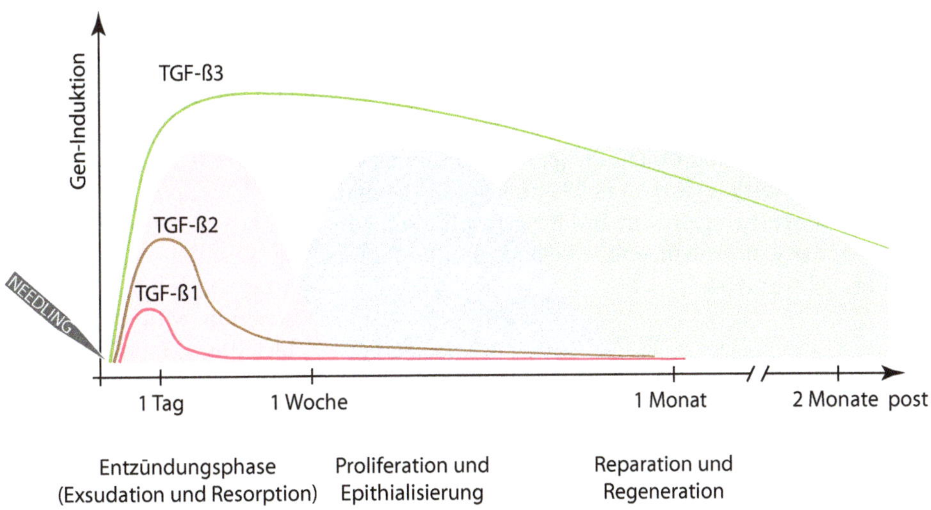

◘ **Fig.** Regulation of transforming and growth factor, TGF-ß3, and scarless healing. Microarray analyses of TGF-ß1, -ß2, and -ß3 expression levels in treated and untreated animals show that the needling treatment stimulates TGF-ß3 to a greater extent than TGF-ß1 or -ß2. Moreover, the induction of TGF-ß3 gene expression continues even beyond the initial wound-healing phase, whereas the two other genes are downregulated during the second week postneedling

Dermal Remodeling

Furthermore, PCI modulates the expression of relevant genes and molecules that are responsible for remodeling the extracellular matrix. The skin appears thicker, more vital, and rejuvenated. Therefore, PCI displays a method that is focused on both quantitative and qualitative improvement of dermal function and appearance. The release of structural proteins, including fibronectin and glycosaminoglycan molecules, as well as the activity of specific enzymes, achieves dermal remodeling. These components of the postneedling cascade stimulate the proliferation of keratinocytes and other skin cells in the basal layer of the epidermis, which changes the physical and biological characteristics of skin. The entire connective tissue framework seems to be thicker and denser. Other endogenous factors contribute toward improved skin elasticity in terms of dermal remodeling, as the amount of elastin is significantly greater after medical needling. A lack of elasticity is typical for HTS and keloids and one reason for their rigid structure, which puts the scar as well as the surrounding healthy skin under a great pressure. Hence, flexibility and mobility of the affected area are compromised, which might be a problem when regions close to joints are affected. Not only for this reason, TGF-ß3 reaches high levels of expression in the initial phases but shows a declining trend in the following phases of proliferation and regeneration. Based on Furguson's work, the initial dominant influence of TGF-ß3 is important for the PCI-related wound-healing mechanisms. However, clinical expertise shows that giving TGF-ß3 additionally in phases of normally low levels can eventually impair regenerative processes. In conclusion, the method of medical needling influences the release and immediate effect of TGF, as well as the synthesis of collagen type I interacting within the process of dermal reorganization and remodeling. Once again, the signal transduction pathway of TGF seems to be one of the most important PCI-related factors. Therefore, the method of PCI has a regulatory function of promoting a controlled activity of growth factors and other regenerative factors as well as cytokines. With regard on HTS and keloids, the main focus is on managing growth and hypertrophy by a controlled activity of growth, epithelial and vascular factors (◘ Figs. 34.6 and 34.7).

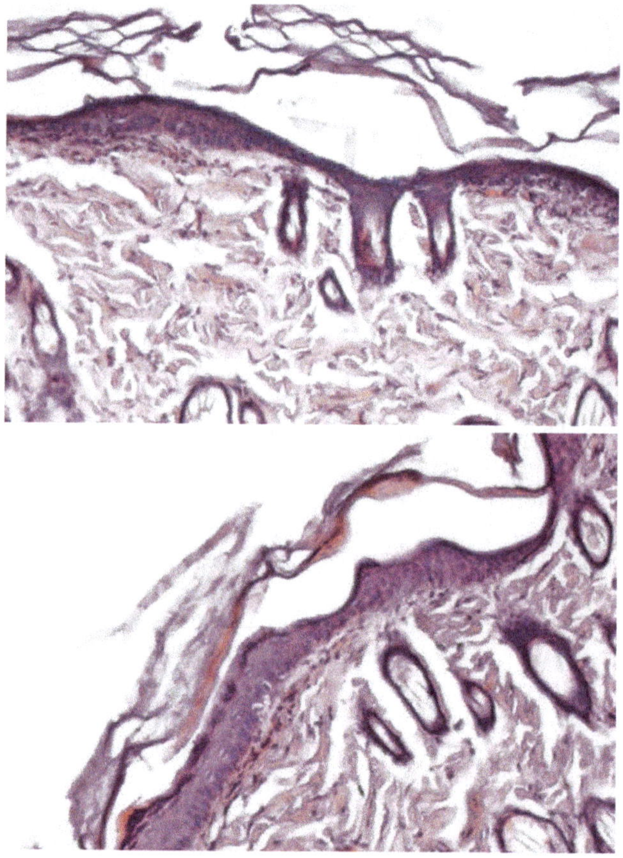

◘ **Figs.** Regenerative effects on the epidermis through needling. One day after the treatment, Masson's trichrome staining shows no injuries in either the epidermis or the dermis. Both skin layers are functionally intact; there are no signs of ablation or cell damage. ◘ Figure 34.6 Untreated animal (control). ◘ Figure 34.7 24 hours postneedling

Improved Perfusion

Another factor showing high concentration during the postneedling regenerative cascade is VEGF. In terms of angiogenesis, its main function of creating new blood vessels and enhancing perfusion accelerates wound-healing processes. The method of PCI provides a controlled and limited release of VEGF in order to prevent dysregulated activity, which can lead to degenerative processes. High levels of VEGF are initially observed in the postneedling cascade, which are again not kept constantly high at all times. Hence, medical needling has a positive effect on subcutaneous structures conveyed by VEGF as an important indicator for active angiogenesis. The expression of this growth factor induces the vascular system by supporting the proliferation and activity of vascular endothelial cells [8]. This process happens after the initial inflammatory response of a vasoconstriction with the primary intention of stopping the bleeding as a typical reaction to an injury. The restricted perfusion is then followed by a massive vasodilatation in the wound-healing phase. The regulative effect on the vascular system explains the intense bleeding after the needling procedure, which is in fact an enhancer of the wound-healing progress. The better the blood perfusion of the skin tissue, the greater the bleeding after mechanical stress induced by PCI, which accelerates healing processes. The limited activity of VEGF for a desired period of time (postinflammation) has the advantage of a rapid wound healing due to a better perfusion and a primary wound closure in a timely and effective way. For this reason, the risk of secondary wound healing can be excluded, as delayed wound-healing processes are very improbable and also not expected after needling. In this context, the development of HTS and keloids is once again kept at minimal risk.

Dermal Thickness and Erythema

An effective wound-healing process implies active vascularization and causes a temporary reddening of the skin, which is not associated with persistent erythema. After needling, the affected area is swollen and reddened due to a better perfusion in the course of effective healing processes. However, the problem of striking discolorations of especially hypertrophic and keloid scars remains a serious one for the affected people, as the scar color differs extensively from the surrounding healthy skin. Discolorations can reach from slightly reddened skin or persistent erythema to dyspigmentation or even hypopigmentation, which is quite typical for HTS. Untreated hypertrophic scars tend to a thin and vulnerable epidermis that is unstable and more transparent for local perfusion. This might support the appearance of erythema through a thin skin texture with a long-term impact. After needling, the intense blood circulation is less prominent and temporarily limited through a thickened epidermis. The entire tissue structure is more compact and makes the great optical difference between scar and surrounding skin less prominent. Either way, medical needling represents a skin-normalizing therapy method and creates a homogenous image of initially reddened scars toward healthy skin. Based on outcomes of objective measurement methods with the Mexameter, medical needling achieves a normalization of the skin color and an almost complete adjustment of the scar tissue toward healthy skin after repetitive treatments. As the method is based on percutaneous collagen induction, the synthesis of collagen improves vital thickness, which is directly associated with less transparency and a low risk for the development of erythematous hypertrophic scars (◘ Fig. 34.8).

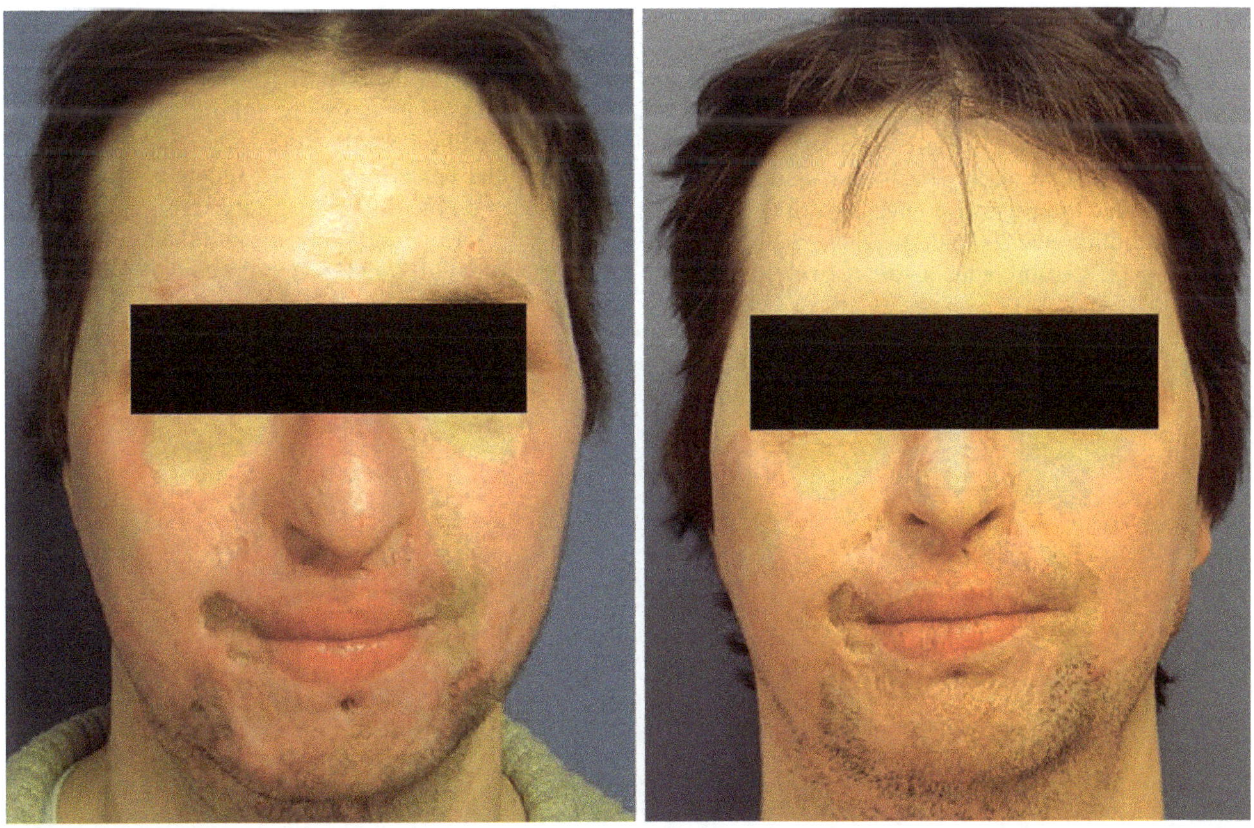

◘ **Fig.** Patient 1, frontal shot, preoperatively (left) and one year postoperatively after needling (right). Areas treated include the entire face. Reduced erythema and hypertrophy of the fibrosis

Richness of Moisture

HTS and keloids are especially characterized by a lack moisture, which combines typical visible anomalies with symptoms of pain and itching. The current difficulty of HTS resides in skin dryness and an insufficient water content of the epidermis [9]. Dehydrated scar conditions are the main cause of pruritus, which is not only considered a sensation disorder but a relevant clinical parameter. In fact, itchy and dry scars are closely related to structural deficits of the typical scar tissue. Fibrous tissue tends to have less skin appendages such as sebaceous and sweat glands and thus produces less moisturizing secretions, which leads to skin dryness, less flexibility, and a rigid scar texture. Moreover, a thin epidermis with parallelly orientated collagen fibers can impair the epidermal barrier function, which is marked by transepidermal water loss (TEWL). Severe and widespread burn scars, for example, hold the risk of an incomplete re-epithelialization of the epidermis due to a lack of stem cell reservoirs. It happens frequently that particularly those skin layers such as the basal layer of the epidermis are impaired by deeper and widespread damage of the skin. However, these components of the skin are able to provide stem cells that differentiate into functional skin or epithelial cells. Thus, a less functional epidermis enhances transepidermal water loss and a reduction of moisture. Therefore, patients suffer from dry, itchy, and painful scars followed by reddened and vulnerable skin. When protective features of epidermal layers are deficient, the skin reacts more sensitively to external factors and is more accessible for various pathogens, which can lead to progressive infections. In this context, medical needling ensures epidermal integrity in terms of regulating TEWL and reducing the risk of dehydration. Measurements with the Corneometer and Tewameter have shown that PCI improves the moisture content of the skin, which is closely related to the regulation of TEWL. Various studies on the effect of medical needling on moisture revealed remarkable improvements regarding skin roughness and rigidity, which both depend on the water content of the skin (◘ Fig. 34.9).

Conservative treatments for scars with deficits in moisture and TEWL include silicone patches or diverse moisturizing creams that are established cosmetic therapy methods. Provided that they are used permanently and several times a day over a longer period of time, they can improve the scar condition to a temporary extent. Concerning the water content of the skin, the fluid silicone gel preserves the moisture content, but does not affect the skin's own potential to produce sufficient moisture [10]. A permanent application of oily creams keeps the skin moist and smooth, but does not improve the scar in quality by itself. TEWL is least affected, as the epidermal barrier function is not influenced by the silicone. Once again, short-term results are frequent and considering TEWL, there are less satisfying results. These kinds of methods have a preventative character and are rather suited for short-term solutions. In the case of HTS or keloids nonablative, conventional treatments can be used in addition to needling or other invasive therapy methods as complementary therapies. Ablative treatments achieve exactly the inverted effect in terms of destroying epidermal structures and holding the risk of degradation. On the contrary, the established method of medical needling preserves the epidermis and improves the epidermal barrier function. The significant impact on the skin's water balance is manifested by regulating moisturizing processes and the passive movement of water (TEWL) through the epidermis.

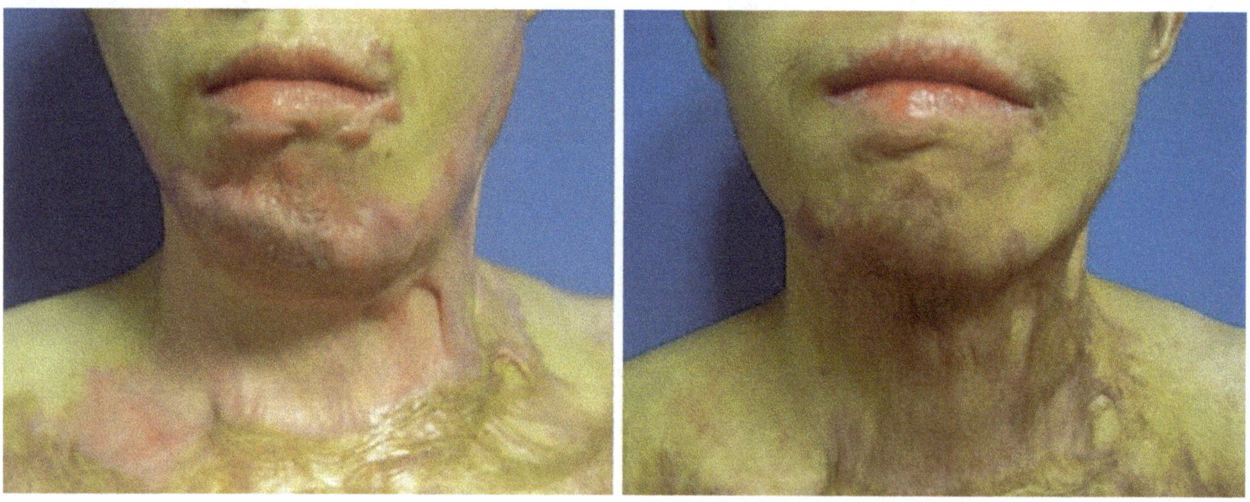

◘ **Fig.** Patient 3, frontal shot, preoperatively (left) and one year postoperatively after needling (right). Areas treated include the face, perilabial, chin, and neck. Reduced erythema and greatness of the scar. Less tension in the fibrotic area

Conclusion

Based on the diverse profile of medical needling regarding different parameters of HTS and keloids, this therapy method is not only an innovative approach, but also rather an effective treatment method of problematic scars. The aim of improving the scar in quality and function is realized by a modified wound-healing cascade, which activates relevant signal transduction pathways for an effective regeneration. After needling, dysfunctional scar tissue gains vital features of healthy skin and shows functional progression months and years after needling. The focus is clearly set on sustainability, which is the major challenge for an effective treatment of HTS and keloids. As underlying causes for the development of these types of scars are various and the clinical research potential on HTS and keloids is still not yet exhausted, medical solutions are required from modern medicine. Common therapy approaches are characterized by different moderate success that does not provide long-lasting outcome. Improvements are temporarily restricted and rather accumulate in the beginning of the therapy. HTS and keloids often tend to reach a nonresponder status in the course of repetitive conventional treatments. Surgical interventions are less attractive for the affected people and are often followed by a structural degradation up to uncontrolled cell death. In terms of not confronting the patients with serious consequences and other complications, medical treatment should be scientifically defined as effective and sustainable. PCI comes very close to what is expected from a medical point of view not only for the supplier side but especially for the demand side. Innovative and patient-friendly therapy approaches aim to be more convenient for patients relative to the required effort. In this context, medical needling seems to be a very promising therapy method that guarantees persistent effect on HTS and keloids. PCI displays a relatively simple and controlled treatment of difficult scars that opens new pathways for modern medicine.

Take-Home Messages

- HTS and keloids are pathological scars with a characteristic histological and clinical profile.
- Persistent lesions to deeper skin layers promote the development of HTS and keloids followed by an inflammatory response.
- Medical approach and success have been quite restricted to minimal outcomes and improvement in the past.
- The greater knowledge of pathomechanisms allows the establishment of targeted intervention.
- Medical needling overcomes deficits of conventional treatment therapies combining minimal invasivity and long-lasting effects at the same time.
- Important clinical endpoints (erythema, pruritus, pain, and moisture) and not only clinical parameters are positively affected by PCI.
- Dysfunctional scar tissue gains vital and healthy features after treatment with PCI.
- Outcomes are up-to-date and underlined by evidence-based clinical research.

References

1. Aust MC, Reimers K, Kaplan HM, et al. Percutaneous collagen induction-regeneration in place of cicatrisation? J Plast Reconstr Aesthet Surg. 2011;64:97–107. https://doi.org/10.1016/j.bjps.2010.03.038.
2. Aust MC, Fernandes D, Kolokythas P, Kaplan HM, Vogt PM. Percutaneous collagen induction therapy: an alternative treatment for scars, wrinkles and skin laxity. Plast Reconstr Surg. 2008;121(4):1421–9. https://doi.org/10.1097/01.prs.0000304612.72899.02.
3. Aust MC, Reimers K, Repenning C, et al. Percutaneous collagen induction: minimally invasive skin rejuvenation without risk of hyperpigmentation – fact or fiction? Plast Reconstr Surg. 2008;122:1553–63. https://doi.org/10.1097/PRS.0b013e318188245e.
4. Aust MC, Bathe S, Fernandes D. Illustrated guide to percutaneous collagen induction. 1st ed. Berlin: KVM; 2013.
5. Aust MC, Knobloch K, Reimers K, Redeker J, Ipaktchi R, Altintas MA, Gohritz A, et al. Percutaneous collagen induction therapy: an alternative treatment for burn scars. Burns. 2010;36:836–43. https://doi.org/10.1016/j.burns.2009.11.014.
6. Laws RA, Finley EM, McCollough ML, Grabski WJ. Alabaster skin after carbon dioxide laser resurfacing with histologic correlation. Dermatol Surg. 1998;24:633–6. https://www.ncbi.nlm.nih.gov/pubmed/9648570. Accessed Jun 1998.
7. Fernandes D. Percutaneous collagen induction: an alternative to laser resurfacing. Aesthetic Surg J. 2002;22:307–9. https://doi.org/10.1067/maj.2002.126195.
8. Mustoe TA, Cooter RD, Gold MH, Hobbs FD, Ramelet AA, Shakespeare PG, Stella M, et al. International clinical recommendations on scar management. Plast Reconstr Surg. 2002;110:560–71. https://www.ncbi.nlm.nih.gov/pubmed/12142678. Accessed Aug 2002.
9. Anthonissen M, Daly D, Peeters R, Van Brussel M, Fieuws S, Moortgat P, Flour M, et al. Reliability of repeated measurements on post-burn scars with corneometer CM 825((R)). Skin Res Technol. 2015;21:302–12. https://doi.org/10.1111/srt.12193.
10. Bernstein LJ, Kauvar AN, Grossman MC, Geronemus RG. The short- and long-term side effects of carbon dioxide laser resurfacing. Dermatol Surg. 1997;23:519–25. https://www.ncbi.nlm.nih.gov/pubmed/9236869. Accessed Jul 1997.

31

Shock Wave Therapy for Wound Healing and Scar Treatment

Peter Moortgat, Mieke Anthonissen, Ulrike Van Daele, Jill Meirte, Tine Vanhullebusch, and Koen Maertens

Contents

Working Mechanism of SWT in Relation to Skin Defects

SWT Dose Effect Relationship

The Effects of Shock Wave Therapy in Soft Tissue Defects
The Effects of SWT in Wound Healing
The Effects of SWT in Scar Management

Conclusion

Bibliography

Background

To influence the evolution of an excessive scar toward a normal scar, several physical treatments exist to manage hypertrophic scarring. Physical treatments include manual and mechanical massage, physiotherapy, thermal therapy, and shock wave therapy. Manual massage has a wide array of beneficial effects on scars such as drainage of edema, reduction of pain, and pruritus and hydration of the skin [1]. Mechanical massage or vacuum massage uses gentle vacuum suction to lift the skin and to create a skin fold [2]. Since scars have a propensity to retract and create contractures in joints, splinting, taping, and posture stretching play a crucial role in the treatment. Thermal therapy includes high pressure showers, thread-like showers, and high pressure water and aims to mobilize the skin, to improve flexibility and to reduce inflammation, pain, and pruritus. All of these techniques are frequently used; however, there is only little supporting evidence [3].

The ideal non-invasive scar treatment should be safe, well tolerated by patients, have low associated complication rates, is easy to apply, cost-effective, and can be used in an outpatient setting. Shock Wave Therapy (SWT) meets all the aforementioned requirements [4–7]. The application of shock wave therapy in scar management (◘ Fig. 55.1) is still in its exploration phase; however, there are some interesting findings [3].

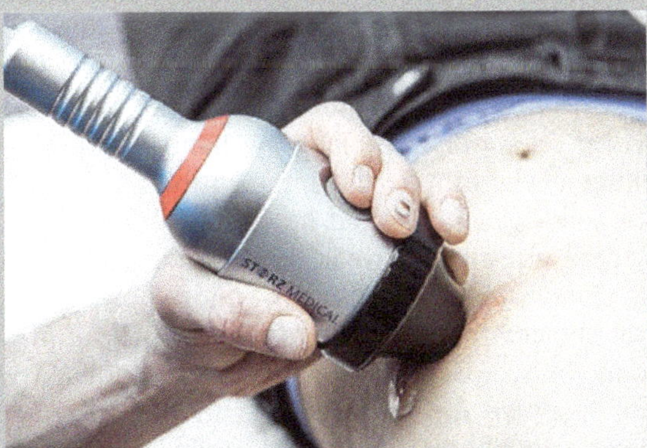

◘ **Fig.** Shock wave application on a scar

Working Mechanism of SWT in Relation to Skin Defects

SWT converts external mechanical stimuli into biochemical cell reactions (e.g., gene transcription leading to collagen remodeling) in living tissue, supported by mechanotransduction pathways, which result in the activation of numerous cellular events, responsible for the positive effects of SWT on cell metabolism and cell cycle [8]. Moreover, as in some other mechanotherapies applied in clinical practice, the main action of SWT seems to focus on inducing tissue regeneration and matrix remodeling *in vivo* [9]. Fibroblasts are the major mechanoresponsive cells in connective tissue, and are therefore the main target of SWT [10, 11]. Fibroblasts play a crucial role in remodeling of the extracellular matrix (ECM) by synthesizing and organizing connective tissue components, and there is a strong believe that SWT has a modulating effect on these actions and could therefore be of interest in scar prevention and management.

Sukubo et al. (2015) described the beneficial effects of SWT on macrophage behavior. SWT does not activate resting macrophages and seems to modulate macrophage activity in the inflammatory phase of wound healing. It inhibits the M1 (pro-inflammatory) activation in the initial inflammatory phase and enhances the M2 (anti-inflammatory) activation in the late inflammatory phase [12]. SWT can also regulate inflammation via TLR3 pathway in three phases. In an initiation phase, it induces a pro-inflammatory reaction mediated by cyclophylin A and IL6. There is a suppression of inflammation in the middle phase and in the limitation phase, there is a late anti-inflammatory effect mediated by IL10 [13]. Both findings indicate that SWT, applied in the wound healing stage or in the early stage of scar development, could prevent pathological scarring.

Non-randomized clinical data suggest that SWT is beneficial in terms of improved skin elasticity and revitalizing dermis in females with cellulite [14]. Fibrillar adipose tissue fibrosis looks very similar to dermal scarring [15], so the outcomes of clinical trials investigating cellulite could be transferred to pathological scarring [2]. MR imaging has shown that fibrous septa, visualized in 97% of the area with cellulite depressions, are markedly thickened in cellulite afflicted areas. Shockwave energy might weaken the fibrous septa, and thus the afflicted skin becomes smoother [14]. There is evolving experimental data suggesting SWT activation pathways in adipose-derived stem cells [14].

Delayed wound healing might be considered as one of the main reasons to develop hypertrophic scars. SWT has repeatedly proven to be effective as a wound-healing modality by decreasing time to full wound closure [4, 5, 16, 17]. From the mechanobiologic point of view, it has been described that the neoangiogenic capacity could be related to the inhibition of endothelial cell apoptosis, occurring in the very early phase after SWT stimulation (first 3 hours), as an initial response to the mechanical stimulus. More in detail, it seems possible to detect some "preparatory" signals, such as downregulation of the genes involved in cell cycle, adhesion and apoptosis, probably correlated to an upcoming detachment of endothelial junction [9]. After a low-energy SWT treatment (800 shocks, 1 Hz, 0.03 mJ/mm^2), mRNA expression and protein levels of vascular endothelial growth factor (VEGF) and endothelial nitric oxide synthase (eNOS) were significantly upregulated. Furthermore, the SW therapy enhanced phosphorylation of caveolin-1 and the expression of HUTS-4 that represents β1-integrin activity. These results suggest that caveolin-1 and β1-integrin are involved in the SW-induced activation of angiogenic signaling pathways [18].

We can summarize that the overall effect of SWT is an improvement of tissue homeostasis, accompanied by an improvement of the tissue self-healing abilities.

SWT Dose Effect Relationship

For a full treatment outline, the energy flux density (EFD), the number of pulses, the pulse frequency, and the number and interval of treatments are the most relevant parameters [5]. Differences in these parameters can lead to varying outcomes, emphasizing the dose dependency of these mechanotransduction events [9]. High-energy SWT can suppress cell growth, while low-energy shock waves might enhance cell proliferation [19]. SWT applied with an EFD of 0.01–0.03 mJ/mm^2 can modulate the inflammatory pathway in which macrophages are involved [12], and with an EFD of 0.08 mJ/mm^2 SWT can regulate inflammation via the TLR3 pathway. The EFD for soft tissue indications is typically in the range of 0.08–0.25 mJ/mm^2 [4], while scars and fibrosis are treated with an EFD ranging between 0.15 and 0.33 mJ/mm^2. SWT settings of 0.22 mJ/mm^2 and 1000 pulses seem to be ideal for fibroblast viability and growth [20]. Fibroblast viability was also influenced by the number of pulses. The higher the number, the more risk for cell destruction [11]. Each cell type seems to be responsive to SWT but probably with different optimal device settings and ranges of mechanical stimulation, thus developing different biochemical effects [8]. A study by Lee et al. showed that the EFD plays an important role in the targeting of specific mechano-signaling pathways, with 0.12 mJ/mm^2 being the optimal dose for activating the mTOR-FAK pathway [21] and 0.10 mJ/mm^2 showed the best results for inhibiting TGF-β1/Smad pathway [22] (◘ Table 55.1).

The Effects of Shock Wave Therapy in Soft Tissue Defects

The Effects of SWT in Wound Healing

Wound healing after SWT is characterized by an upregulation of the angio-active factors such as nitric oxide (NO) and vascular endothelial growth factor (VEGF) leading to induced angiogenesis [17], vasodilatation, increase in vascular and capillary density, and increased local blood flow. NO and VEGF are extremely important, both in early stage and late stage healing [5, 7, 9, 11, 17]. It has been suggested that an aspect of the early gene response of endothelial cells to SWT is characterized by a decreased apoptosis and stimulation of the extracellular matrix metabolism [5, 9]. SWT will lead to reduced tissue necrosis in wound healing by increasing cellular proliferation and procollagen production [11, 23]. In terms of timing, vasodilatation is noticed at an early stage (first 3 days) and neovascularization at late-stage post intervention [17]. In a clinical trial investigating the efficacy of ESWT to heal chronic therapy-refractory ulcers, the underlying molecular mechanisms were also studied *in vitro* [24]. Fibroblasts reorganized in a radial and star-shaped clustered manner and had large "stress" fibers. Cluster formation of fibroblasts was dose dependent, meaning that more applications lead to higher clustering. Shock waves also induce upregulation of 67 genes for keratinocytes and 652 genes for fibroblasts, suggesting that SWT mainly targets fibroblasts [24]. The upregulation of Vimentin on mRNA level leading to a visible reorganization of the cytoskeleton provided yet another proof for mechanotransduction as working mechanism for this intervention.

Besides "general wound healing," SWT has specifically been proven effective in burns. First, SWT applied upon donor site healing burn wounds shows a significantly shorter time to complete epithelialization [25]. Second, burn area perfusion has been evaluated with Laser Doppler Imaging before and after SWT and showed a significantly increased perfusion after extracorporeal shockwave therapy treatment [26]. The review of Antonic et al. suggested that SWT may decrease the need for surgical intervention and associated morbidities in patients with severely deep partial- or full-thickness

◘ **Table** Suggested SWT settings for electro-hydraulic devices when treating wounds or scars

	Energy flux density	Number of pulses	Pulse frequency	Treatment interval	Number of treatments
SWT for wound healing	0.03–0.20 mJ/mm^2	500–1000	4–6 Hz	1× per week	1–3
SWT for scar treatment	0.15–0.33 mJ/mm^2	800–1500	4–6 Hz	1× per week	8–12

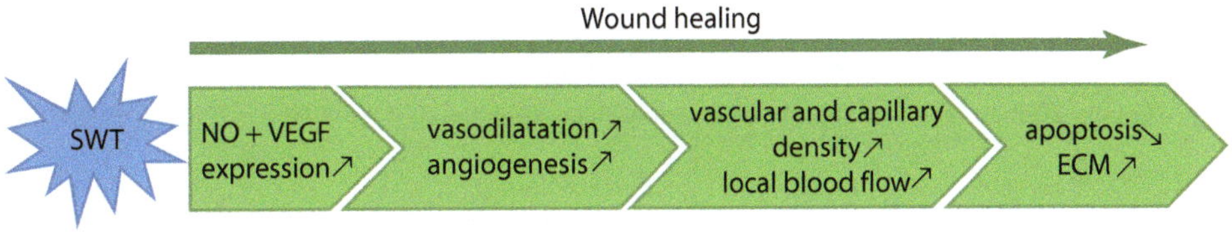

Fig. Cascade of wound-healing processes after SWT

burns [4]. Joo et al. demonstrated that ESWT significantly reduced burn scar pruritus severity and activities-of-daily-living disturbances compared to a control group who received sham treatment. The EFD ranged between 0.05 and 0.20 mJ/mm^2, which seemed useful for pruritus in burn scars [27]. The authors hypothesized that ESWT targeted "neurogenic inflammation," which is an inflammation caused by the release of substances (e.g., SP and CGRP) from primary sensory nerve endings. Nerve fiber loss and the depletion of neuropeptides might decrease inflammation, and thus may decrease itch [28]. A recent meta-analysis showed that ESWT had better therapeutic outcomes on acute and chronic soft tissue wounds when compared to Conventional Wound Therapy (CWT) [29]. The meta-analysis showed that ESWT statistically significantly increased the healing rate of acute and chronic soft tissue wounds 2.73-fold (odds ratio, OR = 3.73, 95% confidence interval, CI: 2.30–6.04, $P < 0.001$) and improved wound-healing area percentage by 30.45% (Standardized Mean Difference (SMD) = 30.45; 95% CI: 23.79–37.12; $P < 0.001$). ESWT reduced wound-healing time by 3 days (SMD = −2.86, 95% CI:-3.78 to −1.95, $P < 0.001$) for acute soft tissue wounds and 19 days (SMD = −19.11, 95% CI: −23.74 to −14.47, $P < 0.001$) for chronic soft tissue wounds and the risk of wound infection by 53% (OR = 0.47, 95% CI: 0.24–0.92, $P = 0.03$) when compared to CWT alone. Serious adverse effects were not reported [29] (■ Fig. 55.2).

The Effects of SWT in Scar Management

Fibrous tissue can be reduced by SWT (at the origin) during wound healing processes, but it can also be remodeled in a second phase of scar formation. Primary data show that height, pliability, vascularity, and pigmentation, all relevant scar parameters, show improvement after SWT [6, 30]. The change in these physical and physiological parameters will probably lead to amelioration in function, which is, for example, demonstrated by an increase of passive ROM reported in a study on retracting hand scars [30]. Subjective pain measures also show a decrease in pain at the scar site after SWT [6, 30].

On a histopathological level, the effects of SWT on fibrosis are plural. A downregulation of alpha-SMA expression, myofibroblast phenotype, TGF-β1 expression, fibronectin, and collagen type I are measured. A significant increase in dermal fibroblast-like phenotype with low contractility and high migratory ability, small vessel density and precursors of extracellular matrix components, probably leads to new and thinner collagen fascicles and parallel orientation to the dermo-epidermal junction [30–32]. Synergistic alterations in pro- and anti-fibrotic proteins (TGF-β1 and MMP-2, respectively) suggest a reduced capsule formation after silicone implantation [33]. One study compared ESWT to triamcinolone injections for the treatment of keloids. ESWT showed comparable functional outcome, together with comparable total sum of scores for POSAS patient scale and POSAS observer scale clinically. A significant reduction in collagen fibers and increased expression of MMP-13 degrading enzyme could be seen when compared to intralesional steroid injection [34]. Zhao et al. demonstrated positive results on planimetric scar characteristics and inhibition of TGF-β1/Smad signaling pathway with Radial Extracorporeal Shockwave Therapy [22], as well as decreased Scar Elevation Index, fibroblast density, and α-smooth-muscle-actin expression in hypertrophic scar tissues of a rabbit model [35].

The most promising results in the research for the effects of SWT on scars were presented as preliminary data of an ongoing randomized placebo controlled trial investigating the effects of SWT in the management of hypertrophic scars. The results of the objective assessments showed a statistically significant better performance of the intervention group for elasticity assessed with cutometry [36] (■ Table 55.2).

Conclusion

All the presented findings are fundamental knowledge for further investigation of SWT to reduce the fibrous component in regenerating and remodeling tissues. The dose dependency of the treatment effects remains understudied. Energy Flux Density, number of shocks, shock frequency, and treatment interval and number are all important parameters in the choice for the most suitable device settings, in relation to the indication. Future studies should include these parameters as covariates to determine the right-specific approach for each scar. The full potential of SWT in wound healing, scar treatment, and cellulite certainly needs further unraveling.

Table SWT effects on wound healing, scar formation + remodeling, and cellulite

Effect of SWT on	Changes in histopathological parameters	Physical and physiological changes
Wound healing	Stimulation of the ECM metabolism Upregulation of cell-cycle regulatory genes Reorganization of the cytoskeleton	Angiogenesis Vasodilatation Increase in vascular and capillary density Increase in local blood flow Decrease in apoptosis Reduction of tissue necrosis
Burn wound healing		Shorter epithelialization time Increase in perfusion
Scar formation and remodeling	Downregulation on alpha-SMA expression, myofibroblast phenotype, TGF-β1 expression, and fibronectin Decrease in collagen type I Upregulation dermal fibroblast-like phenotype Increase small vessel density (ratio type I/type III collagen) Increase in precursors of ECM components Synergistic alterations in pro- and anti-fibrotic proteins	Formation of new and thinner collagen fascicles Reduced capsule formation Decrease in height Increased pliability Normalization of vascularity and pigmentation Amelioration of function (range of motion) Decrease in pain
Cellulite	Decrease of serum malondialdehyde and plasma protein carbonyls Release of lipid peroxidation products influence adipose-derived stem cells	Weakening of the fibrous septae Smoothening of skin

Take-Home Messages

- SWT meets all the requirements for the ideal non-invasive scar treatment.
- Mechanotransduction is the working mechanism behind SWT.
- SWT induces tissue regeneration and remodeling *in vivo*.
- Inflammation can be modulated by SWT.
- Low-energy SWT induces cell proliferation, while high-energy SWT suppresses cell growth.
- SWT can decrease time to full wound closure and reduces the risk for tissue necrosis.
- SWT may improve scar elasticity, which will probably lead to amelioration of function.
- There is a high dose–effect relationship when treating soft tissue defects with SWT.

Bibliography

1. Anthonissen M, Daly D, Janssens T, Van den Kerckhove E. The effects of conservative treatments on burn scars: a systematic review. Manuscr. Submitt. Publ. 2015.
2. Moortgat P, Anthonissen M, Meirte J, et al. The physical and physiological effects of vacuum massage on the different skin layers: a current status of the literature. Burn Trauma. 2016; 4:34.
3. Middelkoop E, Monstrey S, Téot L, Vranckx J. Scar management: practical guidelines. Belgium: Elsene; 2011.
4. Antonic V, Mittermayr R, Schaden W, Stojadinovic A. Evidence supporting extracorporeal shock wave therapy for acute and chronic soft tissue wounds. Wounds Compend Clin Res Pract. 2011;23:204–15.
5. Mittermayr R, Antonic V, Hartinger J, Kaufmann H, Redl H, Téot L, Stojadinovic A, Schaden W. Extracorporeal shock wave therapy (ESWT) for wound healing: technology, mechanisms, and clinical efficacy. Wound Repair Regen. 2012;20:456–65.
6. Fioramonti P, Cigna E, Onesti MG, Fino P, Fallico N, Scuderi N. Extracorporeal shock wave therapy for the management of burn scars. Dermatol Surg. 2012;38:778–82.
7. Romeo P, Lavanga V, Pagani D, Sansone V. Extracorporeal shock wave therapy in musculoskeletal disorders: a review. Med Princ Pract. 2014;23:7–13.
8. Huang C, Holfeld J, Schaden W, Orgill D, Ogawa R. Mechanotherapy: revisiting physical therapy and recruiting mechanobiology for a new era in medicine. Trends Mol Med. 2013;19: 555–64.
9. d'Agostino MC, Craig K, Tibalt E, Respizzi S. Shock wave as biological therapeutic tool: from mechanical stimulation to recovery and healing, through mechanotransduction. Int J Surg. 2015;24:147–53.
10. Wang JH-C, Thampatty BP, Lin J-S, Im H-J. Mechanoregulation of gene expression in fibroblasts. Gene. 2007;391:1–15.
11. Frairia R, Berta L. Biological effects of extracorporeal shock waves on fibroblasts. A review. Muscles Ligaments Tendons J. 2011;1:137–46.
12. Sukubo NG, Tibalt E, Respizzi S, Locati M, d'Agostino MC. Effect of shock waves on macrophages: a possible role in tissue regeneration and remodeling. Int J Surg. 2015;24:124–30.
13. Holfeld J, Tepeköylü C, Kozaryn R, Urbschat A, Zacharowski K, Grimm M, Paulus P. Shockwave therapy differentially stimulates endothelial cells: implications on the control of inflammation via toll-like receptor 3. Inflammation. 2014;37:65–70.

14. Knobloch K, Joest B, Krämer R, Vogt PM. Cellulite and focused extracorporeal shockwave therapy for non-invasive body contouring: a randomized trial. Dermatol Ther (Heidelb). 2013;3:143–55.
15. Kruglikov I. The pathophysiology of cellulite: can the puzzle eventually be solved? J Cosmet Dermatol Sci Appl. 2012;02:1–7.
16. Schaden W, Thiele R, Kölpl C, Pusch M, Nissan A, Attinger CE, Maniscalco-Theberge ME, Peoples GE, Elster EA, Stojadinovic A. Shockwave therapy for acute and chronic soft tissue wounds: a phase II trial. J Surg Res. 2007;137:246.
17. Yan X, Zeng B, Chai Y, Luo C, Li X. Improvement of blood flow, expression of nitric oxide, and vascular endothelial growth factor by low-energy shockwave therapy in random-pattern skin flap model. Ann Plast Surg. 2008;61:646–53.
18. Hatanaka K, Ito K, Shindo T, Kagaya Y, Ogata T, Eguchi K, Kurosawa R, Shimokawa H. Molecular mechanisms of the angiogenic effects of low-energy shock wave therapy: roles of mechanotransduction. Am J Physiol Cell Physiol. 2016;311:378–85.
19. Cai Z, Falkensammer F, Andrukhov O, Chen J, Mittermayr R, Rausch-Fan X. Effects of shock waves on expression of IL-6, IL-8, MCP-1, and TNF-α expression by human periodontal ligament fibroblasts: an in vitro study. Med Sci Monit. 2016;22: 914–21.
20. Berta L, Fazzari A, Ficco AM, Enrica PM, Catalano MG, Frairia R. Extracorporeal shock waves enhance normal fibroblast proliferation in vitro and activate mRNA expression for TGF-beta1 and for collagen types I and III. Acta Orthop. 2009;80:612–7.
21. Lee F-Y, Zhen Y-Y, Yuen C-M, Fan R, Chen Y-T, Sheu J-J, Chen Y-L, Wang C-J, Sun C-K, Yip H-K. The mTOR-FAK mechanotransduction signaling axis for focal adhesion maturation and cell proliferation. Am J Transl Res. 2017;9:1603–17.
22. Zhao J-C, Zhang B-R, Shi K, Wang J, Yu Q-H, Yu J-A. Lower energy radial shock wave therapy improves characteristics of hypertrophic scar in a rabbit ear model. Exp Ther Med. 2018;15:933–9.
23. Kuo Y-R, Wu W-S, Hsieh Y-L, Wang F-S, Wang C-T, Chiang Y-C, Wang C-J. Extracorporeal shock wave enhanced extended skin flap tissue survival via increase of topical blood perfusion and associated with suppression of tissue pro-inflammation. J Surg Res. 2007;143:385–92.
24. Aschermann I, Noor S, Venturelli S, Sinnberg T, Mnich CD, Busch C. Extracorporal shock waves activate migration, proliferation and inflammatory pathways in fibroblasts and keratinocytes, and improve wound healing in an open-label, single-arm study in patients with therapy-refractory chronic leg ulcers. Cell Physiol Biochem. 2017;41:890–906.
25. Ottomann C, Stojadinovic A, Lavin PT, Gannon FH, Heggeness MH, Thiele R, Schaden W, Hartmann B. Prospective randomized phase II trial of accelerated reepithelialization of superficial second-degree burn wounds using extracorporeal shock wave therapy. Ann Surg. 2012;255:23–9.
26. Arnó A, García O, Hernán I, Sancho J, Acosta A, Barret JP. Extracorporeal shock waves, a new non-surgical method to treat severe burns. Burns. 2010;36:844–9.
27. Joo SY, Cho YS, Seo CH. The clinical utility of extracorporeal shock wave therapy for burn pruritus: a prospective, randomized, single-blind study. Burns. 2018;44:612–9.
28. Hausdorf J, Lemmens MAM, Kaplan S, Marangoz C, Milz S, Odaci E, Korr H, Schmitz C, Maier M. Extracorporeal shockwave application to the distal femur of rabbits diminishes the number of neurons immunoreactive for substance P in dorsal root ganglia L5. Brain Res. 2008;1207:96–101.
29. Zhang L, Fu X, Chen S, Zhao Z, Schmitz C, Weng C. Efficacy and safety of extracorporeal shock wave therapy for acute and chronic soft tissue wounds: a systematic review and meta-analysis. Int Wound J. 2018;15:590–9.
30. Saggini R, Saggini A, Spagnoli AM, Dodaj I, Cigna E, Maruccia M, Soda G, Bellomo RG, Scuderi N. Extracorporeal shock wave therapy: an emerging treatment modality for retracting scars of the hands. Ultrasound Med Biol. 2016;42:185–95.
31. Rinella L, Marano F, Berta L, Bosco O, Fraccalvieri M, Fortunati N, Frairia R, Catalano MG. Extracorporeal shock waves modulate myofibroblast differentiation of adipose-derived stem cells. Wound Repair Regen. 2016;24:275–86.
32. Cui HS, Hong AR, Kim J-B, Yu JH, Cho YS, Joo SY, Seo CH. Extracorporeal shock wave therapy alters the expression of fibrosis-related molecules in fibroblast derived from human hypertrophic scar. Int J Mol Sci. 2018; https://doi.org/10.3390/ijms19010124.
33. Fischer S, Mueller W, Schulte M, Kiefer J, Hirche C, Heimer S, Köllensperger E, Germann G, Reichenberger MA. Multiple extracorporeal shock wave therapy degrades capsular fibrosis after insertion of silicone implants. Ultrasound Med Biol. 2015;41:781–9.
34. Wang C-J, Ko J-Y, Chou W-Y, Cheng J-H, Kuo Y-R. Extracorporeal shockwave therapy for treatment of keloid scars. Wound Repair Regen. 2018;26:69–76.
35. Zhao J-C, Zhang B-R, Hong L, Shi K, Wu W-W, Yu J-A. Extracorporeal shock wave therapy with low-energy flux density inhibits hypertrophic scar formation in an animal model. Int J Mol Med. 2018;41:1931–8.
36. Moortgat P, Meirte J, Anthonissen M, Lafaire C, De Cuyper L, Maertens K. Extracorporeal shockwave therapy for management of hypertrophic scars: preliminary results of a randomised placebo controlled trial. Ann Burns Fire Disasters. 2015; https://doi.org/10.13140/RG.2.1.2699.3125.

32

Suture Edge Tension Control Technologies for Scar Improvement

Luc Téot, Sergiu Fluieraru, and Christian Herlin

Contents

Background

Introduction/Objectives

Description of the State of the Art, Historical Evolution, and Recent Data

Silicone Devices

Reinforced Suture Materials

Adjustable Tensors

Closed Incision Negative Pressure Therapy

Conclusion

References

Background

Suture management after closure has been considered as highly important in the prevention of enlargement and infection. The rupture of skin integrity, the surgical dissection, and subsequent trauma of the underlying structures may cause local inflammation, edema, dehiscence, and infection. In this context, new technologies were developed and recently validated. The aim of this chapter is to highlight the role of mechanotherapy in prevention of postoperative complications on the suture line. This chapter is designed for surgeons facing surgical procedures at risk of infection or dehiscence or willing to reduce the scar enlargement after surgery on a visible area.

Introduction/Objectives

The tension exerted on the edges after cutaneous excision surgery has been demonstrated as a source of inflammation and potential complications, like local infection, scar enlargement when skin edges are, even minimally, separated [1, 2]. Keloid generation as well as hypertrophic scarring has been related to mechanical forces in experimental and clinical studies confirming the importance of mechanical control in the prevention of pathological scars especially in Asia [3]. Several techniques have recently been described on the basis of the principle of immobilizing the suture edges after surgery [1].

Globally a better understanding of scar mechanics has been under way for several years [2]. This has made it possible to multiply the compression strategies offered by compression garments or Orlen® (Professional Plastics, Fullerton, CA) plates, particularly in burn scars [4]. Translational research has been stimulated and the optimization of mechanical devices exploiting mechanical forces has been developed, especially in the field of wound healing [5].

A recent study [6] on cadavers measured the forces of tension exerted on the edges of sutured skin and the underlying aponeurosis. These measurements can be considered as a basis for measuring the reapproximation forces of the edges in human clinical practice. A three-dimensional simulation model allowed for reproducing the in vivo tension experienced by the skin, the phenotype of fibroblasts from keloid scars, their matrix synthesis capacity under tension, and in vivo skin tension measured on volunteers. It has been demonstrated that the induction of tension modifies the expression of the genes linked to the mechanical tension of the fibroblasts. This mechanical regulation makes it possible to understand that an increased synthesis of collagen occurs in the scar via the fibroblasts when tension is exerted strongly on the edges. The therapeutic interest of this hypothesis serves as a basis for the development of medical devices opposing edge tension.

Description of the State of the Art, Historical Evolution, and Recent Data

Applying materials over the suture after surgery is a longtime practice.

In the 2000, the first international consensus [7] on scar management emphasized the positive role of silicone but did not pay too much attention to the adhesive tapes, the first cheap device supposed to limit tension on the suture edges.

Silicone Devices

Silicone gels and tapes have been used since 1986 in prevention and treatment of hypertrophic scars and keloids. Although there have been multiple randomized controlled trials evaluating the efficacy of silicone gels [8], the overall quality of evidence is limited [9].

Silicone gels remain the most reported technique in the successive guidelines published since 2002. Silicone is not per se exerting any tension on the skin edges but may contribute to skin moisture.

Reinforced Suture Materials

During recent years a resorbable barb suture was developed, aiming at distribution of tension along the wound, providing a stronger wound edge approximation. The device was made of slowly resorbable material acting as a barber suture, due to obliquely distributed regular cuttings in the core of the device, preventing longitudinal movements on the suture line. The system was proposed as a drastic change in the suturing methods with a single-layer closure facilitated versus a 2-layer closure. Scar revision including large resection, prevention of shearing forces consequence on flap edges, and situations where the suture line may be exposed to mild to moderate tension were indications for the device [10].

Adhesive sutures. Used since decades long term, these paper tapes are placed over the skin edges to maintain a minimal pressure. Forces exerted on the suture are low, the adherence of the paper embedded with glue being solubilized or detached either by the exudation liquids or by the movements. Reiffel could demonstrate some superiority when adhesive sutures were placed longitudinally on the edges instead of transversally as a scale [11].

Self-adherent smart silicone has been proposed as a solution offering a permanent pressure exerted on the skin edges by a smart technology using adherent silicone covering the suture, isolating the suture from any external contamination. A mechanomodulating polymer device was utilized to manipulate the mechanical environment of closed cutaneous wounds in red Duroc swine, by applying tension to the edges through physical means (silicone with pretensioning of axial fibers inserted in the layer) [12]. (EMBRACE®). During a surgical procedure, surgeons strive to make incisions that follow the relaxed tension lines on the body, so-called Langer lines. This strategy is used because tension is well known to increase scarring. The Embrace® device (Neodyne Biosciences, Newark, CA) is designed to shield the healing incision from the natural tension that is inherent in any break in skin that must be pulled together to close a wound. Previous preclinical and first-in-human data initially demonstrated that this mechanism of action was effective in scar mitigation in both pigs and humans.

A prospective RCT in scar appearance was conducted on 36 healthy subjects during the post-operative period after abdominiplasty. Embrace® device was used fon the left part of the scar, and control (surgeon's optimal methods) on the right part. Result was significant on the scar appearance at 12 months after 5 weeks of application (Visual analog scale (VAS) $p = 0.027$, Patient and observer scar assessment scale (POSAS) subject $p = 0.02$, and surgeon $p < 0.001$) [13].

Adjustable Tensors

Another system to reduce skin tension across an incision line is the Zipline® system (ZiplineMedical-Stryker). The originality of the system is its ability to bring the two edges together and set the skin tension. This technique has been used since years in suturing the final epidermal layer as well as in restraining the suture edges movements during the postoperative period, results being linked to the compliance of the patient to wear an hydrocolloid based adhesive, covering the adjustable tensors, with a potential risk of allergy. The system may be used as an alternative to superficial sutures.

The medical device (Zipline®) has been developed and is used clinically as a wound closure technique as an alternative to sutures in many surgical procedures.

The medical device is made up of two adhesive carboxymethylcellulose strips, which have a central reinforcing core made up of polyurethane fibers, placed on the suture edges. These strips are interconnected by tensors formed of a polyurethane thread made up of nodes that are regularly distributed along the wire and finished by collars allowing easy grasping for tensioning. The entire set resembles a ladder with an adjustable length of bars. This tensor is firmly fixed and connected to the central core of polyurethane fibers of one of the two strips and placed transversely to bridge the scar zone. The tensor passes from the opposite side into a collar, and the nodules serve as blockers to maintain the desired tension. The distance between the two strips at rest is 1.5 cm and can be reduced to 0.5 cm. This movement is reversible, allowing for a true adaptation of the tension based on local needs and the wishes of the surgeons. The system can be positioned immediately after surgery and maintained in situ during subsequent weeks (■ Fig. 57.3).

The tension adjustment makes it possible to avoid even minimal edge spacing, which is a source of bacterial penetration and secondary infection. Moreover, the separation movements exerted longitudinally by the natural movements of the body are blocked, and this limitation serves as a transverse but also longitudinal immobilization. This is an essential factor in wound healing, limiting local inflammatory phenomena. Once the tension is stabilized, the loops are cut at their base.

In the author series of 21 clinical cases of skin excision [14], Zipline® was used after tumor resections, scar revision, or flaps. The tension exerted on the edges was variable and Zipline® was able to maintain the suture line outside of the transverse and longitudinal mechanical stresses. The results obtained in this series showed a maintenance of the linear scar measuring less than 0.5 cm permanently after 2 months of application. No local inflammation or secondary enlargement was observed after 2 months.

The anatomical sites were multiple and dependent on the necessities of the surgery. Most areas were located on the shoulders and back, regions known for their dermal fragility and problematic scarring. Maintaining a linear scar on these regions is difficult, especially in young women, after nevus resection. The skin's natural mobility, its thickness, and the forces exerted produce areas of known risk.

All patients underwent cutaneous resection during surgery, with skin loss between 4 cm × 3 cm and 8 cm × 14 cm. The postoperative scars were either straight or slightly curvilinear, and the maximum effect seemed to be obtained when the system was applied to rectilinear scars (■ Figs. 57.1, 57.2, 57.3, and 57.4). ■ Table 57.1 summarizes the population studied and the amounts of skin resected during surgery. The system was applied for an average of 42 days, with three changes on average.

The evaluation of the scar was performed by three independent evaluators. The average follow-up was 6 ±3

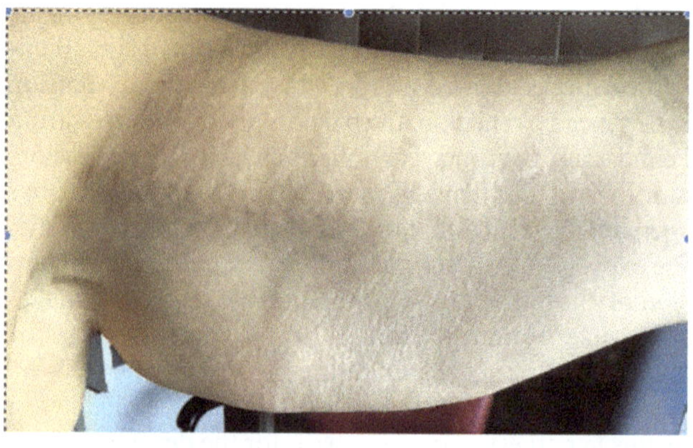

■ **Fig. 57.1** Right arm presenting excessive fat volume (postbariatric surgery)

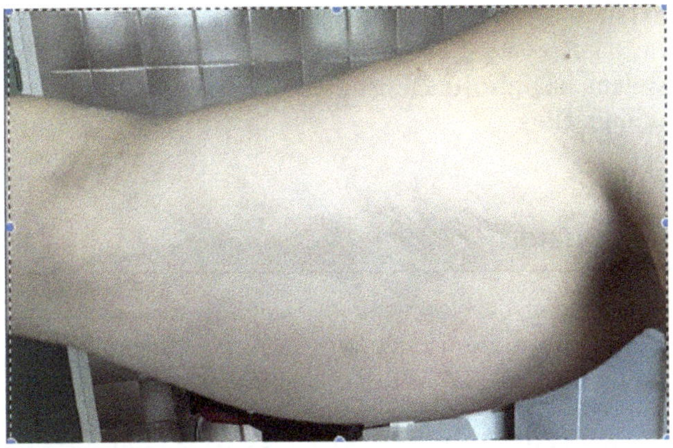

■ **Fig.** Left arm presenting excessive fat volume

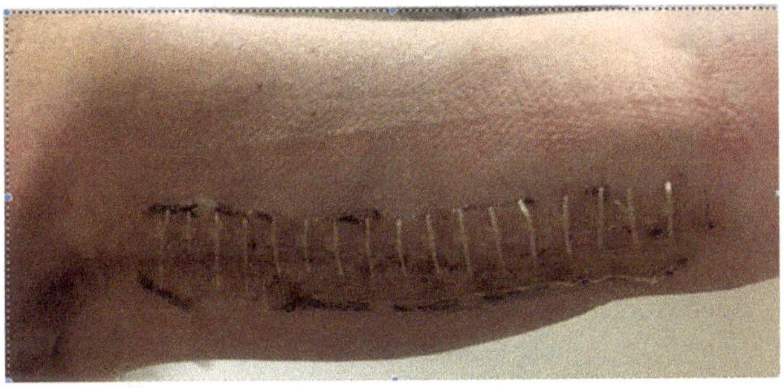

■ **Fig.** Right arm 2 months after fat reduction and suture edge control

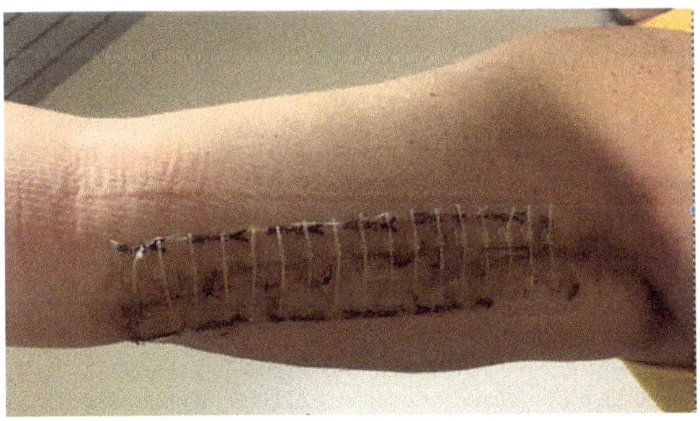

■ **Fig.** Left arm 2 months after fat reduction and suture edge control

months. The results were considered positive when the scar remained linear without secondary enlargement after 6 months.

Zipline® could be proposed as a skin closure system and as an alternative to epidermal suturing. However, it has not yet been used as a tool to maintain mechanical tension after suturing during cutaneous resection.

The distraction forces exerted on a suture line are caused by the patient's movements. The Zipline® system creates an immobilization of the micromovement-generating forces on the suture edges, which are sources of disunion and scar enlargement. Thanks to the polyurethane core and its staggered arrangement on the adhesive strips, any type of movement can be prevented because it opposes both transverse and longitudinal forces. This compression can be considered dynamic, and it prevents the widening of the suture, regardless of the movement to which it is subjected.

Several clinical trials reporting the effects of Zipline® have recently been published [15–19]. These trials report the product's good capacity to be used in the final closure of wounds. In our series, it appears that maintenance in place for several weeks on the skin serves to limit postoperative mechanical tension and to minimize scars, even in areas in tension and after keloid excision.

Zipline® has been proposed in multiple disciplines like orthopedic surgery in mobile areas like knee or shoulders and in plastic surgery after cutaneous excision for scar revision, cutaneous tumor excision, and loss of cutaneous substances due to chronic wounds such as pressure sores.

Closed Incision Negative Pressure Therapy

Several recent studies demonstrate the value of isolating the wound from any source of external contamination and of keeping it under slight tension.

In recent years, the indication for negative pressure wound therapy (NPWT) has been extended to include treatment of closed surgical incisions (incisional NPWT, iNPWT). Some of the first studies were case series and observational studies [20] using one of the exist-

■ **Table** Closed incision NPWT clinical indications

CiNPWT clinical indications	Thoracic surgery	Caesarian section	Orthopedic surgery	Postskin grafting	Pilonidal sinus
PICO®	x	x	x	x	x
Avelle®		x	x		x
Prevena®	x	x	x	x	x
Nanova®	x		x	x	

ing NPWT devices (VAC®; KCI, San Antonio, Texas, USA) [21, 22] designed for open wounds. Two simplified NPWT devices became commercially available in 2010 (Prevena™; KCI) and 2011 (PICO™; Smith & Nephew, Hull, UK). These NPWT devices consist of a single-use battery-powered negative-pressure therapy device, an easy-to-place dressing, and either a very small and easily portable canister, or no canister at all. In the latter case, the liquid is removed by evaporation through a semipermeable dressing. The mechanisms of action of this closed incision management have been supported by biomechanical studies:

Biomechanical testing could experimentally demonstrate that a pressure of 80 mmHg applied over a suture was enough to prevent 55% of tissue deformations compared to a situation when no NPWT dressing is applied [23]. Other authors suggested increased blood flow, decreased lateral and shear stress at the suture lines with decreased risk of wound dehiscence, and increased lymph clearance with reduced formation of hematoma/seroma [24].

A recent meta-analysis was conducted by Strugala et al. [25] on the impact of prophylactic use of a specific design of NPWT device on surgical site complications. Articles were identified in which the specific single-use NPWT device (PICO°, Smith & Nephew) was compared with standard care for surgical site infection (SSI), dehiscence, or length of stay (LOS). Risk ratio (RR) ±95% confidence interval (CI) (SSI; dehiscence) or mean difference in LOS ±95% CI was calculated using RevMan v5.3.

Combining all 16 studies, there was a significant reduction in SSI of 58% from 12.5% to 5.2% with NPWT (RR 0.43, [95% CI 0.32–0.57], $p < 0.0001$). Similar effects were seen irrespective of the kind of surgery (orthopedic, abdominal, colorectal, or cesarean section), although the numbers needed to treat (NNT) were lower in operations with higher frequencies of complications. There was a significant reduction in dehiscence from 17.4% to 12.8% with NPWT (RR 0.71, [95% CI 0.54–0.92], $p < 0.01$). The mean reduction in hospital LOS by NPWT was also significant (−0.47 days, [95% CI −0.71 to −0.23], $p < 0.0001$). The significant reduction in SSI, wound dehiscence, and LOS on the basis of pooled data from 16 studies shows a benefit of the PICO single-use NPWT system compared with standard care in closed surgical incisions (◘ Table 57.1).

Another study focused on the interest of CiNPWT after post-SSI revision of orthopedic implants [26] for total hip arthroplasty (THA) due to septic loosening in the presence of active fistula. They were treated with a PICO® device for NPWT, in combination with the standard treatment for prosthesis infection. Resolution of the infectious process and healing of the surgical wound without complications were considered promising results, confirming the interest of the system in most of the surgical disciplines (plastic surgery, thoracic and cardiac surgeries, and colorectal surgery) [27, 28]. The system has also demonstrated efficiency in stabilizing skin grafting.

Conclusion

The recent development of technologies proposing a mechanical restriction of micromovements on the suture line, with or without negative pressure, tends to demonstrate some evidenced benefits. These techniques are presently used in several surgical disciplines and proposed for at-risk situations in long and difficult procedures and also for minimizing the scar visibility and preventing enlargement as well as volume changes.

Take Home Message

This chapter expoes the interest of mechanotherapy during the post operative period in prevention of pathological scarring and in prevention of postop dehiscence and infection. Several techniques, from adhesive sutures to sophisticated machines applying on the suture edges a negative pressure, have already demosntrated an interest in decreasing the surgical site infection rates. These techniques are exposed and detailed.

Postop mechanotherapy seems adapted in patients at risk of developing local co:plications.

References

1. Lancerotto L, Orgill DP. Mechanoregulation of angiogenesis in wound healing. Wound Repair Regen. 2014;22(5):557–68. https://doi.org/10.1111/wrr.12215.
2. Suarez E, Syed F, Rasgado TA, Walmsley A, Mandal P, Bayat A. Skin equivalent tensional force alters keloid fibroblast behavior and phenotype. Aesthet Plast Surg. 2014;38(4):767–78. https://doi.org/10.1007/s00266-014-0339-x. Epub 2014 Jun 10.
3. Ogawa R, Okai K, Tokumura F, Mori K, Ohmori Y, Huang C, et al. The relationship between skin stretching/contraction and pathologic scarring: the important role of mechanical forces in keloid generation. Wound Repair Regen. 2012;20(2):149–57. https://doi.org/10.1111/j.1524-475X.2012.00766.x. Epub 2012.
4. Roques C. Pressure therapy to treat burn scars. Wound Repair Regen. 2002;10(2):122–5.
5. Kilpadi DV, Lessing C, Derrick K. Healed porcine incisions previously treated with a surgical incision *management* system: mechanical, histomorphometric, and gene expression properties. Biophys J. 2014;106(4):932–43. https://doi.org/10.1016/j.bpj.2013.12.002.
6. Venclauskas L, Grubinskas I, Mocevicius P, Kiudelis M. Reinforced tension line versus simple suture: a biomechanical study on cadavers. Acta Chir Belg. 2011;111(5):288–92.

7. Mustoe TA, Cooter RD, Gold MH, Hobbs FD, Ramelet AA, Shakespeare PG, Stella M, Téot L, Wood FM, Ziegler UE, International Advisory Panel on Scar Management. International clinical recommendations on scar management. Plast Reconstr Surg. 2002;110(2):560–71.
8. Ahn ST, Monafo WW, Mustoe TA. Topical silicone gel: a new treatment for hypertrophic scars. Surgery. 1989;106(4):781–6; discussion 786–7.
9. O'Brien L, Jones DJ. Silicone gel sheeting for preventing and treating hypertrophic and keloid scars. Cochrane Database Syst Rev. 2013;9:CD003826.
10. Reiffel RS. Prevention of hypertrophic scars by long-term paper tape application. Plast Reconstr Surg. 1995;96(7):1715–8.
11. Templeton MM, Krebs AI, Kraus KH, Hedlund CS. Ex vivo biomechanical comparison of V-LOC 180® absorbable wound closure device and standard polyglyconate suture for diaphragmatic herniorrhaphy in a canine model. Vet Surg. 2015;44(1):65–9. https://doi.org/10.1111/j.1532-950X.2014.12201.x. Epub 2014 Jun 24.
12. Gurtner GC, Dauskardt RH, Wong VW, et al. Improving cutaneous scar formation by controlling the mechanical environment: large animal and phase I studies. Ann Surg. 2011;254:217–25.
13. Longaker MT, Rohrich RJ, Greenberg L, Furnas H, Wald R, Bansal V, et al. A randomized controlled trial of the embrace advanced scar therapy device to reduce incisional scar formation. Plast Reconstr Surg. 2014;134(3):536–46. https://doi.org/10.1097/PRS.0000000000000417.
14. Téot L, Boissière F, Bekara F, Herlin C, Fluieraru S. Contrôle de la tension des berges cicatricielles après résection cutanée : un nouveau dispositif médical adhésif réglable. [Control of the skin edge tension after resection: a new adjustable, adhesive medical device.]. Revue Francophone de Cicatrisation. 2017;1(1):46–50.
15. Carli AV, Spiro S, Barlow BT, Haas SB. Using a non-invasive secure skin closure following total knee arthroplasty leads to fewer wound complications and no patient home care visits compared to surgical staples. Knee. 2017;24(5):1221–5.
16. Ko JH, Yang IH, Ko MS, Kamolhuja E, Park KK. Do zip-type skin-closing devices show better wound status compared to conventional staple devices in total knee arthroplasty? Int Wound J. 2017;14(1):250–4. https://doi.org/10.1111/iwj.12596.
17. Tanaka Y, Miyamoto T, Naito Y, Yoshitake S, Sasahara A, Miyaji K. Randomized study of a new noninvasive skin closure device for use after congenital heart operations. Ann Thorac Surg. 2016;102(4):1368–74. https://doi.org/10.1016/j.athoracsur.2016.03.072. Epub 2016 Jun 1. PubMed PMID: 27261084.
18. Mitwalli H, Dolan C, Bacigalupi R, Khorasani H. A randomized, controlled, prospective clinical study comparing a novel skin closure device to conventional suturing. J Am Acad Dermatol. 2016;74(1):173–4. https://doi.org/10.1016/j.jaad.2015.08.004. PubMed PMID: 26702797.
19. Gorsulowsky D, Talmor G. A novel noninvasive wound closure device as the final layer in skin closure. Derm Surg. 2015;41(8): 987–9. https://doi.org/10.1097/DSS.0000000000000399.
20. Reddix RN Jr, Leng XI, Woodall J, Jackson B, Dedmond B, Webb LX. The effect of incisional negative pressure therapy on wound complications after acetabular fracture surgery. J Surg Orthop Adv. 2010;19:91–7.
21. Wilkes RP, Kilpaldi DV, Zhao Y, Kazala R, McNulty A. Closed incision management with negative pressure wound therapy (CIM): biomechanics. Surg Innov. 2012;19:67–75.
22. Kilpadi DV, Cunningham MR. Evaluation of closed incision management with negative pressure wound therapy (CIM): hematoma/seroma and involvement of the lymphatic system. Wound Repair Regen. 2011;19:588–96.
23. Torbrand C, Anesäter E, Borgquist O, Malmsjö M. Mechanical effects of negative pressure wound therapy on abdominal wounds – effects of different pressures and wound fillers. Int Wound J. 2018;15(1):24–8. https://doi.org/10.1111/iwj.12810. Epub 2017 Nov 23.
24. Hyldig N, Birke-Sorensen H, Kruse M, Vinter C, Joergensen JS, Sorensen JA, Mogensen O, Lamont RF, Bille C. Meta-analysis of negative-pressure wound therapy for closed surgical incisions. Br J Surg. 2016;103(5):477–86.
25. Strugala V, Martin R. Meta-analysis of comparative trials evaluating a prophylactic single-use negative pressure wound therapy system for the prevention of surgical site complications. Surg Infect. 2017;18(7):810–9. https://doi.org/10.1089/sur.2017.156. Epub 2017 Sep 8.
26. Miyahara HS, Serzedello FR, Ejnisman L, Lima Allm Vicente JRN, Helito CP. Incisional negative-pressure wound therapy in revision total hip arthroplasty due to infection. Acta Ortop Bras. 2018;26(5):300–4. https://doi.org/10.1590/1413-785220182605196038.
27. Conde-Green A, Chung TL, Holton LH III, et al. Incisional Negative-Pressure Wound Therapy versus conventional dressings following abdominal wall reconstruction. A comparative study. Ann Plast Surg. 2013;71(4):394–7.
28. Stannard JP, Volgas DA, McGwin G, et al. Incisional negative pressure wound therapy after high-risk lower extremity fractures. J Orthop Trauma. 2012;26(1):37–42.

Permissions

All chapters in this book were first published in TSM, by Springer; hereby published with permission under the Creative Commons Attribution License or equivalent. Every chapter published in this book has been scrutinized by our experts. Their significance has been extensively debated. The topics covered herein carry significant findings which will fuel the growth of the discipline. They may even be implemented as practical applications or may be referred to as a beginning point for another development.

The contributors of this book come from diverse backgrounds, making this book a truly international effort. This book will bring forth new frontiers with its revolutionizing research information and detailed analysis of the nascent developments around the world.

We would like to thank all the contributing authors for lending their expertise to make the book truly unique. They have played a crucial role in the development of this book. Without their invaluable contributions this book wouldn't have been possible. They have made vital efforts to compile up to date information on the varied aspects of this subject to make this book a valuable addition to the collection of many professionals and students.

This book was conceptualized with the vision of imparting up-to-date information and advanced data in this field. To ensure the same, a matchless editorial board was set up. Every individual on the board went through rigorous rounds of assessment to prove their worth. After which they invested a large part of their time researching and compiling the most relevant data for our readers.

The editorial board has been involved in producing this book since its inception. They have spent rigorous hours researching and exploring the diverse topics which have resulted in the successful publishing of this book. They have passed on their knowledge of decades through this book. To expedite this challenging task, the publisher supported the team at every step. A small team of assistant editors was also appointed to further simplify the editing procedure and attain best results for the readers.

Apart from the editorial board, the designing team has also invested a significant amount of their time in understanding the subject and creating the most relevant covers. They scrutinized every image to scout for the most suitable representation of the subject and create an appropriate cover for the book.

The publishing team has been an ardent support to the editorial, designing and production team. Their endless efforts to recruit the best for this project, has resulted in the accomplishment of this book. They are a veteran in the field of academics and their pool of knowledge is as vast as their experience in printing. Their expertise and guidance has proved useful at every step. Their uncompromising quality standards have made this book an exceptional effort. Their encouragement from time to time has been an inspiration for everyone.

The publisher and the editorial board hope that this book will prove to be a valuable piece of knowledge for researchers, students, practitioners and scholars across the globe.

List of Contributors

Fiona M. Wood

F. W. Timmermans

E. Middelkoop

Luc Téot

F. Bassetto

Rei Ogawa

Matteo Tretti Clementoni

Clarisse Ganier

Julian Poetschke

Huidi Tchero

E. de Bakker

Hester Colboc

Wouter B. van der Sluis

Peter Moortgat

Alexandra Chambers

Anne Le Touze

Vincent Hunsinger

Ursula Mirastschijski

Nancy E. E. Van Loey

Joëlle Nonni

Roohi Vinaik

Juhee Lee

M. Tretti Clementoni

Sun Hyung Kwon

Wei Liu

Antigona Aliu

V. Vindigni

Ernest Azzopardi

C. Scarpa

Sonia Gaucher

Gerd G. Gauglitz

M. C. E. van Leeuwen

Sylvie Meaume

Johan P. W. Don Griot

Jill Meirte

Martin Lhuaire

Joel Fish

Jihee Kim

E. Azzopardi

Jagannath Padmanabhan

Matthias Aust

Mieke Anthonissen

O. W. M. Meijer

Ulrike Van Daele

Ibrahim Dagher

Marc G. Jeschke

Dominic Henn

F. B. Niessen

Laurent Lantieri

Kellen Chen

Tine Vanhullebusch

Geoffrey C. Gurtner

Koen Maertens

Sergiu Fluieraru

Christian Herlin

Index

A

Acne Inversa, 133-134, 147, 151
Adjacent Skin, 63, 66, 186
Adjustable Tensors, 222, 224
Allogeneic Cell Therapy, 50, 52
Anterior Lamella, 56-57

B

Blistering, 66, 110, 175, 186
Bone Marrow, 51
Botulinum Neurotoxin, 108, 110

C

Carnosus Muscle, 135
Cartilage, 109, 135
Cell Based Therapies, 5
Chemical Peels, 3, 41, 207
Chronic Ulcers, 50
Collagen Matrix, 11, 51
Cryotherapy, 64, 66-67, 73, 75, 90-91, 115, 122, 173, 177, 191

D

Dartos Fascia, 135-137
Deprodone, 165-170
Dermabrasion, 3, 5-6, 42, 48, 123, 207
Dermal Scaffolds, 10
Dermal Substitutes, 8, 11-12, 49-51, 58, 60
Diabetes, 2, 78-80, 105, 210
Dorsum, 58-60
Dupuytren's Disease, 25, 27-28, 191
Dyschromia, 40, 46, 66, 187

E

Ecchymosis, 161, 207
Embryonic Stem Cells, 52
Epidermolysis, 50-51, 66

F

Fascia, 15-17, 135-137, 141
Fludroxycortide Tape, 166-167, 169
Full-skin Substitutes, 7, 11-12

G

Genital Tissue, 133, 137
Genitalia, 132-139, 142-145, 147-148, 150-152
Good Manufacturing Practice, 51

H

Hair Transplantation, 57, 60-61
Human Donor, 15

I

Infection Control, 3, 5, 133

J

Juvidex, 109, 192-194

K

Keloids, 29-30, 38, 42, 63-68, 70-75, 77-78, 80, 91, 112, 116, 123-124, 165-167, 169-170, 173-175, 180, 182-185, 187-189, 195, 205-215, 219, 223

L

Lagophthalmos, 55, 57, 61
Laser Techniques, 3, 5

M

Macrophages, 10, 22, 52-53, 63, 118, 140, 193, 217-218, 220
Mechanical Stress, 66, 99, 191, 193, 210
Mental Disorders, 135, 154
Mesenchymal Stromal Cells, 49-50, 53
Microplasma Treatment, 197, 203

N

Necrotic Tissue, 2, 28, 134, 147, 210
Neutrophils, 63, 193, 210

O

Occupational Therapy, 55, 58, 186
Oncological, 21, 29, 83, 85, 134
Oral Hygiene, 27, 55

P

Pathological Scars, 29, 88, 91, 110, 117, 119-122, 166-167, 206, 215
Plastic Surgery, 22, 30, 75, 104, 112, 154, 225-226
Post-therapy Wound Care, 197
Pre-therapy Preparation, 197
Psoriasis, 161, 191, 193, 199

R

Radiotherapy, 25, 27-28, 64-65, 67-75, 83, 85, 110, 168

S

Safety Issues, 7, 12
Scar Appearance, 13, 60, 104, 109, 195, 224

Scar Management, 1-2, 5, 7, 9, 11, 13, 21, 23, 25, 27, 29-30, 39-41, 43, 45, 47, 49-55, 57, 59, 61, 68-69, 71, 73, 75, 88, 115, 118, 123, 131, 153, 176-177, 179, 181, 184, 188, 195-197, 199, 201, 203, 223, 227

Scar Pliability, 175, 184-186, 188

Scar Resurfacing, 1-3, 5

Scarred Area, 2, 59

Severe Scarring, 45, 55, 59, 133-134, 148, 155, 202

Sharp Dissection, 3, 5

Silicone Gels, 191, 223

Skin Architecture, 57, 132, 137, 141

Skin Equivalent, 49, 51, 226

Skin Expansion, 15-17, 20

Skin Fibrosis, 27, 30, 68, 102, 196

Skin Substitutes, 4, 7-13, 51, 108, 172

Skin Texture, 21, 24-25, 28, 47, 148, 213

Split Skin, 9

Subcutaneous Fat, 8, 11, 15, 28, 135-137

Subcutis, 11, 209

U

Umbilical Cord, 51, 136

V

Viral Infections, 133, 207

Visible Scar, 198, 203

W

Wound Closure, 8, 108, 112, 139-140, 148, 151, 196, 200, 202-203, 206, 213, 217, 220, 224, 227

Wound Healing, 2, 5-6, 8-10, 12, 22, 24, 28, 30, 51-53, 59, 72-73, 76-79, 106, 108-109, 117-118, 123, 126, 129, 132-133, 137, 140-141, 143, 151-152, 154, 206-211, 213, 216-221, 223, 226

CPSIA information can be obtained
at www.ICGtesting.com
Printed in the USA
LVHW060851030122
707669LV00002B/90

9 781639 871148